Withdrawn

ESSENTIAL ENDOCRINOLOGY

A Primer for Nonspecialists

ESSENTIAL ENDOCRINOLOGY
A Primer for Nonspecialists

C. R. Kannan, M.D.

Chairman
Division of Endocrinology and Metabolism
Department of Medicine
Cook County Hospital
and Clinical Associate Professor of Medicine
University of Illinois at Chicago
Chicago, Illinois

PLENUM MEDICAL BOOK COMPANY
New York and London

Library of Congress Cataloging in Publication Data

Kannan, C. R. (Charkravarthy R.), 1943–
  Essential endocrinology.

  Includes bibliographies and index.
  1. Endocrinology—Outlines, syllabi, etc. 2. Endocrinology—Handbooks, manuals, etc. I. Title. [DNLM: 1. Endocrine Diseases. WK 100 K16e]
RC648.K35   1986   612′.4   86-4925
ISBN 0-306-42172-0

© 1986 Plenum Publishing Corporation
233 Spring Street, New York, N.Y. 10013

Plenum Medical Book Company is an imprint of Plenum Publishing Corporation

Printed in the United States of America

This work is dedicated to Cook County
Hospital, still the last bastion of
hope for many.

Preface

This work, *Essential Endocrinology: A Primer for Nonspecialists,* is written with dual purposes in mind: first, to provide a framework of basic endocrinology and diabetology to the medical student, and second, to provide a quick, concise, and handy "guide" to the junior residents in their early years of training who wish to obtain a working knowledge about endocrine disorders that affect their patients. One of the outstanding advantages of being a teacher of endocrinology to students and junior residents is that it bestows a perspective from a unique vantage point. Books written for the junior members of our profession have suffered from extremes of caliber, ranging from excellence beyond their comprehension to insufferable mediocrity. Textbooks in endocrinology that are simple enough to cover the principles of that speciality and yet comprehensive enough without treading into controversial quicksand are few and far between. This book is aimed at filling that gap and is written with no other criterion than simplifying a complex subject matter. From this touchstone, the work has never really departed.

A decade of experience as a teacher and physician in the field of endocrinology has impressed on me that the process of "simplification" rests on four basic principles: an understanding of endocrine concepts, the application of these concepts to the understanding of diseases, the transference of knowledge to clinical situations, and the integration of the patient with the laboratory, the ultimate testing ground where clinical diagnoses stand or fall. A brief overview of the method in the making of this text seems appropriate.

An understanding of endocrine concepts is the common thread that is woven throughout the book. Each part begins by emphasizing the basic anatomic and physiological considerations that govern the proper functioning of each gland. The importance of understanding physiology is fostered by my firm belief that unless normal physiology is understood, disease states cannot be completely understood, nor can laboratory tests be clearly interpreted. Endocrine concepts can be divided into three classes: "core concepts" (concepts that are so vital that failure to understand these concepts precludes further comprehension), "primary concepts" (which include basic dogma that has been passed down in every edition of every standard textbook), and "current concepts" (concepts that are believed to be true given the "state-of-the-art" information of the times). This last category of concepts is somewhat controversial, often enigmatic, and always intriguing. This text, at the risk of being labeled simplistic, has strived to focus on the "core concepts" and "primary concepts" that have stood the tests of time and weathered many a storm of controversy.

The controversial concepts have been kept to a minimum, since they matter very little to the student of basics, although they have enormous impact in stimulating the mind of the student who has mastered the basics. For instance, the beginner who is learning about insulin should first know the core concepts about that hormone: the source, the actions as they pertain to glucose transport, adipose tissue, and the liver, etc. After these are understood, the "primary concepts" constitute the regulation of the synthesis and release of the hormone as well as the major factors that modify these phenomena and the role of the hormone in maintaining glucose homeostasis. The "current concepts" in this context would be the speculative hypotheses on the possible mediators that express insulin action. Although the student will find all three types of concepts discussed, the proportion of core concepts and primary concepts far exceeds that of controversial concepts. This has been done deliberately to avoid overwhelming the student physician with trivia or confusing concepts. A list of references provided at the end of each section should satisfy the appetite of those who want more.

The second cornerstone of simplification is the application of the above-mentioned concepts to the understanding of diseases. This is done in the following manner: the book has been divided into nine sections: the pituitary gland (adenohypophysis and neurohypophysis), the thyroid gland, the parathyroids, the adrenal glands, the testes, the ovaries, the disorders of sexual differentiation, diabetes, and a section on miscellany. Each section involving individual endocrine organs, begins with a discussion of salient anatomy and physiology, followed by laboratory methods of testing glandular function; disorders involving hyperfunction, hypofunction, and other specific diseases affecting each gland are subsequently discussed. The inevitable physical limitations to what can be compressed between the boards of a book force every author to decide how much space to devote to each topic. The decision to devote maximal allotment to the pituitary gland, the thyroid gland, and diabetes is based on three facts: first, the pituitary, by virtue of the numerous hormones that it secretes, forces the author (and the reader) on a long sojourn with several detours; second, thyroid disorders are the most frequent ones that find a place in the general internist's practice (as well as in the Board Examination); third, diabetes is a subspeciality within a subspeciality demanding attention (and space) by its commonality and far-reaching effects that penetrate every discipline of internal medicine.

Unlike the standard treatises in endocrinology and diabetes, this book does not have the space to tell all, which is why the focus is at all times aimed at being direct, simple, uncomplicated, and above all, on clinically oriented topics. For the reader who thirsts for more, the concise but comprehensive references at the end of each section or the standard voluminous textbooks in endocrinology would prove quite quenching. The incorporation of important concepts into diseases has been accomplished by juxtaposing the principles with the clinically established facts. Several tables have been used to indicate to the reader the reasons and logic underlying endocrine phenomena. Several of these tables are "thumbnail sketches" of entire paragraphs and are meant to serve as "instant replays" of the more detailed paragraphs in the text. This is especially so in the chapters on the gonads and sexual differentiation, topics that are justifiably perceived to be particularly difficult ones to comprehend.

Having conveyed the importance of endocrine concepts and their incorporation in the understanding of diseases, the third facet in the process of simplifying clinical endocrinology is the transference of knowledge to clinical situations. This is particularly important for the student physician, who must learn to think of symptoms rather than "disease labels." Whenever possible, the reader is provided with tables that correlate symptoms and signs of a certain disease with other disorders that cause identical symptoms or signs. The section on diagnostic studies in each chapter provides further correlations between established facts and several relevant diseases.

Finally, integration of the endocrine laboratory with the clinical presentations constitutes the fourth, and perhaps the conclusive, ingredient in the diagnostic process. This is approached in this book by providing the reader with two interconnected perspectives. First, at the beginning of each section, a chapter is devoted to testing function of a specific gland with particular reference to the important tests employed to assess functional integrity of the gland. Second, under individual diseases, the principles behind each test used, the indications for performing the tests (or study), and, more importantly, what the tests can and cannot reveal are outlined. Although it is true that endocrine studies do not always conclusively "make or break" a clinical diagnosis, in the interest of clarity, the student is shielded from these uncertainties. For the same reason, therapeutics of endocrine disorders is also dealt with in noncontroversial terms. In most instances, the therapeutic principles are broadly outlined. These principles do not include the beleaguering heterogeneity in patient responses.

Limitation on space, curiously enough, is a double-edged sword; on one hand, it impedes the amount an author wishes to offer (and all authors initially write more than what they intended), but on the other hand, when the time comes to "trim" (or edit), the limitations enforce focus on vital issues and reduce redundancy. Like most authors I have participated in both processes, and during the painful process of self-editing, the only determinant of what stays and what goes is the relevance and importance of the subject to the medical student and junior house staff. The constant questions, "Can a student afford to not know this fact?" and "Is this a core concept?" have dominated the editing process. For example, several paragraphs on human thyroid stimulators (a topic close to the author's heart) were sacrificed to make room for principles underlying the T_3 resin uptake test—a basic core concept that needed expounding. The final product is a work trimmed to the bare essentials.

From the aforementioned, it should become evident that the student who sets out to learn the fundamentals of endocrinology and diabetes and goes to the well with this purpose will not come away dry. For the student who wishes to wander the academic vistas of molecular or research endocrinology, this book is but a window to that world. If either goal is accomplished, this book would have served its purpose. This work is meant to be a guide, not a reference work; a short story, not a novel; a song, and not a symphony.

ACKNOWLEDGMENT. The support and well wishes of several friends have made this work possible. The single authorship of the book notwithstanding, I have heavily relied on a "little help from my friends." Most notably, I am deeply grateful to Ms. Gayla Blake who has played several crucial roles as a supporter, as a typist, and as a graphic illustrator. Her incessant zeal has had a galvanizing effect on the making of this book. I am deeply indebted to my medical editor, Mrs. Janice Stern, and the entire staff of the Plenum Publishing Corporation. It is indeed my good fortune to have a publishing house that takes great pride in enhancing an author's work. Finally, without the patience and fortitude of my wife Molly and son Ashley, this work would not have been accomplished.

C. R. Kannan, M.D.

Cook County Hospital
Chicago, Illinois

Contents

Part III. The Parathyroids

Part IV. The Adrenal Glands

Part V. The Testes

Part VI. The Ovaries

Part VII. Disorders of Sexual Differentiation

Part VIII. Diabetes and Glucose Intolerance

Part IX. Miscellany

ESSENTIAL ENDOCRINOLOGY

An Introduction to Endocrinology

1. Background

Endocrinology is the study of hormones. The term *hormone* is derived from the Greek word *harmao* (I excite) and was used by the legendary physiologist E. H. Starling in his Croonian lectures at the Royal College of Physicians in 1905. He proposed, with remarkable prophecy, that these substances are secreted by one organ and are transported by the bloodstream ("ductless transport") to other organs at distant sites, on which they exert their diverse effects. It was further speculated at that time, again with remarkable accuracy, that these "chemical messengers" had a rather rapid onset of action and excited their target organs even in extremely small quantities. Since then, endocrinology has evolved into an extremely sophisticated branch of internal medicine. A brief historical review of the events that have bridged the past and the present is pertinent, since it illustrates how the echoes of the past have been profoundly visionary.

Although the science of "hormonology" had its origins at the turn of this century, the existence of hormones was suspected as early as the 16th century. In 1690, Fredrick Ruysch, the celebrated Dutch anatomist, suggested that the thyroid gland "poured important substances into the bloodstream." Historians of medicine regard Theophile Bordeu as the founder of endocrinology. This famous French physician from Montpellier (which was the citadel of research in the 17th century) wrote in his masterpiece, *Recherches sur les Maladies Chroniques* (*Research on Chronic Diseases*), that several parts of the body gave off "emanations" that had profound effects on other parts of the body. His concepts, however, remained as speculations that lacked experimental proof.

In 1849, two events occurred that were destined to affect the concept of hormones forever. First, Arnold Berthold reported the first documented experimental evidence of hormonal deficiency; he demonstrated that castration

1

of the rooster resulted in atrophy of its comb and that such atrophy can be prevented if the testes are transplanted to another part of the rooster's body. He proposed that an "internal secretion" from the testes prevented the atrophy of the rooster's comb. The second event was a much more celebrated and memorable one; on a gray afternoon in the autumn of 1849, Thomas Addison read to an audience of the London Medical Society about his 11 patients with a fatal condition. All of these cases were characterized by "anemia, increasing weakness, feebleness of the heart, a smoky pigmentation and disease of the suprarenal glands at autopsy." Thus, the first link between a disease entity and a diseased gland was established. This condition, which Addison termed "melasma suprarenale," was renamed Addison's disease (by his friend Trosseau). In 1855, Claude Bernard introduced the tern "internal secretion" ("*secretion interne*"), and the science of endocrinology took off at a very high pitch. Between 1860 and 1900, the existence and functions of the thyroid, pituitary, adrenals, gonads, parathyroids, and even the islets of Langerhans had become established with reasonable clarity.

The discoveries in this century have unraveled several secrets and mysteries of hormonal disorders. The most exciting discovery of the 1920s (and perhaps the century) was the discovery and chemical synthesis of insulin by the collaborative efforts of Banting, Best, Macleod, and Collip. The major breakthroughs of the 1930s were the characterization of the catecholamines and the synthesis of desoxycorticosterone; the concept of neurotransmitters was born in this decade, and yet the surface of Pandora's box had only been scratched; more was to come. The 1940s witnessed a lull in endocrine research, when the world went to war. Yet this period saw the systematic description of various endocrine disorders. Fuller Albright described, for the first time, three important concepts that were to revolutionize endocrine thought: he showed that the bone disease of hyperparathyroidism disappeared on removal of the parathyroid adenoma; he proposed that tumors can ectopically secrete a parathormonelike substance; and he introduced the concept of target organ resistance by describing pseudohypoparathyroidism. These concepts, taken for granted today, were conceived by the sheer genius of intellect at a time when laboratory proof for such phenomena were, at best, rudimentary. Also in the 1940s two therapeutic events occurred quietly in widely separated parts of the globe: a French scientist accidentally discovered an oral hypoglycemic agent, and in Boston radioactive iodine was administered for the first time to a thyrotoxic patient.

The 1950s and 1960s filled the pages of endocrine literature with the description of several new hypersecretory and hyposecretory syndromes. Gut hormones, prostaglandins, and calcitonin became new members in the "hormone club." Sutherland's concept that the actions of several hormones are mediated by that omnipotent second messenger cyclic AMP revolutionized the understanding of syndromes of target organ resistance. But the event that singlehandedly catapulted endocrinology into an extremely sophisticated sphere was the emergence of the radioimmunoassay. This tool permitted measurement of practically every hormone in blood, conferring a sacrosanct status to the endocrine laboratory.

The 1970s and 1980s have witnessed a whole new realm of hypothalamic releasing factors that have had an enormous impact on diagnosis and therapy. The "high-tech" era has permeated endocrinology with marvels such as high-resolution computerized tomographic scans (which see everything), selective catheterization techiques (that can reach anywhere), sophisticated insulin-delivery pumps (that can be worn anywhere), and microsurgery. This remarkably dynamic subspeciality is still growing. Before embarking on a systematic description of disorders that involve the individual glands, it is important to outline some basic principles common to all endocrine glands. The focus is on four areas: hormonal secretion, hormonal feedback regulation, hormonal circulation, and hormonal action.

2. Hormonal Secretion

The secretory cells of the endocrine glands actively secrete, store, and release hormones. These cells are endowed with complicated synthetic machinery, histologically represented by an intense granular cytoplasm. Many hormones (ACTH, insulin, etc.) are synthesized as prohormones that are biologically inactive. Several enzyme systems within the cytoplasm are responsible for cleaving these prohormones at proper sites, converting them into active hormones. Very little is known regarding basal secretion of hormones by endocrine glands. Basal secretion is defined as the secretory activity of the endocrine gland in the absence of provocative or suppressive factors. It is believed that basal secretion of hormone by endocrine cells is under neuroregulatory control. The "bursts" of secretory activity of certain hormones (prolactin, growth hormone, etc.) and the diurnal rhythm of several hormones, particularly ACTH, are perhaps mediated by neuroregulation from the cortex or hypothalamus.

In contrast to the basal secretory rate of hormones, the stimulated output of endocrine glands has been studied extensively. Both physiological and chemical factors stimulate increased hormonal output. It is believed that hormones are stored within endocrine cells in two pools: a labile preformed pool, which is the moiety that is immediately released in response to provocative stimuli, and a synthetic pool, from which new hormone is actively synthesized, packaged, and released in response to continuous or chronic stimulation. The provocative factors that cause increased hormonal output can be hormonal, chemical, or neural or can be the circulating levels of certain metabolites. Examples of these four categories of provocative factors are outlined in Table 1 for growth hormone as an example.

There are several mechanisms by which trophic factors stimulate hormonal output, but the most dominant and frequent mechanism is the stimulation of membrane-bound adenylate cyclase, which catalyzes the conversion

TABLE 1
Provocative Stimuli for Growth Hormone Release

Type of stimulus	Example
Hormonal	Growth hormone-releasing hormone
Chemical	L-Dopa serotonin
Neural	α-Adrenergic stimulation
Metabolites	Hypoglycemia

of ATP to cyclic AMP. This is the mechanism that governs the trophic effect of TSH on the thyroid, the trophic effect of ACTH on the adrenal cortex, etc. This simplistic concept becomes more complex when one evaluates the role of metabolites in controlling hormone release. For instance, the mechanism of glucose-mediated insulin release belongs in this category and is discussed in Chapter 44. The magnitude of response of the same endocrine cell to different stimuli can have an impressive range. For instance, the response of prolactin release from the lactotroph can be quite variable, depending on the stimulus employed; stimulation of the nipple causes a much more brisk and profound increase in serum prolactin than chemical stimuli such as chlorpromazine or metoclopramide.

Suppressive factors are those that inhibit the release of glandular secretions. These factors are important in the day-to-day maintenance of constant hormonal levels and in avoiding hypersecretion. These suppressive factors, again, can be hormonal, chemical, neural, or metabolites themselves. Table 2 illustrates the variety of suppressive factors with growth hormone again used as an example.

Understanding the stimulatory and suppressive factors that govern the release of each hormone has tremendous diagnostic impact. The dictum, "when hypofunction is suspected the gland should be tested by stimlation, and when hyperfunction is suspected the gland should be tested by suppression," is a basic endocrine dogma. Table 3 outlines the multitude of provocative and suppressive factors for some of the frequently tested hormones.

TABLE 2
Suppressive Factors for Growth Hormone Release

Type of suppressive factor	Example
Hormonal	Somatostatin
Chemical	Chlorpromazine, progesterone, serotonin antagonist
Neural	β-Adrenergic stimulation
Metabolites	Hyperglycemia

TABLE 3
Provocative and Suppressive Factors That Affect Hormone Release

Hormone	Provocative factors	Suppressive factors
ACTH	Hypoglycemia, stress, CRF	Cortisol
TSH	TRH	Thyroid hormones
Growth hormone	Hypoglycemia, stress, dopamine, sleep, GHRH	Glucose, somatostatin
Prolactin	Stimulation of nipple or areola, chlorpromazine, TRH, sleep	Dopamine and dopamine agonists
LH, FSH	GnRH (gonadoptropin-releasing hormone)	Sex steroids
Thyroid hormone	TSH	
Cortisol	ACTH	
Aldosterone	Renin–angiotensin system, ACTH, hyperkalemia	Volume expansion, hypokalemia
Catecholamines	Stress, hypoglycemia	
Sex steroids	LH, FSH	
Insulin	Hyperglycemia, amino acids	Hypoglycemia
Glucagon	Hypoglycemia, amino acids	Hyperglycemia
PTH	Hypocalcemia	Hypercalcemia

3. Feedback Regulation

The term *feedback regulation* (or feedback loop) refers to the delicate relationship between ambient concentrations of the target gland hormone and its respective trophic hormone. With the notable exception of the parathyroids and pancreatic islet cells, almost all other endocrine glands participate in feedback loops involving the hypothalamic–pituitary unit. Thus, the functions of the thyroid, adrenal cortices, testes, and ovaries are modulated and fine-tuned by an intimate servo feedback mechanism involving the hypothalamic–pituitary unit. The term *negative feedback* implies a reciprocal relationship between target gland hormone and its trophic hormone; i.e., an increase in the concentration of target gland hormone will result in suppression of its spective trophic hormone, whereas decreasing concentrations of target gland hormone cause an increase in its respective trophic hormone level. Such is the relationship between the thyroid hormones and thyrotropin (TSH), glucocorticoids and cotricotropin (ACTH), as well as between testosterone and luteinzing hormone (LH). The effects of estrogens on the hypothalamic–pituitary unit in normal females is dichotomous, consisting of both negative and positive feedback regulatory mechanisms. The term *positive feedback* implies a linear relationship between target gland hormone and its trophic hormone; i.e., an increase in the circulating levels of target gland hormone results in stimulating its respective trophic hormone. The most illustrative physiological example of positive feedback between hormones is the "LH surge" that occurs during the midmenstrual cycle caused by a progressive increase in circulating concentrations of 17 β-estradiol. Notably, this response is restricted only to females.

Feedback loops have also been categorized as "long," "short," and "ultrashort" feedback loops (Table 4):

1. *Long feedback loops* are exemplified by the feedback regulation between the hypothalamus and glucocorticoids or gonadal steroids. In the case of cortisol and testosterone, this feedback loop is exclusively a negative feedback loop, whereas in the case of 17β-estradiol this long feedback loop is both negative as well as positive under different circumstances.

2. *Short feedback loops* denote the servo feedback relationship between the pituitary gland and the hormones secreted by several of its target glands. The most impressive example of such a short feedback loop is the relationship between the pituitary TSH and the thyroid hormones. A similar situation is seen between ACTH and cortisol as well as between LH and gonadal steroids. Cortisol and the gonadal steroids feed back on both the hypothalamus (long negative feedback) as well as the pituitary (short negative feedback), whereas the thyroid hor-

TABLE 4
The Feedback Regulatory Loops

Type of loop	Target gland hormone	Trophic hormone
I. Long feedback		
A. Negative feedback	Cortisol	CRH[a]
	Testosterone or 17β-estradiol	GnRH[b]
B. Positive feedback	17β-Estradiol	GnRH
II. Short feedback		
A. Negative feedback	Thyroid hormones	TSH
	Testosterone or 17β-estradiol	LH
	Cortisol	ACTH
B. Positive feedback	None	None
III. Ultrashort feedback		
A. Negative feedback	ACTH	CRH
	?TSH	TRH
B. Positive feedback	Growth hormone	Somatostatin
	Prolactin	Hypothalamic PIF[c] (dopamine)

[a] CRH, corticotropin-releasing hormone.
[b] GnRH, gonadotropin-releasing hormone.
[c] PIF, prolactin inhibitory factor.

mones predominantly exert their negative feedback effect on the pituitary gland (short negative feedback loop).

3. The term *ultrashort feedback* refers to the intimate relationship between the pituitary gland and its hypothalamic master. These loops can be negative or positive. Thus, a negative ultrashort feedback loop exists between ACTH and corticotropin-releasing hormone (CRH) of the hypothalamus. A similar loop perhaps also exists between TSH and TRH. In contrast, a positive ultrashort feedback loop operates between growth hormone and somatostatin and perhaps between prolactin and hypothalamic dopamine.

4. Hormonal Circulation

In general, there are three major types of hormones secreted by endocrine glands, steroid hormones, polypeptide hormones, and amino acid (or short peptide) hormones. The steroid hormones (exemplified by cortisol, testosterone, estradiol, and aldosterone) circulate in blood bound to carrier proteins. The bound hormone is biologically inactive, and their circulating levels in plasma can be altered by quantitative or qualitative alterations in their respective carrier proteins. These carrier proteins are usually globulins (cortisol-binding globulin, sex-hormone-binding globulin, etc.) and are synthesized by the liver. An important concept to understand is that although the bound moiety of hormone is biologically inactive, it maintains equilibrium with its free, biologically active counterpart, for it is from this "reservoir" of bound hormone that the body draws up free hormone as and when the need arises. Generally, the bound hormone levels parallel the free hormone levels as long as there are no abnormalities in the binding proteins. The bound hormones circulate longer in plasma and are infinitely easier to measure than the free hormones.

The polypeptide hormones (exemplified by growth hormone, ACTH, PTH, and insulin) circulate in blood as such and are characterized by an extremely short half-life, usually in minutes. Some polypeptide hormones (insulin, PTH, ACTH, etc.) are derived from longer (or larger) precursor molecules with longer half-lives.

The third class of hormones, amino acid (or short peptide) hormones, are represented by thyroid hormones and catecholamines. There is extreme variability among these hormones in terms of their half-lives in the circulation. For instance, thyroxine circulates bound to several binding proteins (thyroxine-binding globulin, thyroxine-binding prealbumin, and albumin) and has a long half-life, whereas catecholamines circulate as such with an extraordinarily short half-life. Even among thyroxine and triiodothyronine, two seemingly identical iodoproteins, significant differences exist in binding, transport, and half-life.

The ambient level of a given hormone depends on two major factors, the production rate by the gland and the metabolic clearance rate of the hormone. The clearance of a hormone from the circulation depends on its metabolic degradation (usually carried out by the liver or the kidneys) as well as on internalization within its target cells.

The emergence of the radioimmunoassay has enabled measurement of even minute quantities of hormones in the circulation. The principle of the radioimmunoassay is simple, and it is performed in a sequence of two steps. The first step involves the reaction among a known quantity of antigen ("cold" standard), its respective antibody, and a known amount of radiolabeled ("hot") antigen. The standard ("cold") antigen and the radiolabeled, quantified "hot" antigen compete for the same antibody. The first step is to derive a standard curve, illustrating the degree of binding of various dilutions of cold antigen with the antibody. During the second part of the procedure, the unknown serum is substituted for the cold standard, and the degree of competition with the labeled antigen for the same antibody is now determined. Since the hot (labeled) antigen and the antibody used are constant, the determination of the degree of binding between the antigen in serum tested and the antibody permits projection of the quantity of hormone in the serum; this is done by reading the percentage of bound versus free from the standard curve obtained earlier. The precision of the radioimmunoassay lies in the specificity of the reaction between antigen and antibody. However, when the hormone measured demonstrates immunoheterogeneity, the fragment measured is a reflection of the fragment "seen" by the antibody employed. Immunoheterogeneity is a particularly inherent problem with PTH. The purity of standards used, the heterogeneity of the hormone tested, the pulsatile nature of secretion, as well as possible impairment in clearance (as in renal failure) are all factors to be considered in interpreting hormone levels obtained by immunoassay.

5. Hormonal Action

The classification of hormones into steroid hormones, polypeptide hormones, and amino acid (or short peptide) hormones assumes significance in terms of their action as well. All hormones express their action on receptors in their target tissues. There is a great deal of variability in the methods by which hormones exert their actions on their target tissue. Regardless of the ultimate differences in hormonal expression, all hormones must first interact with some part of their target cells. As a group, steroid hormones bind to specific cytosol receptor proteins in the cytoplasm. The polypeptide hormones, on the other hand, generally bind to receptors located in the membrane of the target cell to stimulate the membrane-bound enzyme adenylate cyclase. The short peptide hormones, particularly thyroxine and triiodothyronine, bind to receptors located in the nuclei of their target cell. The locus of attachment of hormone appears to have some clinical impact on the diseases characterized by target organ receptor insensitivity: disorders of peripheral resistance to hormones that bind to receptors can be modified, an example

TABLE 5
Spectrum of Disorders Characterized by Target Organ Resistance

Hormone	Disease
I. Polypeptide hormones	
PTH	Pseudohypoparathyroidism
Insulin	Non-insulin-dependent diabetes mellitus
Growth hormone	Laron dwarfism
ADH	Nephrogenic diabetes insipidus
II. Steroid hormones	
Testosterone and dihydrotestosterone	Testicular feminization syndrome (complete) Reifenstein's syndrome (partial)
III. Amino acid hormones	
Thyroid hormones	Hypothyroidism

of such a pheonmenon being receptor insensitivity to insulin. In contrast, disorders of peripheral resistance to hormones that bind to cytoplasmic receptors tend to be fixed and in many instances complete (testicular feminization).

The mechanism of action of steroid hormones following binding of hormone to specific cytolsol receptor proteins involves transport of the hormone–cytosol protein complex to the nuclear chromatin. The resultant formation of new messenger RNA with transcription of the coded message results in the metabolic expression of hormonal action. A prototypic steroid hormone is testosterone. The intricacy of phenomena involved in the expression of testosterone action on its target cell is outlined in Chapter 33.

The mechanism of action of polypeptide hormones following binding to cell membrane involves activation of adenylate cyclase, formation of cyclic AMP (the second messenger, cyclic adenosine monophosphate) from ATP (adenosine triphosphate), and the formation of protein kinases that express the hormonal action. A prototypic polypeptide hormone is parathormone. The complexity of the phenomena involved in the expression of PTH action on its target cell is described in Chapter 20.

Short peptide hormones have widely differing mechanisms of action. Thus, thyroid hormones bind to the nucleus, whereas catecholamines bind to receptors in the membrane of the target cells.

Regardless of the exact mechanism, the sensitivity of the target cell is the most crucial factor required for expression of hormonal action. Target organ receptor sensitivity encompasses several facets: recognition of hormone, binding of hormone to specific loci within the target cell, activation of chemical events (e.g., cyclic AMP formation, messenger RNA formation), and facilitation of postreceptor events (e.g., protein kinase formation). Target organ resistance can occur as a consequence of breakdown in any of these facets. Down-regulation and enhancement of receptor sensitivity appear to be limited to hormones that express their action by binding to membrane receptors on target cells (insulin, calcitonin, PTH, catecholamines, etc.). The spectrum of disorders characterized by target organ resistance is outlined in Table 5.

Endocrinopathies can occur as a result of hyperfunction or as a consequence of hypofunction of a particular gland. In the latter situation, the disorder can result from either decreased production of hormone or decreased sensitivity at the receptor level.

The general framework outlined above permits understanding of the specifics of endocrine disorders discussed in this book.

I

The Pituitary Gland

1

The Anatomy of the Pituitary Gland

The pituitary gland (hypophysis ceribi) is a small organ housed in a bony cavity called the sella turcica. The sella is contained in the sphenoid bone at the base of the skull. The sella turcica is separated from the rest of the cranial cavity by a thick reflection of dura called the diaphragma sella. This membraneous structure has a small central aperture through which the infundibulum (stalk) passes. This stalk connects the pituitary gland to the brain and serves as an important avenue for transport of the hypothalamic peptides to the pituitary.

The pituitary gland measures approximately 10 mm × 13 mm × 6 mm, weighs about 500 mg, and occupies most of the volume of the sella turcica. The gland itself is basically divided into two parts, adenohypophysis and neurohypophysis. These two portions have different embryological, morphological and functional characteristics. The adenohypophysis has its origin from the Rathke's pouch, an ectodermal diverticulum from the roof of the stomadeum, whereas the neurohypophysis is derived from the diencephalon. The adenohypophysis is divided into the pars anterior (anterior lobe) and the pars intermedia (intermediate lobe). The neurohypophysis consists mainly of the "pars posterior" (posterior lobe), part of the infundibular stem, and the median eminence. The adenohypophysis secretes several hormones (somatotropin, gonadotropins, thyrotropin, adrenocorticotropin, prolactin, lipotropic hormones, and endorphins), whereas the posterior pituitary essentially stores vasopressin and oxytocin, secreted by the supraoptic and paraventricular nuclei of the hypothalamus.

Anatomically, the pituitary gland is related superiorly to the optic chiasm, inferiorly to the sphenoid sinus, and laterally, on either side, to the cavernous sinus and the structures contained within. The pituitary gland enjoys dual blood supply. The arterial supply is derived from the superior hypophyseal arteries, which branch off from the internal carotid artery. In addition, the

13

CHAPTER 1

TABLE 6
Anatomic Dimensions of the Sella

Dimension	Definition	Normal values
Length	The greatest AP diameter of sella	Mean 11.9 mm (range 9–19)
Depth	The perpendicular of the line drawn from the tuberculum sellae to the top of the dorsum sellae	Mean 8 mm (range 6.5–10.5)
Width	Distance between the highest points of the lateral edges of the floor	Mean 13.1 mm (range 9–19)
Volume	$L \times D \times W/2$	Mean 594 mm³ (range 240–1092)

pituitary is supplied by a portal system of venous blood that originates from the median eminence of the hypothalamus and reaches the capillary plexus of the adenohypophysis. This portal system carries important hypothalamic peptides from the median eminence of the hypothalamus.

Histologically, the cell types of the anterior pituitary can be divided into acidophils, basophils, and chromophobe cells, depending on the presence and staining properties of granules within the cytoplasm. The cells can also be classified on the basis of their appearance by electron microscopy into somatotrophs, gonadotrophs, lactotrophs, thyrotrophs, and corticotrophs.

For clinical purposes, it is important to recognize the appearance and dimensions of the normal sella turcica on lateral skull films. The anterior and posterior clinoids can easily be recognized as the prominent tips of the anterior and posterior walls of the sella turcica. The tubercalum sellae is the bony prominence below and anterior to the anterior clinoid. The dorsum sellae is the bony posterior continuation of the posterior clinoids. The length, depth, width, and volume of the normal sella are variable, but the definition and mean values of the parameters are outlined in Table 6.

The dimensions of the sella vary with age and body height. In addition to size, the sella turcica should be evaluated for the shape and the symmetry of contours. Erosions of the clinoids, the wall, or the floor are better visualized by polytomography. The presence of suprasellar calcification is a notable feature of craniopharyngiomas. Intrasellar calcification has less diagnostic significance and can be encountered with tumors, aneurysms, cysts, or, rarely, tuberculosis.

The emergence of high-resolution computerized tomography has rendered plain films and polytomography obsolete. The CT image in the coronal projection at the plane of the sella effectively outlines the sellar size, the pituitary size, and the presence of masses within the sella or the sphenoid sinus. The CT image obtained at the level of planum sphenoidale outlines the sphenoid sinus. An image obtained at the level of the dorsum sellae detects suprasellar extension of pituitary tumors, since the technique readily distinguishes the density of soft tissue from CSF. The upper border of the contents of the sella is usually concave, with the suprasellar cistern usually dipping a few millimeters into the sella. When this concavity is lost or replaced by convexity (upward bowing), suprasellar extension can be diagnosed.

2

Physiology
The Secretion, Regulatory Control, and Actions of Pituitary Hormones

2.1. Introduction

The characteristics of the various hormones secreted by the anterior pituitary, the regulatory mechanisms governing their secretion and release, and the actions of these trophic hormones should be viewed individually. The ability of the anterior pituitary to secrete diverse hormones with far-reaching effects on other endocrine glands had once earned it the title "the master of the endocrine orchestra," a title that rightfully belongs to the hypothalamus. Together, the hypothalamic–pituitary unit controls growth, regulates thyroid function, stimulates the adrenals to secrete hormones necessary for life, and plays a dominant role in preserving sexuality. Since each trophic hormone functions as an independent hormonal unit with individual control mechanisms and different target organs, it is necessary to review the physiology of each hormone separately. The aspects that are focused on include the chemistry, control, release, circulation, and actions of each trophic hormone.

2.2. Growth Hormone

Human growth hormone is a polypeptide containing 191 amino acids with two intramolecular S–S bonds. Growth hormone is secreted by the somatotrophs, which are acidophilic, resembling lactotrophs. On electron microscopy, the somatotrophs can be distinguished from lactotrophs by their uniformity and by the size of the electron-dense granules contained in the somatotrophs.

The growth hormone secretion of anterior pituitary is controlled by the

17

hypothalamus and other parts of the brain. The control of growth hormone is mediated by stimulatory and inhibitory mechanisms. The stimulatory (provocative) influences on growth hormone release are mediated by three neurotransmitters: adrenergic (norepinephrine), dopaminergic, and serotoninergic.

It is believed that all three neurotransmitters are involved in the mediation of growth hormone-releasing factor. The recent isolation of this releasing factor from pancreatic tumor tissue has resulted in the characterization of this peptide, which contains 40 to 44 amino acids. A homologous peptide has been isolated from rat hypthalamus. The availability of synthetic growth hormone-releasing hormone ($GH-RH_{1-40}$ and $GH-RH_{1-44}$), which effectively releases growth hormone in normal subjects, indicates that these peptides are identical to human growth hormone-releasing hormone of the hypothalamus.

The role of neurotransmitters in the release of growth hormone is mediated by adrenergic, dopaminergic, and serotoninergic mechanisms. The adrenergic release of growth hormone is mediated by the ventromedial nucleus of the hypothalamus. This nucleus contains glucoreceptors that are exquisitely sensitive to a lowering of blood glucose. This is the reason for the marked increases in growth hormone levels in response to hypoglycemia. The adrenergic mediation of this phenomenon is supported by the fact that α-adrenergic blockade can abolish the response to hypoglycemia. The dopaminergic mediation for growth hormone release is centered around the arcuate nucleus. The fact that growth hormone levels increase following the oral adminstration of L-dopa and decreases after phenothiazines supports the dopaminergic mediation of growth hormone control. The third neurotransmitter, serotonin, works through the limbic system. The fact that growth hormone levels dramatically increase during deep sleep (which increases the serotonin content of certain parts of the CNS) and are found to be elevated in the carcinoid syndrome support the serotoninergic mediation of growth hormone control.

Besides these three well-known neurotransmitters that stimulate release, there are other unclear mechanisms involved in growth hormone release. The growth hormone release secondary to exercise, stress, and morphine belong in this category.

In addition to exerting a stimulatory control on growth hormone release, the hypothalamus also exerts an inhibitory influence on somatotrophs. This is mediated by the peptide somatostatin, which, incidentally, is found throughout the CNS and some parts of the GI tract, especially the pancreas. Administration of somatostatin results in profound lowering of growth hormone as well as in abolition of the provoked responses of growth hormone to all stimuli. In addition to lowering growth hormone, somatostatin consistently lowers TSH, insulin, glucagon, and gastrin. Somatostatin is ideally suited for studying suppressibility of growth hormone but is not widely available for study purposes. Therefore, suppressibility is studied by using glucose, which is a potent suppressor of growth hormone.

The factors that stimulate and suppress growth hormone release are outlined in Table 7.

TABLE 7
Factors Controlling GH Release

Factors that stimulate HGH release	Factors that suppress HGH release
Hypoglycemia	Somatostatin
L-Dopa	Glucose
Arginine	α-Blockade
Sleep	Corticosteroids
Serotonin	
Exercise	
Stress	
Morphine	

Growth hormone circulates in the plasma mostly unbound. The basal levels range from 0.5 to 5 ng/dl.

The main action of growth hormone is to promote longitudinal growth. In addition, growth hormone has significant effects on carbohydrate, protein, and fat metabolism. The growth-promoting, diabetogenic, anabolic, and lipolytic effects need brief mention.

The growth-promoting effects of growth hormone are mediated by intermediary peptides called somatomedins. Originally, the mediator of growth hormone was called sulfation factor (SF) because of its ability to incorporate sulfate into the chondroitin sulfate of the actively proliferating cartilage. Currently called somatomedins, these peptides do more than incorporate sulfate: they influence leucine incorporation into protein, uridine incorporation into RNA, and thymidine incorporation into DNA. The somatomedin family incorporates an array of peptides with growth-promoting and insulinlike activity (insulinlike growth factors). Several peptides (somatomedins A, B, and C) belong to the generic family of somatomedins, with somatomedin C demonstrating the most intense cartilage-stimulating ability.

Physicochemically, the molecular weight of somatomedins ranges between 3,900 and 12,400. The sources of somatomedins are the liver and, to a lesser extent, skeletal muscle. Following the injection of growth hormone, there is a brisk rise in somatomedin C that reaches a peak in 3 hr and has effects lasting from 9 to 24 hr. Although growth hormone specifically stimulates somatomedin generation, occasionally other hormones, particularly prolactin, can stimulate somatomedin generation. A negative feedback relationship between somatomedin and growth hormone may exist. Somatomedins cannot stimulate the longitudinal growth of the skeleton once the epiphyses have fused. Somatomedins are also involved in the other metabolic effects of growth hormone.

The effects of growth hormone on carbohydrate metabolism are three-fold:

1. Growth hormone is a counterinsulin hormone, antagonistic to the peripheral action of insulin. Thus, growth hormone decreases the

peripheral utilization of glucose by tissues. In this sense, growth hormone is diabetogenic.

2. Growth hormone is β-cytotropic, i.e., stimulates the β cell to secrete more insulin. This insulinotropic effect is evidence by the fact that prior administration of growth hormone results in a vastly enhanced insulin response of β cell to glucose.

3. The third effect of growth hormone on glucose homeostasis is seen only when supraphysiological doses of growth hormone are administered. This glucose-lowering effect is paradoxical and resembles the action of insulin. It is believed that this early action is seen only when very high tissue levels are attained, and it is transient. It is unclear which somatomedin, if any, mediates this effect.

The effect of growth hormone on adipose tissue is also antiinsulinlike. Growth hormone is lipolytic, in contrast to the lipogenic effects of insulin. Following the injection of growth hormone, there is a prompt increase in free fatty acids (FFA). This lipolytic effect can be attenuated by concomitant administration of glucose or by administering insulin, which is antilipolytic.

The effect of growth hormone on protein metabolism is anabolic. Growth hormone enhances incorporation of leucine into muscle protein. This is reflected best when the muscle tissue of acromegalics is examined. Increase in muscle fiber size and increased mitochondria are strikingly obvious. The incorporation of amino acid into muscle is also mediated by somatomedins and is probably brought about by enhancing the tissue permeability.

The clinical indications that require evaluation of growth hormone dynamics are discussed in Chapter 3.

2.3. Thyrotropin

Thyrotropin (TSH) is secreted by the pituitary thyrotrophs. These cells represent 3% to 5% of the pituicyte population and can be recognized by their angular or polyhedral shape and by the small size of their secretory granules. Thyrotropin is a glycoprotein consisting of two peptide chains, an α and a β subunit. The α subunit is identical to α subunit of other glycoprotein hormones (LH, FSH, HCG). The β subunit confers hormonal specificity. The β chain *per se* does not possess any biological activity.

The TSH in the plasma can be measured by a sensitive radioimmunoassay. The level of circulating TSH in the plasma ranges between 0.5 to 8 μu/ml. The level of TSH in the plasma is affected by the rates of production and of degradation by the kidney. In the basal state, the TSH is relatively constant and nonpulsatile, in contrast to other pituitary hormones such as growth hormone, ACTH, and prolactin.

The secretion and release of TSH by the pituitary gland are controlled by two opposing forces, the negative effect of circulating thyroid hormones on one hand and the stimulatory effects of the hypothalamic tripeptide thyrotropin-releasing hormone (TRH) on the other. Physiologically, in the presence of a normal hypothalamic–pituitary–thyroid (HPT) axis, the plasma TSH bears a striking reciprocal relationship to the free thyroid hormone levels. The level of TSH in the plasma at any time is determined by the interaction between the negative feedback of thyroid hormones on the thyrotroph and the positive trophic effect of TRH on the thyrotroph.

Feedback regulation by thyroid hormones is the dominant force involved in control of TSH secretion. Administration of T_4 or T_3 to euthyroid patients is characteristically associated with two changes: first, a decrease in the resting level of TSH, and second, a blunting of the provocative effect of TRH on TSH. Conversely, a decrease in the circulating level of thyroid hormones is associated with a rise in the resting level of TSH as well as an exaggerated response of TSH to the administration of TRH. Thus, it appears that both the basal TSH level and the ability of the thyrotroph to respond to exogenous TRH are modified by the circulating level of thyroid hormones.

It is believed that the suppressive effects of thyroid hormones on TSH secretion and release are mediated primarily at the level of the pituitary gland rather than at the hypothalamic level. Whereas short-term administration of thyroid hormones decreases the release of TSH, longterm administration suppresses synthesis of TSH by the thyrotroph. The exact mechanism involved in the negative feedback effect of thyroid hormones on the thyrotroph is unclear, but four experimental lines of evidence provide some insight into the yet-unclear mechanisms.

1. Experiments in thyroidectomized rats indicate an important role for intrapituitary conversion of T_4 to T_3. When T_4 is given to thyroidectomized rats previously treated with iopanoic acid (a drug that inhibits the intrapituitary conversion of T_4 to T_3, no acute decrease in TSH occurs.

2. Several *in vitro* studies have demonstrated the ability of normal pituitary homogenates to convert T_4 to T_3. It is hypothesized that the binding of T_3 to the nuclear receptors of the thyrotroph is important in initiating the acute suppression of TSH release following T_4 or T_3 administration.

3. There is also *in vitro* experimental evidence to indicate that the administration of thyroid hormones is associated with a reduction of TRH receptors in the thyrotrophs.

4. Finally, there is the possibility that the nuclear-bound T_3 induces the formation of a protein that interferes with the response of the thyroptroph to TRH.

Whatever the mechanism, administration of thyroid hormones consistently lowers the TSH level and impairs the response of the thyrotroph to exogenous TRH.

The hypothalamic control of TSH secretion and release is maintained by thyrotropin-releasing hormone (TRH). The identification, chemical characterization, and synthesis of the hypothalamic tripeptide TRH has clearly established the tonic stimulatory control of the hypothalamus on the thyrotroph. Thyrotropin-releasing hormone is a modified tripeptide (pyroglutamyl-histidyl-prolinamide) that is synthesized by the hypothalamus. It reaches the anterior pituitary via the hypophyseal portal blood vessels and binds to specific receptor sites on the thyrotroph membrane. It causes an increase in the synthesis and release of TSH by activating adenylate cyclase, resulting in an increase of intracellular cyclic AMP. The importance of TRH in preserving the functional integrity of the thyrotroph is evidenced in "tertiary hypothyroidism," a condition characterized by failure of the hypothalamus to generate TRH. In this disorder, hypothyroidism develops as a consequence of failure of the thyrotroph deprived of its hypothalamic drive.

The relative influences of TRH and the thyroid hormones on the pituitary are balanced in a delicate fashion. Although the thyrotroph depends on TRH for stimulation and secretion of TSH, an excess of thyroid hormones can obliterate the effect of TRH on the secretion and release of TSH by the pituitary. This principle forms the basis of several dynamic tests using TRH (Chapter 3).

The action of TSH is to stiumlate thyroid function. Thyrotropin stimulates function and growth of the thyroid gland. The acute effects of TSH enhance and stimulate all facets of thyroid hormonogenesis as well as release. The effect of TSH on iodide transport is biphasic. In the early phases, there is an efflux of iodide out of the gland, but later there is a tremendous enhancement of iodide uptake by the gland. Thyrotropin greatly activates organification, iodide binding, coupling, and formation of thyroxine and triiodothyronine. Histologically, colloid droplet formation is the hallmark of thyroid stimulation by TSH (or any other thyroid stimulator). The delayed effects of TSH on the thyroid gland relate to effects on growth, resulting in increased volume and number of cells as well as increased protein and nucleotide synthesis by the thyroid follicular cells.

The exact mechanisms involved in the thyroid regulation by TSH have been extensively studied. The predominant mechanism is by activation of the adenylate cyclase, cyclic AMP system. In addition, the cyclic GMP system (coupled with calcium ions) is also intimately involved in the mediation of TSH action. The role of iodide in modifying the action of TSH has also been well studied. It is recognized that in the presence of iodine deficiency there is enhancement of trapping (of iodine), a TSH-mediated effect, and in the presence of excess iodide there is an inhibition of several effects of TSH on the thyroid gland. It is believed that following its trapping and oxidation, part of oxidized iodide is transformed into a compound called compound XI. This compound XI inhibits adenylate cyclase (or activates phosphodiesterase, which degrades cyclic AMP) and thus negatively controls TSH-induced cyclic AMP accumulation. In addition to the iodine-mediated thyroregulation, the thyroid gland probably possesses alternate autoregulatory mechanisms including changes in TSH receptors. For example, after maximal stimulation by TSH, the thyroid cells resist further stimulation by TSH but respond to other stimulators such as prostaglandin E_1. Thus, it appears that although thyroid function is predominantly regulated by pituitary TSH, this can be modified at a local level by autoregulatory mechanisms that involve iodine and to a lesser extent other substances such as prostaglandins.

In summary, pituitary thyrotropin is controlled by dual mechanisms: negative feedback regulation by the circulating thyroid hormones and positive trophic regulation by hypothalamic TRH. Physiologically, TSH bears a reciprocal relationship to the level of thyroid hormone. The negative feedback exerted by thyroid hormones is a direct effect on the pituitary, probably dependent on the conversion of T_4 to T_3 within the pituitary gland. The trophic effect of TRH on the thyrotroph is blunted or lost in the presence of excess circulating thyroid hormones. The primary effect of TSH on the thyroid is to enhance function and promote growth under certain circumstances. Although the thyroid gland is driven mainly by TSH, there are built-in autoregulatory mechanisms that modify the effect of TSH on the thyroid. The utility of the TSH assay and the clinical indications to obtain a basal TSH and for performing a TRH test are discussed in Chapter 3.

2.4. Adrenocorticotrophic Hormone

Pituitary ACTH is secreted by the corticotrophs, cells that densely populate the pars distalis and the pars intermedia of the adenohypophysis. The corticototrophs take basophilic stains and can be recognized by electron microscopy by the presence of secretory granules (100–150 μu in diameter) with a characteristic halo.

Recent studies have recognized that several peptides with structural similarity to ACTH exist in the anterior pituitary. These include β-lipotropin (β-LPH), α- and β-melanocyte-stimulating hormones (α-, β-MSH), and the endorphins. All of these peptides are derived from one common precursor, proopiomelanocortin. This is a glycoprotein with a molecular weight between 30,000 and 36,000. If one visualizes the proopiomelanocortin as a trisegmented molecule, the midregion is occupied by ACTH, with a molecular weight of 4500 (hence termed 4.5K ACTH). The ACTH molecule is flanked by β-LPH at the carboxy terminal and by pro-γ-MSH at the amino terminal (see Figure 1). The actual sequence of processing of the proopiomelanocortin into the hormonally active subfragments begins in the anterior pituitary. The first cleavage results in formation of two fragments, β-LPH and the pro-γ-MSH–ACTH residue (or 21K ACTH). Further cleavage of the latter results in the formation of two residues, pro-γ-MSH and ACTH, both of which are active. The subsequent processing takes place in the intermediate lobe of the pituitary gland. The first step is the cleavage of 4.5K ACTH to form α-MSH and CLIP (corticotropinlike intermediate lobe peptide), which represents the C-terminal portion of the ACTH (Figure 2). The β-LPH subunit is further cleaved into LPH and endorphins; pro-γ-MSH is broken to smaller fragments of MSH.

The above scheme highlights several points:

1. There are significant differences in the processing methods of the anterior lobe and the intermediate lobe of the pituitary.

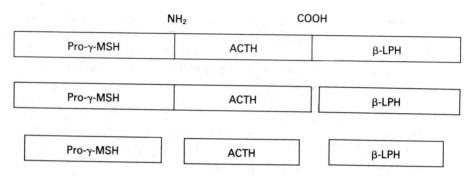

FIGURE 1. Initial processing of proopiomelanocortin in the anterior lobe.

2. The glycoprotein proopiomelanocortin is the common precursor for ACTH, β-LPH, and endorphin. The terms "big ACTH" and "big-big ACTH" represent this precursor, which does not possess the biological activity of ACTH unless further cleaved.

3. The intermediate lobe possesses a unique ability in processing the three fragments derived from proopiomelanocortin (pro-γ-MSH, ACTH, and β-LPH) into much smaller fragments. Thus, detection of these cleavage products (γ-MSH, α-MSH, CLIP, γ-LPH, and endorphins) from the "big three" indicates a pituitary origin. This is of relevance in cases of ectopic secretion of ACTH-like peptides by tumors. These tumors secrete the same type of precursors as the anterior pituitary (ACTH or β-lipotropin) but do not possess the enzymatic machinery of the intermediate lobe to cleave these big molecules into smaller cleavage products.

Human ACTH is a linear polypeptide containing 39 amino acids. The basal level in the circulation ranges between 0 and 80 pg/ml. The ACTH secretion follows a diurnal rythm with a peak in the early hours of the morning, resulting in the diurnal rhythm of cortisol secretion. However, the diurnal rhythms of ACTH and cortisol secretions should be viewed in light of the fact that cortisol is secreted in episodic, pulsatile bursts, and, therefore, the level in the blood at a given time can be impressively variable.

The regulation of ACTH secretion is controlled by trophic stimuli from above and by negative feedback from glucocorticoids. Both of these factors significantly influence the secretion and release of ACTH. The trophic factor

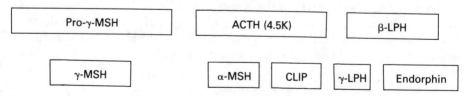

FIGURE 2. Intermediate lobe processing.

involved in stimulating ACTH release is corticotropin-releasing factor (CRF), which is a hypothalamic peptide containing 41 amino acids that provokes the release of ACTH. The release of CRF from the hypothalamus is initiated by several factors, the two notable ones being stress and hypoglycemia. The main factor that suppresses CRF is the level of glucocorticoids in the circulation. There also exists a short feedback loop between the hypothalamus and the pituitary whereby increasing concentrations of ACTH suppress the secretion of CRF.

The negative feedback exerted by glucocorticoids on ACTH secretion is directed against both the hypothalamus and the pituitary. This negative feedback can be overcome by stress. For instance under continued stress the pituitary continues to secrete ACTH despite elevated cortisol levels. In the nonstressed person, adminstration of even small amounts of dexamethasone is associated with a prompt decrease in ACTH (and cortisol) secretion, forming the basis of a variety of dexamethasone suppression tests (Chapter 27).

The main action of ACTH is to stimulate the adrenal cortex to secrete glucocorticoids almost instantly. ACTH also plays a role in the regulation of aldosterone secretion, albeit a secondary one to the renin–angiotensin–aldosterone system. The adrenal androgens are also stimulated by ACTH. All of the actions of ACTH are mediated by increasing the cyclic AMP level within the adrenal tissue.

The utility of the ACTH assay as well as the clinical indications for testing ACTH reserve are discussed in Chapter 3.

2.5. Follicle-Stimulating Hormone and Luteinizing Hormone

Although the two gonadotropins LH and FSH possess different actions, they are considered together since they are probably secreted by the same cell type (the gonadotroph) and are controlled by regulatory mechanisms that are not too dissimilar. Both FSH and LH are secreted by the gonadotrophs, which constitute approximately 5% of the population of the pituitary cells. These cells are PAS positive and have been referred to as the "castration cells," since they enlarge with striking vacuolation following the removal of the gonads. Electron microscopic studies have suggested the existence of two types of gonadotrophs, one for FSH and one for LH, but this issue is far from settled.

Both LH and FSH are glycoproteins consisting of an α and a β chain. The α chains of LH, FSH, TSH, and HCG are identical, containing 96 amino acids in the same sequence. The β chain is the unique part of these glycoproteins, conferring hormonal specificity.

The control of gonadotropin secretion and release is modulated by dual mechanisms: trophic influence from the hypothalamus and negative feedback by the sex steroids in the circulation. Before each of these dual aspects is discussed, three fundamental statements require emphasis: first, in both sexes, both gonadotropins are controlled by a single hypothalamic peptide called gonadotropin-releasing hormone (GnRH); second, in both sexes, the respective sex steroids (testosterone or 17β-estradiol) exert a negative feedback on the hypothalamic–pituitary unit; third, the hypothalamic–pituitary unit of females is uniquely capable of responding to positive feedback by estrogens, whereas males never do. It is believed that the exposure of the fetus (or neonate) to aromatizable androgens such as testosterone or androstenedione forever abolishes the ability of the hypothalamus to respond to positive feedback with estrogens. This phenomenon (lack of hypothalamic positive feedback to estrogen) is called "defeminization" of the hypothalamus.

Hypothalamic control over gonadotropin secretion is mediated by GnRH. There are several impressive lines of evidence to support the important role of this hypothalamic peptide.

1. The LH and FSH levels of prepubertal children are extremely low, and the pituitary gland does not begin to secrete significant quantities of gonadotropins until puberty. Although the hormonal events of puberty are far from clear, it is believed that the release of GnRH by the hypothalamus and the establishment of gonadotroph sensitivity to GnRH represent the two major steps. The prepubertal pituitary gonadotroph characteristically fails to show an LH peak in response to a bolus of synthetic LHRH. However, at the time of puberty, the gonadotrophs become sensitive and "tuned in" to respond to GnRH. This "LH programming," as it is called, may be a consequence of improved receptor sensitivity of the gonadotrophs or may be a response to the pulsatile release of GnRH by the hypothalamus.
2. Failure of the hypothalamus to generate GnRH results in classic Kallmann's syndrome with hypogonadotropic hypogonadism.
3. The exogenous administration of synthetic LHRH to a normal adult results in a four- to tenfold rise in LH and a two- to fourfold rise in FSH over the basal level, indicating the provocative influence of this hypothalamic peptide.

The negative feedback of the sex steroids on gonadotropin secretion is exerted at the hypothalamic and pituitary levels. In the male, LH secretion is negatively controlled by the serum testosterone level;, i.e., a high testosterone level suppresses and a low testosterone level stimulates LH, the hormone responsible for testosterone production. The FSH secretion by the gonadotroph is negatively controlled by the protein inhibin. This substance, secreted by the Sertoli cells of the testes, correlates with spermatogenesis. A low sperm count is associated with a low level of inhibin, which stimulates the synthesis and release of FSH and spermatogenesis (Figure 3). Although the feedback mechanism is compartmentalized in the above manner, persistent adminstration of testosterone will suppress the hypothalamus (GnRH), resulting in a lowering of both LH and FSH (Chapter 33).

The negative feedback of sex steroids on the control of gonadotropin secretion in the female is more complex. Three aspects are to be underscored.

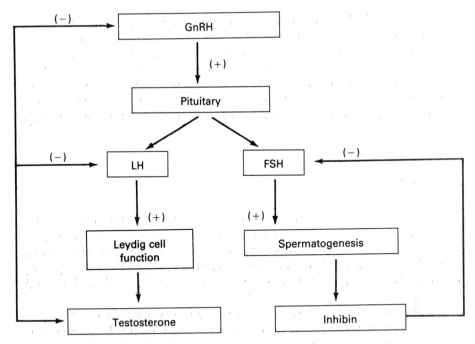

FIGURE 3. Feedback regulation of gonadotropins in the male.

1. In contrast to males, there are no separate feedback mechanisms for LH and FSH.
2. Estrogens exert their negative feedback effect on the pituitary as well as the hypothalamus. The suppressive effect of estrogens on the pituitary is evidenced by the fact that the administration of ethinyl estradiol is associated with a lowering of the basal concentrations of FSH and LH as well as a blunted response of these two hormones to exogenous LHRH. (The situation is analogous to the response of the thyrotroph to increasing thyroid hormone levels.)
3. The effects of estrogen on the hypothalamus are rather paradoxical. The hypothalamus can be visualized as consisting of a tonic portion and a cyclic portion. The tonic hypothalamus responds to negative feedback from estrogens, whereas the cyclic part responds to positive feedback from estrogens. This concept helps in explaining the hormonal events during a normal menstrual cycle. At the beginning of the cycle, the low estrogen level stimulates the tonic hypothalamus to secrete GnRH, with consequent increases in LH and FSH. During the midcycle, the high estrogen level stimulates the cyclic portion to release GnRH, which in turn results in an abrupt surge of LH. This preovulatory surge of LH is responsible for rupture of the mature graafian follicle, resulting in ovulation.

The levels of LH and FSH in the circulation range from 5 to 20 mU/ml depending on the phase of the menstrual cycle. Since these hormones fluctuate considerably, results from a single sample should be interpreted carefully. The action of LH and FSH in the male is to promote testosterone synthesis and spermatogenesis. In the female, LH and FSH stimulate the granulosa cell to synthesize estrogens, and the LH surge is responsible for ovulation.

The clinical utility of measurement of LH and FSH is discussed in Chapter 3.

2.6. Prolactin

Prolactin, a polypeptide with a molecular weight of 22,500 and an amino acid sequence of 198 amino acids, is secreted by the lactotrophs of the anterior pituitary. The lactotrophs, which populate predominantly the lateral wings of the adenohypophysis can be identified by immunoperoxidase staining using specific antisera and are believed to arise directly from the acidophil stem cell line.

The secretion and release of prolactin by the lactotrophs is totally controlled by the hypothalamus and is mediated by inhibitory (prolactin inhibitory factor, PIF) and stimulatory [prolactin-releasing factor(s) and thyrotropin-releasing hormone] influences. Each of these three is briefly discussed.

2.6.1. Prolactin Inhibitory Factor

Although the hypothalamus exerts dual control, i.e., trophic and inhibitory control, on the pituitary lactotroph, prolactin secretion and release are predominantly mediated by a negative tonic inhibitory mechanism from the hypothalamus. The hypothalamic inhibition of prolactin control is evidenced by a large body of experimental and clinical data. For instance, when the pituitary of the rat is transplanted under the renal capsule, the lactotrophs of the transplanted pituitary "escape," as it were, from the negative control of the hypothalamus, resulting in hypersecretion of prolactin. Similarly, when the pituitary stalk is transected, there is a prompt and dramatic increase in circulating prolactin levels along with a slow decline in other pituitary hormones that are under trophic control from the hypothalamus.

Clinically, convincing data to implicate the hypothalamic tonic inhibitory control over prolactin secretion are provided by several observations: lesions that infiltrate the hypothalamus (metastases, sarcoidosis, histiocytosis, or tumors) are often associated with hyperprolactinemia; drugs that deplete the hypothalamic inhibitory factor are associated with hyperprolactinemia with or without galactorrhea. Even nonsecretory pituitary adenomas may be associated with hyperprolactinemia when the tumor extends above the sella and compresses the stalk, thus interrupting the hypothalamo–hypophyseal connection that serves as the avenue of transport for the hypothalamic inhibitory factor. Thus, it is clear that the hypothalamus secretes a substance that keeps the lactotrophs under tonic inhibitory control.

It has become increasingly clear in the last few years that the hypothalamic prolactin inhibitory factor (PIF) is in fact the neurotransmitter dopamine. The release of prolactin from cultured pituitary cells can be abolished completely by dopamine and its agonists. Further, the inhibitory effect of dopamine on prolactin release can be abolished by dopamine antagonists. Several drugs, particularly the phenothazines, increase prolactin, presumably by depleting hypothalamic dopamine. In addition, these drugs may also have a direct effect on the pituitary by blocking dopaminergic receptors on the lactotrophs. In contrast, levodopa and dopamine agonists such as bromocriptine lower prolactin by virtue of their dopaminergic effects.

The interrelationship between prolactin secretion by the lactotrophs and hypothalamic dopamine is intricate and complicated. There is evidence to suggest the existence of a short feedback loop between pituitary prolactin and hypothalamic dopamine. Systemic adminstration of prolactin to animals is known to increase the turnover of dopamine in the hypothalamic median eminence, suggesting the presence of a short positive feedback loop wherein increasing prolactin concentrations result in an increase of hypothalamic dopamine (PIF), thus autoregulating prolactin secretion by the lactotroph.

2.6.2. Prolactin-Releasing Factors

In addition to exerting a tonic negative influence on the lactotrophs via dopamine, the hypothalamus also exerts trophic control over the pituitary through a prolactin-releasing factor (PRF) and thyrotropin-releasing hormone (TRH). The prolactin-releasing factor is presumably involved in the mediation of prolactin release in response to suckling. The act of suckling initiates a reflex arc involving the axons from the nipple and areola, the cerebral cortex, the hypothalamic PRF, and the lactotrophs. It has been suggested that serotonin may be involved in this mediation. Vasoactive intestinal polypeptide (VIP) is gaining exerimental acceptance as the prolactin-releasing factor of the hypothalamus. Although thyrotropin-releasing hormone (TRH) consistently releases prolactin when administered to humans and is extensively used as a stimulus for testing prolactin reserve, it probably has no physiological significance in the day-to-day control of prolactin secretion.

Prolactin can be measured in the serum by a sensitive radioimmunoassay. The indications to obtain prolactin level in the serum are outlined in Chapters 3 and 4.

3

Testing Pituitary Function

3.1. Introduction

The regulatory control of secretion and release of pituitary hormones is discussed in Chapter 3. The specific tests involved in the evaluation of each hormone of the pituitary gland form the subject of this chapter. In evaluating the pituitary gland, it is essential to determine whether all hormones need to be evaluated. Depending on the circumstance, one, more than one, or all trophic hormones may require evaluation. Also, the choice of tests depends on whether hypo- or hyperfunction is suspected. Provocative tests are used when hypofunction is suspected, and suppression tests are employed when hyperfunction is suspected. In the following discussion, each hormone is discussed separately, focusing on specific indications, methods of testing, and the types of tests involved; following this, collective testing of all pituitary hormones (total pituitary workup) is outlined.

3.2. Human Growth Hormone

3.2.1. The Indications

The two circumstances in which growth hormone dynamics require specific evaluation are when hyperfunction and hypofunction are suspected.

3.2.1.1. Hypersomatotropism

When acromegaly or gigantism is suspected, the tests available are (1) measurement of basal growth hormone levels, (2) response of human growth hormone (HGH) to an oral load of glucose, and (3) response of HGH to intravenous administration of thyrotropin-releasing hormone (TRH). Measurement of basal growth hormone does not always permit separation between normals and acromegalics. There are several causes for an elevated basal growth hormone level, and these are outlined in Table 13 of Chapter 4.

A good screening test for hypersomatotropism is the evaluation of the growth hormone response to an oral load of glucose. This is based on the principle that physiologically the somatotrophs are suppressed by elevated glucose levels following an oral load of glucose. The test is performed by measuring HGH levels basally and 30, 60, and 90 min following an oral load of 100 g glucose. A normal response is characterized by a decline in the growth hormone level to below 5 ng/dl regardless of how high the basal level was. The test is a good screening test since nearly all acromegalics demonstrate an inability to drop their HGH levels to below 5 ng/dl post-glucose. The limitation of the test is that several other conditions are also characterized by failure to completely suppress (see Table 12 of Chapter 4).

The HGH response to TRH is striking in acromegaly. Normally, there is no increase in the HGH level following administration of TRH. In contrast, approximately 70–80% of acromegalics demonstrate a brisk increase in their growth hormone levels following an intravenous bolus of TRH. The test is performed by obtaining HGH levels basally and 15, 30, and 60 min following the administration of 500 μg of intravenous TRH. The only conditions other than hypersomatotropism in which a HGH response to TRH may be seen are chronic renal failure and a rapid adolescent growth spurt.

The confirmatory test for hypersomatotropism, of course, is the measurement of circulating somatomedin C levels in the plasma (Chapter 4).

3.2.1.2. Hyposomatotropism

Hyposomatotropism, growth hormone deficiency, assumes primary importance in the evaluation of the child with growth retardation. Assessment of the growth hormone reserve also assumes importance in the hormonal evaluation of pituitary tumors, since this hormone is one of the earlier ones to be lost by tumor encroachment. The adequacy of growth hormone secretion cannot be established by measuring basal levels, since there is considerable overlap in the basal level of normals and hypopituitary patients. (The range of basal hormone levels in normals is 0.5–5 ng/dl.) Thus, the adequacy of growth hormone reserve can be established only by evaluating the response of this hormone to provocative stimuli. There are several physiological and pharmacological provocative stimuli that release growth hormone: exercise, deep sleep, hypoglycemia, L-dopa arginine, glucogon, etc. Of these stimuli, the two important ones that are practically used are insulin-induced hypoglycemia and L-dopa.

The hypoglycemia test is performed on the overnight-fasted patient by intravenously administering 0.1 U of regular insulin per kilogram body weight. The growth hormone levels are measured basally and 30, 60, and 90 min following insulin, with simultaneous glucose determinations. The degree of reduction in the blood glucose needed to stimulate growth hormone is variable, but, in general, a reduction by 50% of the base-line level is considered optimal. The reserve of growth hormone is considered normal when the level exceeds an absolute value of 10 ng/dl. In addition to hypopituitarism, causes for a blunted growth hormone response include obesity, depression, and hypothyroidism. Occasionally, a normal person who fails to respond to hypoglycemia on one occasion may demonstrate a perfectly normal response on a subsequent day. The reason for such a phenomenon is unclear.

L-Dopa is also a reasonably good provocative test to assess growth hormone reserve. The test is performed by assaying growth hormone in a basal sample and 30, 60, and 90 min following 1 g of orally administered L-dopa. The criteria are the same as for the hypoglycemia challenge.

Insulin hypoglycemia and L-dopa stimulate growth hormone via the mediation of different neurotransmitters, i.e., hypoglycemia by adrenergic and L-dopa by dopaminergic mediation. Failure to respond to both hypoglycemia and L-dopa usually indicates hyposomatotropism, i.e., loss of growth hormone reserve. The only exception to this is the child with growth retardation secondary to emotional deprivation syndrome. This person is characterized by loss of growth hormone responses to pharmacological stimuli but preservation of the sleep-related growth hormone surge, which is mediated by serotoninergic mechanisms.

Table 8 summarizes the clinical indications and applications of the growth hormone assay.

3.3. Thyroid-Stimulating Hormone

The clinical circumstances that require assay of TSH can be divided into indications in which basal TSH alone is required and those in which dynamic testing of TSH, i.e., evaluating the TSH response to TRH, is required.

TABLE 8
Assessment of Somatotroph Function

Condition	Basal level	Dynamic study	Comment
Hyperfunction	Elevated	Glucose suppression	Failure to suppress <5 ng is suggestive
Acromegaly Gigantism		HGH response to TRH	Abnormal response to TRH highly suggestive of acromegaly
Hypofunction Short		Insulin hypoglycemia	Failure to increase HGH above 10 ng by
stature	Nondiagnostic	L-Dopa	dual stimuli indicates impaired HGH
Tumor			reserve
Emotional deprivation syndrome		Sleep	Nycthemeral response preserved but response to chemical stimuli impaired

The indications to obtain measurement of basal TSH level are:

1. To establish the etiology of hypothyroidism. Primary hypothyroidism is associated with elevated TSH level, whereas pituitary or hypothalamic hypothyroidism is associated with a lack of elevation of TSH. In the latter situation, even the demonstration of a "normal" TSH is indicative of a breakdown in the normal reciprocal relationship between thyroid hormones and TSH.
2. To demonstrate adequacy of therapy with levothyroxine for replacement or suppressive purposes. In patients receiving replacement therapy for primary hypothyroidism, the maintenance dose of levothyroxine is that which normalizes the elevated basal TSH before initiation of therapy. When levothyroxine is used for suppressive purposes, the aim is to achieve complete suppression of TSH below normal.
3. In the evaluation of "euthyroid goiters." Compensated thyroid function can account for euthyroidism and a goiter at the expense of an elevated TSH. Such is the situation in patients with compensated Hashimoto's thyroiditis, iodine-deficient goiters, defects in thyroid hormonogenesis, and certain instances of peripheral resistance to thyroidal hormones.

It should be noted that measurement of basal TSH is seldom indicated in the evaluation of the hyperthyroid patient unless unusual disorders are suspected, e.g., hyperthyroidism secondary to excessive secretion of pituitary TSH or hypothalamic TRH. The conditions characterized by abnormal basal TSH levels are outlined in Table 9. The indications for TRH study are:

1. To establish the diagnosis of hyperthyroidism in general and Graves' hyperthyroidism in particular. When the clinical features of hyperthyroidism are mild and the laboratory data are borderline, the demonstration of an absent or blunted TSH response to TRH establishes the diagnosis of hyperthyroidism.

TABLE 9
Disorders Characterized by Abnormal Basal TSH Levels

Elevated basal TSH	Decreased basal TSH
Primary hypothyroidism	Hyperthyroidism
Compensated euthyroidism	Hypopituitarism
Neonatal period (first day)	Depression
TSH-secreting tumors	Anorexia nervosa
Peripheral resistance to thyroid hormones	Drugs: thyroid hormones, L-dopa, dopamine, glucocorticoids
Malnutrition	

2. To evaluate TSH reserve. In the presence of an intrasellar tumor, the demonstration of loss of TSH response to TRH is indicative of compromised thyrotroph reserve. Since TRH also stimulates release of prolactin, the adequacy of two hormones (TSH, prolactin) can be assessed by a single stimulus.
3. To establish the diagnosis of primary hypothyroidism. The TRH test has found application when hypothyroidism is mild or compensated with only marginal changes in the thyroxine or T_3 values. In such instances, even when the TSH level is equivocal, the response of TSH to TRH is exaggerated, establishing the diagnosis of subtle, subclinical primary hypothyroidism.
4. To differentiate between pituitary (secondary) and hypothalamic (tertiary) hypothyroidism. The TSH response to TRH in pituitary hypothyroidism is blunted or absent, whereas in hypothalamic hypothyroidism the response is delayed but sustained.
5. To ensure adequacy of suppressive therapy with levothyroxine. This situation is especially important in patients with differentiated thyroid carcinoma on suppressive doses of levothyroxine. The adequacy of dosage can be determined by demonstrating abolition of the TSH response to intravenous TRH.
6. To establish the gravesian nature of ophthalmopathy in euthyroid Graves' disease. Patients with euthyroid Graves' disease (EGD) often demonstrate an abnormal TSH response to TRH. The usual abnormality is an impaired or blunted TSH response to TRH. This abnormality is encountered in approximately 60% of patients with euthyroid Graves' disease.
7. To provide strong supportive evidence for hypersomatotropism. The TRH test has diagnostic and prognostic value in acromegaly. Nearly 80–85% of acromegalics demonstrate an abnormal HGH response to TRH administration (normally TRH does not cause release of growth hormone). There is often a dramatic and temporally related increase in the growth hormone levels of acromegalics 30–60 min following an intravenous bolus of TRH. When positive, the test strongly supports the diagnosis of acromegaly and can be used as a diagnostic tool and a parameter to predict response to therapy. Restoration of eusomatotropism following surgery or radiation is associated with normalization of this abnormal response. Finally, acromegalics with the abnormal HGH response to TRH tend to respond more favorably to drug therapy with the ergot alkaloid bromocriptine.

The sampling of blood for hormone determinations following TRH depends on the indication for which the test is performed. In its most simplistic form, when the test is done to document hyperthyroidism, all that are needed are a sample for TSH before and one 30 min after an intravenous bolus of TRH (short TRH test). If the test is performed to assess the pituitary reserve, samples are required at 30, 60, 90, and 120 min, and the samples are assayed for TSH as well as prolactin. If the test is performed to differentiate between

TABLE 10
Indication for TRH Study

To establish the diagnosis of hyperthyroidism
To evaluate the TSH reserve in the presence of pituitary tumors
To establish the diagnosis of compensated primary hypothyroidism
To differentiate secondary from tertiary hypothyroidism
To ensure adequacy of suppressive therapy with levothyroxine
To support the diagnosis of euthyroid Graves' disease
In the evaluation of acromegaly

pituitary and hypothalamic disease, the sampling may have to be extended to 180 min.

The test is generally well tolerated. Nausea, desire to micturate, and lightheadedness are the usual side effects.

The indications requiring dynamic testing of TSH, i.e., evaluating the TSH response to TRH, are several. The TRH test evaluates the ability of the thyrotroph to respond to the intravenous administration of TRH. Thyrotropin-releasing hormone is an extremely effective stimulus for the release of TSH from the pituitary gland. Although TRH is effective orally, subcutaneously, or intramuscularly, the peak levels are achieved by the intravenous route following a bolus of TRH. The peak response occurs between 20 and 40 min after a bolus and is usually evident in the plasma 30 min following TRH. The normal response in our laboratory is a 14- to 20-μU/ml increment over the basal TSH value or at least a threefold rise of TSH over the basal value. The magnitude of the response of TSH to TRH is logarithmic and dose related up to the 400-μg dose; most laboratories use 200 to 400 μg of TRH. The magnitude of the TSH response is directly related to the basal concentration of TSH in plasma. The indications to perform a TRH study are outlined in Table 10.

3.4. Adrenocorticotropic Hormone

The indications for measuring pituitary ACTH can also be divided into those circumstances in which a basal sample is drawn for diagnostic purposes and those involving studies that evaluate ACTH dynamics.

3.4.1. Indications for Obtaining Basal ACTH

There are two circumstances in which measurement of plasma ACTH can provide diagnostic assistance:

1. In the evaluation of patients with hypoadrenalism. The measurement of basal plasma ACTH in hypoadrenal patients can help differentiate primary from secondary adrenal insufficiency. The demonstration of an elevated basal ACTH in the presence of a low serum cortisol is

diagnostic of primary adrenal insufficiency (Addison's disease), whereas the demonstration of a low serum ACTH in the presence of hypocortisolemia is indicative of secondary adrenal insufficiency (hypopituitarism).

2. In the evaluation of patients with hypercortisolism. The measurement of basal plasma ACTH in patients with hypercortisolism (Cushing's) is an adjunctive test to delineate the etiology in the following manner: (a) the combination of a high serum cortisol and a normal or minimally elevated plasma ACTH is suggestive of pituitary-dependent Cushing's disease; (b) the combination of a high serum cortisol and a low (or undetectable) ACTH is suggestive of adrenal tumor causing Cushing's syndrome; (c) the combination of a high serum cortisol and a high plasma ACTH is highly indicative of ectopic ACTH secretion causing Cushing's syndrome.

Although measurement of basal plasma ACTH can be helpful in evaluating patients with hypo- and hypercortisolism, the assay is useful only when the results are classic. Most often, when the results are borderline high or low, difficulties in interpretation preclude diagnostic assumptions.

3.4.2. Indications for ACTH Dynamic Studies

There are three studies that evaluate the dynamics of ACTH: the hypoglycemia test, the metyrapone test, and the ovine CRF (corticotropin-releasing factor) test.

3.4.2.1. The Insulin Hypoglycemia Test

Hypoglycemia is a powerful provocative stimulus for the release of ACTH, probably mediated by adrenergic mechanisms via release of hypothalamic CRF. The principle and method of testing are the same as those for growth hormone release and have been oulined in Section 3.2.1.2. The hormones measured are ACTH and cortisol before and 30, 60, and 90 min following the intravenous administration of insulin. Although the definition of a "normal response" is variable, in general a twofold increase in ACTH is desirable. The cortisol response lags behind the ACTH response. An absent ACTH response to adequate hypoglycemia is supportive of ACTH deficiency, either as a result of intrinsic pituitary pathology or secondary to hypothalamic dysfunction.

3.4.2.2. The Metyrapone Test

Metyrapone is a drug that inhibits the conversion of 11-deoxycortisol (compound S) to cortisol (compound F) by inhibiting the enzyme 11β-hydroxylase within the adrenal cortex. As a result, there is a decrease in compound F level, which stimulates the hypothalamic–pituitary axis to secrete more ACTH. The increased amounts of ACTH stimulate the adrenal cortex with resultant activation of steroidogenesis. However, because of the block in the final step, the steroidogenesis stops short of synthesizing increased amounts of compound S.

Therefore, the triple response of a normal person, i.e., one with normal adrenals and an intact hypothalamic–pituitary axis, to the oral administration of metyrapone is as follows: a decrease in cortisol (F), an increase in ACTH, and an increase in deoxycortisol (S), which is the precursor product proximal to the block created by metyrapone. This is reflected in the normal person as an increase in the urinary 17-hydroxycorticosteroids, which measure compound-S. (The 17-OHCS normally measure both compound F and compound S, but metyrapone precludes formation of compound F, and hence most of the 17-OHCS consists of the precursor, compound S.)

The proper interpretation of the metyrapone test depends on three prerequisites:

1. The completeness of the enzymatic block created by the drug. Unless the block is significant enough to lower the cortisol level, the subsequent phenomena will not take place. Adequacy of the block should always be confirmed by demonstrating a significant lowering of cortisol level in plasma.
2. The integrity of the hypothalamic–pituitary axis, since the ACTH response to declining cortisol levels is the key phenomenon.
3. The integrity of the adrenal cortex to respond to the endogenous ACTH drive. The metyrapone test cannot be interpreted without knowing whether the adrenal glands are viable or not. For instance, a failure to increase urinary 17-OHCS following metyrapone can be indicative of either hypopituitarism (ACTH lack) or Addison's disease (primary adrenal disease). However, if the presence of adrenal responsiveness has been established prior to performing the metyrapone test, then the failure to increase the 17-OHCS following metyrapone can only mean hypopituitarism. Therefore, it is essential to perform an adrenal stimulation test by the administration of exogenous ACTH before doing the metyrapone test. If the adrenal glands are shown to respond to exogenous ACTH, one can assume that a similar response can be expected with increases in the endogenous ACTH, and, hence, attempts to stimulate the endogenous ACTH reserve by metyrapone are valid. If, on the other hand, the adrenals fail to respond to exogenous ACTH, the metyrapone test is not indicated, since a lack of response to metyrapone can no longer be interpreted.

The test is performed by measuring basal levels of urinary 17-hydroxycorticosteroids, serum cortisol, and ACTH before and following the oral administration of 750 mg of metyrapone every 4 hr for six doses. A failure to increase the 17-OHCS in the urine collection on the day after metyrapone is indicative of either inadequate block, ACTH lack, or primary adrenal insufficiency. Adequacy of block can be ensured by demonstrating a significant lowering of cortisol in the serum, and adequacy of adrenal function can be ensured by prior assessment of the adrenal response to exogenous ACTH. With these two prerequisites satisfied, a failure to increase the 17-OHCS following metyrapone is diagnostic of ACTH deficiency.

Patients receiving anticonvulsant therapy and patients who are hypothyroid or depressed may also demonstrate blunted responses to metyrapone.

Although metyrapone challenge is used primarily to diagnose ACTH deficiency, it can also be employed in the differential diagnosis of hypercortisolism (Cushing's). Patients with pituitary-dependent Cushing's disease increase their 17-OHCS following metyrapone, whereas those with suppressed ACTH secondary to an autonomous adrenal tumor show no response.

3.4.2.3. The CRF Test

The response of ACTH to the intravenous administration of ovine CRF has recently found application in two areas: in the etiological diagnosis of hypercortisolism and as a provocative stimulus to evaluate ACTH reserve. Patients with hypercortisolism from pituitary-dependent Cushing's disease respond to the intravenous CRF with a brisk, even supranormal, increase of plasma ACTH levels, whereas patients with Cushing's syndrome secondary to adrenal tumor or ectopic ACTH secretion by a nonendocrine tumor do not demonstrate an increase in plasma ACTH levels following the administration of CRF.

3.5. Follicle-Stimulating Hormone and Luteinizing Hormone

The pituitary gonadotropins, FSH and LH, are often evaluated together. Like growth hormone and ACTH, the pituitary gonadotropins are also pulsatile. Especially in the female, the pituitary gonadotropins demonstrate significant fluctuation depending on the phase of the menstrual cycle, rendering the interpretation of an isolated sample quite difficult and often meaningless. The clinical indications for obtaining basal FSH and LH levels and for performing dynamic studies of these hormones are mostly in the evaluation of hypogonadal patients.

3.5.1. Indications for Obtaining Basal LH and FSH Levels

1. Male and female hypogonadism. In both sexes, measurement of basal LH and FSH with concomitant measurement of the respective sex steroids constitutes the first step in the hormonal evaluation of hypogonadism. Three possible combinations can be encountered, depending on the etiology of hypogonadism (Table 11). It should be pointed out that in patients with marked lowering of sex steroids, even the demonstration of "normal" LH and FSH should be considered as a poor, suboptimal pituitary response indicating a blunted output of FSH and LH to hypotestosteronemia or hypoestrogenemia.

TABLE 11
Gonadotropin Levels in Hypogonadism

LH, FSH	Testosterone or 17β-estradiol	Interpretation	Condition
↑	↓	Hypergonadotropic hypogonadism	Primary gonadal failure
↓	↓	Hypogonadotropic hypogonadism	Hypothalamic or pituitary disease
Normal	↓	"Normogonadotropic"	Hypothalamic or pituitary disease

2. Secondary amenorrhea. In patients with secondary amenorrhea, the basal measurements of LH and FSH are likely to help only if these gonadotropins are elevated (which indicates a primary gonadal disorder). It is difficult to interpret "low" or "normal" LH and FSH in a single sample since the ranges seen in normal and hypopituitary patients do overlap considerably.

3. Hirsutism. In patients with hirsutism, the demonstration of an elevated basal LH : FSH ratio is suggestive of polycystic ovarian disease. However, this abnormality may not be evident unless multiple samplings are done, preferably on different phases of the menstrual cycle.

3.5.2. Indications for Evaluating Gonadotropin Dynamics

The gonadotropin dynamics can be evaluated by studying the LH and FSH response to the administration of exogenous synthetic LH-RH. Theoretically, the two indications for doing such a study are the evaluation of gonadotroph reserve and the differentiation between pituitary and hypothalamic hypogonadism.

1. Evaluation of the gonadotropin reserve by the use of LH-RH. Adults respond to the intravenous administration of LH-RH by a four- to tenfold increase in LH and a two- to fourfold increase in FSH. The vast degree of variability in the normal response does pose difficulties in interpreting marginal responses. A clearly flat response of both LH and FSH to LH-RH is indicative of compromised gonadotropin reserve.

2. The differentiation between hypothalamic and hypopituitary hypogonadism with the use of LHRH has not proven to be as effective as originally thought. Theoretically, hypopituitary patients do not respond to LHRH, whereas those with hypothalamic hypogonadism demonstrate a delayed, diminutive response to LHRH. In practice, however, such clear-cut patterns of separation have not emerged, minimizing the application of a single bolus of LHRH as a diagnostic test for this purpose.

3.6. Prolactin

The main indications to obtain basal serum prolactin are (1) galactorrhea, (2) secondary amenorrhea with or without galactorrhea, (3) infertility, and (4) impotence. In all of these instances, the underlying problem can be related to a prolactin problem. When the hyperprolactinemia is mild, the abnormality can be missed in a single sample because of the pulsatile nature in prolactin secretion. This can be obviated by drawing three blood samples 20 min apart, pooling the serum, and assaying prolactin in a single pooled sample.

As far as dynamic studies of prolactin, the response of this hormone to a bolus of intravenous TRH is used as an indicator of lactotroph reserve. Thus, when hypopituitarism, especially Sheehan's syndrome, is considered, the prolactin response to TRH is used to test prolactin reserve. In contrast, in the evaluation of the hyperprolactinemic patient, dynamic studies of prolactin secretion yield inconsistent results and do not have practical application.

3.7. Total Pituitary Work-up

The secretory output of the entire pituitary gland can be evaluated by simultaneously using three stimuli to release six hormones. Thus, insulin (for HGH and ACTH), TRH (for TSH and prolactin), and LH-RH (for LH and FSH) can be concomitantly administered without significant interference. The total reserve testing is indicated under the following circumstances: (1) when panhypopituitarism is considered, (2) when a pituitary tumor is demonstrated and the degree of functional compromise needs to be established, and (3) when pituitary surgery has been performed and replacement therapy is considered.

The total pituitary reserve testing can be performed within 3 hr. The basal samples of HGH, ACTH, cortisol, TSH, prolactin, FSH, and LH are drawn, following which 250 μg of TRH, 150 μg of LH-RH, and 0.1 U of regular insulin per kilogram are administered intravenously, one at a time. Blood is drawn at 30, 60, and 120 min after the boluses for measurement of the same hormones. Blood glucose should be determined to ensure that hypoglycemia has occurred. An adequate drop in blood glucose is required to provoke the release of ACTH and HGH. Since hypoglycemia can pose a serious problem in patients with hypopituitarism, who often have blunted counterregulatory hormones, the patient must be supervised very closely. The persistence of hypoglycemic symptoms or the development of CNS symptoms should necessitate immediate intravenous 50% dextrose. The total pituitary reserve testing thus demands the presence of a physician at the bedside of the patient and hence should only be performed in special units where such facilities are present.

4

Pituitary Hyperfunction

4.1. Introduction

Pituitary hyperfunction usually involves hypersecretion of a single pituitary hormone. The three common examples of pituitary hypersecretion involve growth hormone, ACTH, and prolactin, resulting in the clinical syndromes of acromegaly, Cushing's disease, and galactorrhea, respectively. Rarely, hypersecretion of TSH may result in hyperthyroidism. Hypersecretion of gonadotropins, β-lipotropins, or endorphins is extremely rare, often diagnosed by extracting these hormones from tumor tissue. Occasionally, plurihormonal hypersecretion can be encountered, usually exemplified by hyperprolactinemia in conjunction with acromegaly or Cushing's disease.

The three most common clinical syndromes—acromegaly, Cushing's disease, and galactorrhea—are reviewed in this chapter.

4.2. Acromegaly and Gigantism

Acromegaly and gigantism are conditions caused by sustained hypersecretion of growth hormone by the pituitary gland. The term gigantism denotes onset of hypersomatotropism prior to epiphyseal closure, whereas acromegaly refers to the onset of disease after epiphyseal fusion. Both disorders are characterized by their insidious onset and relentless progression. Untreated, both disorders result in considerable morbidity and even mortality as a consequence of cardiovascular compromise or perisellar expansion.

4.2.1. Etiology

Acromegaly and gigantism are nearly always caused by secretory pituitary tumors. These tumors originate from the somatotrophs, which histologically contain eosinophilic granules. Hence, on gross section these tumors are called eosinophilic adenomas. However, hypersomatotropism can also be caused by tumors arising from pituicytes with nongranular cytoplasm. Thus, chromophobe adenomas represent an important etiology for acromegaly. Anatomically, the tumor can be a microadenoma (size less than 10 mm), a noninvasive macroadenoma (confined to the sella), or an invasive macroadenoma (expanding superiorly and laterally with destruction of the walls of the sella turcica). Rarely, acromegaly may be a result of nontumorous hyperplasia of the somatotrophs. Also rare are instances in which acromegaly occurs as a consequence of ectopic secretion of growth hormone by a nonpituitary tumor. The most illustrative examples of such a phenomenon are carcinoid tumors of the bronchus or islet cell tumors of the pancreas secreting growth hormone.

4.2.2. Clinical Features

The onset of acromegaly is so insidious and the progression so slow that the disease evolves gradually, causing subtle changes that often go unnoticed by the patient. The disease literally creeps under the skin of its victims; the change in appearance can be strikingly demonstrable only on comparison of serial photographs taken over a period of time. Although acral enlargement and prognathism are the hallmarks of the process, acromegaly is in reality a systemic disease with protean manifestations.

4.2.2.1. Acral and Soft Tissue Changes

In its fully evolved form, acromegaly can be recognized at a glance. Enlargement of the hands and feet and prognathism are often striking. The soft tissue hypertrophy of the enlarged, sweaty hands impart an unmistakable feeling during a handshake with the patient. The profile of the prognathous face is aptly termed "lantern jaw." The acromegalic facies, when complete, is characterized by the prognathism, thickening of the cartilages of the nose and earlobes, overhanging supraorbital ridges, coarsening of the facial features by furrows, and thick oily skin over the malar region. The facial expression is very often constant, seemingly incapable of change ("wooden expression").

4.2.2.2. Skin Changes

Characteristic changes in the skin occur in over 90% of patients with acromegaly and consist of a thickened, coarse, oily skin firmly attached to the subcutaneous tissue. Hypertrichosis and pronounced sweating are often present. Less frequent changes in skin include increased pigmentation, acanthosis nigricans, and development of fibrous skin tags or papilloma.

4.2.2.3. Heart and Cardiovascular System

The four important cardiovascular sequelae of chronic hypersomatotropism are hypertension, cardiomegaly, cardiomyopathy, and cardiac arrythmias. It is not entirely clear if any or all of these are completely reversible. Hypertension is encountered in 30% to 50% of patients with acromegaly. The characteristics of the hypertension are identical to those seen in essential hypertension with volume expansion. An occasional association between aldosteronoma and acromegaly has been reported. Although cardiomegaly is a sriking postmortem finding in acromegalic patients, the incidence of this finding in the absence of congestive failure is relatively low. The high prevalence of echocardiographic abnormalities (septal hypertrophy, abnormal wall motion, etc.) in acromegalics without cardiac symptoms or radiological evidence of cardiomegaly indicates significant cardiac involvement in this disease. Acromegalic cardiomyopathy is a unique entity that deserves special emphasis. Affecting a small percentage of acromegalics, especially young males with no prior heart disease, this devastating complication is characterized by the development of rapidly progressive biventricular failure, usually resistant to conventional therapy. In these patients, a correlation between the degree of growth hormone elevation and the presence of cardiac failure has been demonstrated, and, hence, such patients are deemed candidates for rapid correction of the hypersomatotropism. Cardiac arrhythmias in acromegalics, especially supraventicular, should invoke the suspicion of concomitant hyperthyroidism, a not infrequent association.

4.2.2.4. Articular and Neuromuscular Manifestations in Acromegaly

The two articular manifestations of acromegaly are acromegalic arthropathy and chondrocalcinosis (pseudogout). The arthropathy of acromegaly resembles closely that of degenerative joint disease. The involvement of the major joints as well as the severity and clinical progression are identical to osteoarthritis. Radiologically, the widening of joint spaces as a result of cartilaginous hypertrophy is a striking finding. Unfortunately, the articular sequelae remain as permanent stigmata of acromegaly even after attainment of eusomatotropism. Pseudogout can be recognized by the demonstration of calcification of the menisci or by documenting calcium pyrophosphate crystals in the joint aspirate.

The neuromuscular manifestations of acromegaly are several. Entrapment neuropathies (such as carpal tunnel symdrome) are present in more than 60% of patients. Hypertrophy of the nerves can sometimes be clinically detected. Very rarely, vertebral root pain can be experienced as a result of the thickened spinal roots being entrapped in the vertebral foramena. Muscle weakness, especially of the proximal muscles, is seen in fewer than 10% of patients but occasionally can be pronounced. Abnormal nerve conduction velocities may be demonstrable even in asymptomatic individuals and are considered a sign of active disease.

Visceromegaly in acromegaly is a consistent autopsy finding. Thus, hepatomegaly, splenomegaly, renomegaly, and cardiomegaly are frequently seen post-mortem. For clinical purposes three aspects are pertinent. First, sialomegaly (especially enlargement of the submaxillary gland) is extremely frequent in acromegaly, being encountered in more than 90% of patients in some series; second, although hepatomegaly can be caused by hypersomatotropism *per se,* a second etiology may be operative in a small but significant number of acromegalics; third, thyromegaly, diffuse as well as nodular, may be seen in 25% to 30% of acromegalics, mostly euthyroid.

The other manifestations of acromegaly are related to those of a tumor growing in a strategic intracranial location. When acromegaly is caused by an enlarging and invasive pituitary tumor, the pressure effects can result in destruction of the pituitary gland (resulting in hypopituitarism) or in chiasmal compression (resulting in visual field defects).

4.2.3. Differential Diagnosis

Acromegaly may have to be distinguished from an entity called pachydermoperiostosis, a hereditary condition characterized by hypertrophy and thickening of skin, subcutaneous tissue, and bone. This entity can be differentiated from acromegaly by the lack of systemic involvement and by the normal hormone data.

4.2.4. Complications

The complications of acromegaly are several. In addition to cosmetic disfigurement, the following complications may develop:

1. Pituitary apoplexy or sudden bleeding into the tumor. This is an important complication, often lethal if unrecognized. Acromegaly represents the single most common underlying predisposing disorder for pituitary apoplexy, which is a very rare phenomenon. The condition is characterized by the sudden development of severe headache and vomiting with rapid visual deterioration. The two immediate complications are blindness and adrenal failure secondary to acute loss of ACTH. This intrasellar castastrophe can be readily recognized by the "core-and-ring" appearance in computerized tomograms. Unless emergency decompression is carried out, the condition carries an extremely high mortality. In those who survive the episode without surgery, residual visual loss and panhypopituitarism are certain sequelae. Ironically, the development of apoplexy is curative for the acromegaly except in rare instances where the hypersomatotropism may recur years after the apoplexy.
2. Hypopituitarism as a result of encroachment of normal tissue by the enlarging tumor.
3. Visual field defects as a result of upward extension of the pituitary tumor.
4. Cardiac failure secondary to chronic hypersomatotropism, an extremely disabling complication.

4.2.5. Diagnostic Studies

The laboratory studies in patients with hypersomatotropism can be classified into four types of tests: screening tests, confirmatory tests, topographical tests, and nonspecific tests.

4.2.5.1. Screening Tests for Hypersomatotropism

In addition to the serial photographs taken over a protracted period of time, which can be strikingly illustrative, the major screening test for acromegaly is the evaluation of growth hormone response to an orally administered load of glucose in a fashion similar to the oral GTT.

In normal subjects, oral glucose, following absorption, promptly suppresses the growth hormone level to below 5 ng/dl regardless of the basal level. In contrast, patients with acromegaly demonstrate one of the following three abnormal response patterns to glucose administration. The first and the most frequent one is called "partial response pattern" in which the elevated basal level declines, but not to under 5 ng/dl (indicating that the hyperactive somatotropes are still capable of partially responding to physiological cues). The second response is termed "nonresponse pattern," in which no change is seen following glucose; the third pattern, referred to as the "paradoxical response pattern," is seen when the growth hormone paradoxically increases following glucose. Care should be taken in interpreting the growth hormone levels in acromegalics because of the high degree of spontaneous fluctuation in growth hormone levels encountered in these patients. Also, it should be realized that several conditions may be characterized by an abnormal suppression test (Table 12). Very rarely, acromegaly can occur in the presence of a normal suppression test. Therefore, the glucose suppression test is, at best, a screening test.

Measurement of basal growth hormone levels does not consistently sep-

TABLE 12
Inadequate Growth
Hormone Suppression to
Glucose

1. Acromegaly, gigantism
2. Unstable ("brittle") diabetes
3. Chronic renal failure
4. Cirrhosis
5. Pubertal growth spurt
6. Carcinoid syndrome
7. Protein–calorie malnutrition
8. Anorexia nervosa
9. Primary hypothyroidism

arate normals from those with acromegaly. This is because of the extremely pulsatile nature of growth hormone and the extreme perturbations in the circulating levels of growth hormone that can be caused by numerous physiological factors; further, several disease states can be associated with elevated growth hormone level in the circulation. The various causes for an elevated basal growth hormone level are outlined in Table 13.

4.2.5.2. Confirmatory Tests

The confirmatory test for establishing the diagnosis of acromegaly is the measurement of the level of somatomedin C in the circulation. Somatomedin C belongs to a family of peptides referred to as growth-promoting factors with insulinlike activity. Somatomedins are generated by the liver under the trophic effect of growth hormone. These peptides mediate the growth-promoting effect of growth hormone and in that sense can be considered as "messengers" that mediate the somatotrophic effect of the hormone. The multitude of assay systems that have been developed in recent years to facilitate measurement of these peptides has created a great deal of confusion in terminology as well as in interpretation of results. Nevertheless, the immunoassay for somatomedin C closely reflects the level of circulating growth hormone and is considered to be the confirmatory test to document the presence of chronic, sustained hypersomatotropism. A normal somatomedin C level in the plasma clearly excludes acromegaly. In addition to its diagnostic utility, somatomedin C is one of the best parameters to assess response to therapy.

The growth hormone response to the intravenous administration of thyrotropin-releasing hormone (TRH) is also considered diagnostic for acro-

TABLE 13
Causes for Elevated
Growth Hormone

Pathological
1. Acromegaly, gigantism
2. Unstable diabetes
3. Carcinoid syndrome
4. Cirrhosis with portocaval shunt
5. Anorexia nervosa
6. Protein–calorie malnutrition
7. Hypoglycemia
8. Drugs: β blockers

Physiological
1. Pubertal growth spurt
2. Exercise
3. Stress

megaly. Approximately 70–80% of patients with active acromegaly demonstrate a prompt increase in growth hormone following an intravenous bolus of TRH, in contrast to normal subjects who do not show a growth hormone increase in response to TRH. In conjunction with somatomedin C levels, the growth hormone response to TRH is employed in the diagnosis and follow-up of patients with acromegaly.

4.2.5.3. Topographical Tests

The topographical tests in the evaluation of acromegaly include plain lateral films of the skull, computerized tomography of the sella (and suprasellar area), and perimetry for visual fields. The aims of these tests are (1) to document enlargement of the sella turcica or the pituitary gland, (2) to delineate extension of tumor above or laterally, and (3) to detect encroachment on the optic chiasm.

4.2.5.4. Nonspecific Tests

The nonspecific, nonhormonal tests merely provide supportive evidence for the presence of hypersomatotropism. Thus, the heel pad thickening in soft tissue films of feet, the sesamoid index in the hand X rays, the hyperphosphatemia (from increased tubular reabsorption of phosphorus), and abnormal glucose tolerance (or even overt diabetes) belong in this category.

The interhormonal relationship between growth hormone excess and other hormones merits mention. Three in particular are worth focusing on:

1. The abnormal glucose tolerance occurs for several reasons. Growth hormone is an antagonist to the peripheral action of insulin. In the early stages of disease, growth hormone actually stimulates the secretion of insulin by the β cell, but eventually this results in β-cell exhaustion. ("Growth hormone tickles the β cell, eventually tickling it to death.")
2. The serum calcium is usually normal in acromegaly. The presence of persistent hypercalcemia associated with acromegaly should evoke the suspicion of concomitant hyperparathyroidism (and the possibility of the multiple endocrine adenomatosis, type I).
3. Interpretation of thyroid function in acromegaly should be viewed in light of the fact that chronic hypersomatotropism alters the thyroxine-binding proteins (decrease in TBG and increase in TBPA). Also, interpretation of the TSH response to TRH should take into consideration the fact that chronic hypersomatotropism blunts the TSH response to TRH. This reversible phenomenon obviously poses difficulty in a diagnosis of thyrotropin deficiency consequent to tumor encroachment

as well as concomitant hyperthyroidism, which may be present in some acromegalics.

4.2.6. Course and Prognosis

Untreated acromegaly carries a high morbidity, usually as a consequence of cardiac disease, local pressure effects of the encroaching tumor, and hypopituitarism. Mortality from acromegaly is usually from cardiac failure or apoplexy. The so-called "burnt-out acromegaly" merely represents instances of pituitary apoplexy developing during the course of acromegaly, resulting in "auto cure." The price to pay in those surviving the apoplectic episode is usually panhypopituitarism.

4.2.7. Treatment

The therapeutic options for acromegaly and gigantism have broadened in the past decade. Of the three available options—surgery, radiation, and drug therapy with dopamine agonists—medical therapy with drugs is at best only adjunctive. Thus, definitive therapy for acromegaly revolves around surgery and radiation therapy. The ideal method for treating acromegaly should be one that effectively removes all hyperfunctioning tissue with preservation of normal pituitary function and one that is associated with very little morbidity or mortality and carries a low recurrence rate. Theoretically, all the above goals can be attained by carefully performed transsphenoidal microadenectomy. However, the single most important factor determining the outcome of transsphenoidal microadenectomy is the surgical expertise and track record of the institution in "curing" acromegaly by this surgical modality.

Despite controversy regarding the "single most effective" means of therapy, certain principles are well accepted. First, surgical intervention is clearly indicated in the presence of large tumor, visual compromise, and supra- or parasellar extension. Similarly, when rapidly progressive or refractory congestive failure is present, surgical therapy provides a rapid method of lowering growth hormone. Second, conventional radiation to the pituitary gland is a safe and nonmorbid modality to deliver 5000 rads to the pituitary over a 3- to 4-week period. The low rate of complications (such as hypopituitarism) with this form of therapy should be tempered by the long duration taken to achieve a "cure" as well as the relatively low cure rates (ranging from as low as 30% to as high as 60%). Third, proton beam radiation to the pituitary may work faster (6 months) but is associated with an unacceptably high rate of development of subtle or overt hypopituitarism. Besides, such therapy is limited to few centers in the United States. Fourth, drug therapy with ergot derivatives—bromocriptine and, more recently, pergolide—is at best adjunctive, since the growth hormone-lowering effect of these drugs, although impressive, is seldom complete or permanent. Besides, tumor progression can occur even while the patient is on therapy, the cost of which on a long-term basis can be considerable.

4.3. Pituitary-Dependent Cushing's Disease

Cushing's disease (bilateral adrenal hyperplasia, central Cushing's) is characterized by the development of hypercortisolism secondary to inappropriate ACTH secretion by the pituitary gland.

4.3.1. Etiology

Pituitary tumors are the most important and frequent anatomic etiology for Cushing's disease. Thus, microadenomas (tumors under 10 mm), noninvasive macroadenomas (tumors larger than 10 mm but confined to the sella), and invasive macroadenomas are all known to cause Cushing's disease. Rare cases of Cushing's disease secondary to hyperplasia of the corticotrophs probably represent the early stages in the evolution of the disease. Histologically, basophilic as well as chromophobe adenomas can cause excess ACTH production.

Although the anatomic etiology of Cushing's disease is rather clear, the pathophysiological basis for the development of the disease is far from explicit. It is believed that an abnormality in the hypothalamo–pituitary–adrenal (HPA) axis sets the stage for the development of this disorder. The characteristic hallmark of a normal HPA axis is the prompt recognition and brisk suppression of even minor increases in circulating cortisol levels. This unique ability to suppress in response to negative feedback is blunted in pituitary-dependent Cushing's. Consequently, the hypothalamic–pituitary threshold for suppression is raised, and the ACTH secretory rate is consistently inappropriate relative to the circulating cortisol levels at any given time. The raised threshold to negative feedback is evidenced by the response of patients with Cushing's disease to the standard dexamethasone suppression test: lack of physiological suppression to low-dose dexamethasone but preservation of suppression to higher doses. The degree of abnormality is variable from patient to patient, some requiring a higher dose than that used in the conventional test. Nevertheless, they do suppress, denoting preservation of physiological cues, albeit operating at a higher threshold. This response pattern is classic for pituitary-dependent Cushing's disease.

As to whether the loss in corticotroph sensitivity to negative feedback reflects an intrinsic problem within the pituitary cells or a more central problem in the hypothalamus is a much-debated issue. The bulk of evidence favors the notion that the intrinsic abnormality in this disorder is an increased production of CRF or enhanced sensitivity of the corticotrophs to the hypothalamic peptide.

4.3.2. Clinical Features

4.3.2.1. Hypercortisolism

The hallmark of pituitary-dependent Cushing's disease is hypercortisolism, which evolves slowly and progresses gradually. The clinical features of hypercortisolism are easily recognized when chronic. The classic truncal obesity with thin extremities may be seen only in longstanding cases. The violaceous striae and thinning of skin can be seen in approximately 60% of patients. The many features that are customarily associated with Cushing's—moon face, buffalo hump, and supraclavicular fat pads—are seen only when the disease has been long standing and may also be encountered with gross exogenous (noncushinghoid) obesity. Hypertension is frequently present and is caused by volume expansion and sodium retention, effects attributable to excessive glucocorticoids. Subjective muscle weakness and even myopathy are frequent features, seen in more than two-thirds of patients with hypercortisolism, and reflect the catabolic effects of excessive glucocorticoids. Backache and bone pain from osteoporosis are late sequelae. Menstrual irregularities and hirsutism result from excessive secretion of adrenal androgens, but virilization is not a feature of pituitary-dependent Cushing's disease. A varity of psychiatric disturbances ranging from depression or paranoid ideation to suicidal tendencies may dominate the course of patients with Cushing's disease.

There are a few clinical features that may permit recognition of patients with pituitary-dependent Cushing's disease. These include increased generalized skin pigmentation (because of concomitant hypersecretion of β-lipotropin), galactorrhea (as a result of hyperprolactinemia, which is seen in 30% of patients with pituitary-dependent Cushing's), and the presence of headaches or visual field cuts (caused by the enlarging pituitary mass). However, when these features are not evident, it may be difficult to distinguish this entity from hypercortisolism of other causes.

4.3.2.2. Parasellar Symptoms

Headaches or visual field cuts may be encountered when pituitary-dependent Cushing's is secondary to macroadenomas, especially when these are invasive.

4.3.3. Diagnostic Studies

The diagnostic studies in patients with pituitary dependent Cushing's may be classified into five categories: tests to establish hypercortisolism, dynamic tests to indicate the pituitary origin, adjunctive hormonal tests, topographical studies, and nonspecific metabolic abnormalities (Table 14).

4.3.3.1. Tests to Establish Hypercortisolism

Measurement of the 24-hr urine free cortisol is a reliable index of glucocorticoid hypersecretion by the adrenal cortex. It ranks second only to the measurement of cortisol production rates. The free cortisol in the 24-hr urine is not affected by alterations in the cortisol-binding globulin, a phenomenon that affects and therefore limits the measurement of serum cortisol. Since

TABLE 14
Diagnostic Studies in Pituitary-Dependent Cushing's Disease

Test	Diagnostic	Suggestive
1. Test to establish hypercortisolism	24-Hour urine free cortisol	Random serum cortisol 8 a.m., 4 p.m. serum cortisol 24-Hour urine 17-OHCS
2. Dynamic tests	Standard dexamethasone suppression test (high dose)	ACTH stimulation test Metyrapone test
3. Adjunctive hormonal tests	Plasma ACTH level	CRF stimulation test
4. Topographical tests	CT scan of the pituitary Selective venous sampling of the inferior petrosal sinus when indicated	CT scan of both adrenals
5. Nonspecific		Hypokalemic alkalosis; abnormal skull X-ray

significant amounts of free cortisol are detectable in the urine only after near-total saturation of the binding sites in the cortisol-binding globulin, an elevation of "free" cortisol denotes increased production by the adrenal gland. The only situations other than true hypercortisolism that are associated with elevated urinary free cortisol are stress and endogenous depression. The increased free cortisol in these situations is reversible on treatment of the mental illness or after correction of the stressful situation.

Measurement of serum cortisol and the 24-hr urinary 17-OHCS are less specific as definitive screening tests. As indicated above, immunoassay of the serum cortisol measures only the cortisol that is bound to the serum proteins and, hence, is altered in such diverse states as obesity, pregnancy, alcoholism, and drug therapy with estrogens or diphenylhydantoin. When the cortisol levels are markedly elevated, the diagnosis of hypercortisolism can readily be made, but in nearly one-third of patients with hypercortisolism, the serum cortisol is in the range compatible with other states characterized by increased cortisol-binding globulin.

The 24-hr urinary 17-hydroxycorticosteroids (17-OHCS) measure the metabolites of glucocorticoids. Although the 17-OHCS do reflect the integrated secretion of cortisol in a given 24-hr period, the test is affected by the same variables that affect the serum cortisol and hence is not a screening procedure with significant diagnostic value. The 17-OHCS assume importance during the performance of the standard dexamethasone suppression test, since this test has been standardized by the 17-OHCS in the urine.

4.3.3.2. Dynamic Studies

The standard dexamethasone test involves evaluation of the response of the 24-hr urinary 17-OHCS to the oral administration of a low (0.5 mg q.i.d.) and a high (2 mg q.i.d.) dose of dexamethasone. Patients with hypercortisolism, regardless of etiology, fail to suppress to the low-dose dexamethasone, suppression being defined as a postdexamethasone 17-OHCS below an absolute value of 3.5 mg in 24 hr. The classic response pattern of patients with pituitary-dependent Cushing's disease is nonsuppression to the low dose but preservation of suppression to a high dose, i.e., a decline in 17-OHCS to below 50% of the base line. Patients with Cushing's syndrome secondary to adrenal tumors and those with the syndrome of ectopic ACTH secretion caused by tumors do not demonstrate suppression to the high dose. Thus, the high-dose dexamethasone suppression test provides the first line of delineation between pituitary-dependent and -nondependent varieties of hypercortisolism.

Classic as the response to the high-dose dexamethasone test is, there are rare exceptions to the diagnostic interpretation of this test. For instance, approximately 10–20% of patients with pituitary-dependent Cushing's disease may not suppress to a high-dose dexamethasone. Such patients may respond to a "high-high dose" dexamethasone (indicating a markedly elevated threshold) or to hydrocortisone (indicating receptor insensitivity to dexamethasone). Occasionally an adrenal tumor may demonstrate suppression to the high-dose dexamethasone. Rarely, bronchial carcinoids with ectopic ACTH secretion may demonstrate suppression to high-dose dexamethasone, mimicking pituitary-dependent Cushing's.

The ACTH stimulation test, i.e., the response of the adrenal steroids to intravenous administration of ACTH, is predictable in patients with pituitary-dependent Cushing's. The hyperplastic adrenal glands respond in an exaggerated fashion when 40 U of ACTH are infused intravenously over 8 hr. This response, however, is variable from patient to patient, minimizing the diagnostic impact. Similarly, patients with pituitary-dependent Cushing's disease respond to metyrapone in an exaggerated, supranormal pattern.

4.3.3.3. Adjunctive Hormonal Tests

The basal ACTH level is an excellent adjunctive test in the evaluation of patients with hypercortisolism. The basal ACTH level in the plasma is normal to minimally elevated in pituitary-dependent Cushing's, whereas it is low to undetectably suppressed in Cushing's syndrome secondary to adrenal tumors. Patients with ectopic ACTH secretion are the ones with very high ACTH levels in the plasma. The ACTH assay is a difficult one to perform and requires better standardization. The extremely pulsatile nature of this hormone also poses problems in interpreting an isolated result of a sample drawn at a single time.

The recent availability of ovine CRF has introduced another dimension to the etiologic diagnosis of hypercortisolism. The ACTH response to ovine CRF in pituitary-dependent Cushing's disease is characterized by a brisk, even supranormal response, whereas the endogenous ACTH, already suppressed by an adrenal tumor or one ectopically secreting ACTH, shows minimal or no response to administration of ovine CRF.

4.3.3.4. Topographical Tests

Computerized tomography of the pituitary may or may not be abnormal in pituitary-dependent Cushing's disease. The computerized tomography of the adrenal will often demonstrate bilaterally enlarged adrenals.

In the rare patient with hypercortisolism and dynamic data suggestive of pituitary dependent Cushing's but in whom the pituitary imaging is normal or equivocal, selective venous catheterization of the inferior petrosal sinus and measurement of ACTH in the effluent may help to establish or exclude a pituitary origin.

4.3.3.5. Nonspecific Tests

Several nonspecific abnormalities may be noted in patients with hypercortisolism; hypokalemic alkalosis, mild polycythemia, widened mediastinum from fat pad thickening, hyperglycemia (or an abnormal glucose tolerance), lymphopenia, and an abnormal thyroid profile (low T_4, high T_3R, and low triiodothyronine) belong in this category.

The algorithmic approach for the evaluation of the patient with hypercortisolism is outlined in Figure 4.

4.3.4. Treatment

The ideal treatment for pituitary dependent Cushing's disease is extirpation of the tumor mass in the pituitary with preservation of other pituitary hormones. The choice among surgical therapy, conventional radiation to the pituitary, and drug therapy depends on numerous factors such as (1) the size of the tumor, (2) the presence or absence of suprasellar extension, (3) the degree of hypercortisolism (fulminant versus nonfulminant), (4) the surgical expertise in performing transsphenoidal microadenectomy, and (5) the presence of steroid-related complications (e.g., vertebral fractures).

When Cushing's disease is caused by an ACTH-secreting microadenoma, the ideal therapeutic recommendation is transsphenoidal microadenectomy. Performed properly, this method satisfies the dual goals of removing the tumor tissue with preservation of pituitary function. However, even in patients who respond well, there is a significant recurrence rate, possibly because the underlying mechanism of this disorder, at least in some patients, is predominantly hypothalamic.

When Cushing's disease is caused by an ACTH-secreting macroadenoma, especially one that is invasive, the therapeutic reommendation is again surgery

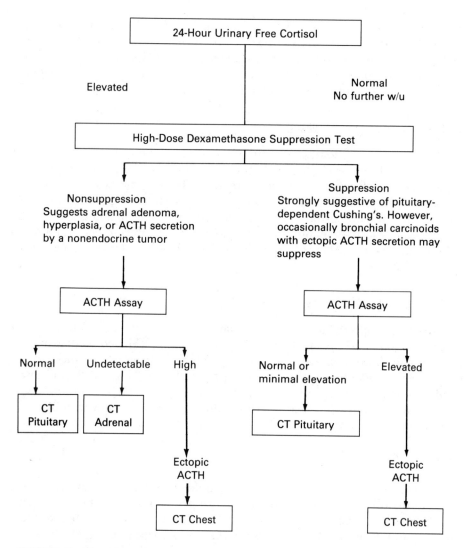

FIGURE 4. Algorithmic approach for evaluating hypercortisolism. Note that ACTH assay is not 100% standardized yet.

on the pituitary gland. The route of entry (sphenoidal versus frontal), the extent of normal rim of tissue surrounding the tumor that should be concomitantly removed, and the decision to recommend a postsurgical course of radiation to the pituitary are highly individual neurosurgical decisions.

Conventional radiation to the pituitary as an isolated modality of therapy for Cushing's disease is being recommended less frequently in centers with considerable expertise in transsphenoidal microsurgery. Conventional radiation involves the delivery of 5000 rads to the pituitary gland over a 3- to 4-week period. The low incidence of complication rates associated with this form of therapy should be tempered by the relatively low cure rates and the long duration to achieve a cure. Conventional radiation to the pituitary gland for Cushing's disease is not indicated in the presence of suprasellar extension or large tumors. Because of the long duration needed to achieve remission, radiation is not recommended when hypercortisolism is fulminant and its sequelae (bone disease, fractures, severe diabetes or hypertension, cardiac involvement, severe myopathy, and psychiatric problems, particularly suicidal tendencies) demand quick restoration of eucortisolism. Radiation therapy as an adjunct to surgery for large adenomas is recommended by some.

Drug therapy for pituitary-dependent Cushing's disease is limited to three types of drugs: those that act centrally to reduce ACTH secretion (cyprohep-tadine, L-dopa, reserpine), adrenolytic agents (o,p-DDD and aminogluteth-emide) and drugs, such as metyrapone, that interfere with conversion of 11-deoxycortisol (compound S) to cortisol (compound F). Experience with cen-trally acting drugs, in particular cyproheptadine, indicates a rather hetero-geneous response that is often only partial and is at best only adjunctive. The short-term use of adrenolytic agents that block steroidogenesis is indicated only when rapid correction of hypercortisolism is needed; these agents are employed widely in the treatment of Cushing's syndrome secondary to adrenal carcinoma.

The role of bilateral total adrenalectomy in the treatment of pituitary-dependent Cushing's disease is questionable at best. This form of therapy, although possessing the advantage of a reasonably fast cure, does not correct the basic pathology, which has its origins in the hypothalamic–pituitary locus. Following the removal of both adrenal glands, therefore, the pituitary tumor continues to grow, sometimes at a faster rate than before, despite replacement glucocorticoid therapy. The development of an enlarging pituitary tumor, increased pigmentation, and elevated serum ACTH levels despite glucocor-ticoid supplementation is called Nelson's syndrome. The incidence of this syndrome developing after bilateral total adrenalectomy for Cushing's disease is 30% to 60%. It is unclear if concomitant radiotherapy to the pituitary gland would prevent the occurrence of this syndrome following bilateral total ad-renalectomy for Cushing's disease. It should be pointed out that Nelson's syndrome develops only when bilateral total adrenalectomy has been per-formed for pituitary-dependent Cushing's disease. This underscores the fact that the prerequisite, in this circumstance, is the presence of an underlying hypothalamic–pituitary abnormality. Arguably, the only place for performing bilateral total adrenalectomy is in the patient who needs very rapid correction of hypercortisolism (fulminant hypercortisolism). Even in this circumstance, the availability of effective adrenolytic agents (medical adrenalectomy) has rendered bilateral total adrenalectomy a superfluous procedure.

In summary, the therapy for pituitary-dependent Cushing's disease should be aimed at the pituitary gland. Pituitary surgery dominates the choice of options. In the past decade conventional radiation has become a less-preferred alternative. The availability of adrenolytic agents has added a new dimension in attempting rapid restoration of eucortisolism when short-term measures are needed. Bilateral total adrenalectomy has no role in the management of pituitary-dependent Cushing's disease.

4.4. Galactorrhea

Galactorrhea or the expression of milk from the nipples in the absence of a physiological stimulus such as suckling usually indicates an underlying problem with prolactin hypersecretion. Prolactin, the lactotrophic hormone of the pituitary lactotrophs, is physiologically responsible for the mammary glands secreting milk for lactation during puerperium. The occurrence of lactation in nulliparous or nonpuerperal females or in males should invoke the suspicion of an underlying dysfunction in prolactin dynamics.

4.4.1. Etiology

The control of prolactin secretion by the pituitary gland is discussed in Chapter 2. In essence, prolactin secretion by the lactotroph is under a tonic inhibitory control by the hypothalamic prolactin inhibitory factor (PIF). The PIF is, in fact, the neurotransmitter dopamine. Thus, any mechanism that depletes hypothalamic dopamine or diminishes the sensitivity of the lactotroph to dopamine would result in "escape" of the lactotrophs from the tonic inhibitory control of PIF, with hypersecretion of prolactin. Although most patients with galactorrhea demonstrate hyperprolactinemia, in approximately 5% of patients the prolactin level may be normal. In these patients, the galactorrhea may be related to hypersensitivity of the breast tissue to normal circulating prolactin levels.

The etiologic considerations involved in hyperprolactinemic galactorrhea may be classified into five categories: hypothalamic mechanisms, pituitary disorders, chest wall diseases, miscellaneous conditions, and ectopic secretion of prolactin. Each of these categories needs brief mention.

4.4.1.1. Hypothalamic Mechanisms

Since the hypothalamus exerts a dominant negative control on the lactotrophs, it is not surprising that several conditions cause hyperprolactinemia by interfering with the hypothalamic PIF. There are three important causes in this category; drugs, infiltrative diseases of the hypothalamus, and disorders that interfere with the functional integrity of the hypothalamo–pituitary connection. Drug-induced galactorrhea (with phenothiazines as the prototype) represents a substantive etiology of hyperprolactinemia. In addition to phenothiazines, antihypertensives (reserpine, methyldopa), antidepressants, benzodiazepines, and estrogens may also induce hyperprolactinemia. These drugs cause hyperprolactinemia either by depleting hypothalamic dopamine or by decreasing dopamine receptors on the lactotrophs. The infiltrative disorders that may involve the hypothalamus are metastatic disease, sarcoidosis, and

Hand–Schuller–Christian disease. Finally, disorders that interrupt the hypothalamo–hypophyseal connection by stalk section are suprasellar tumors and pituitary tumors with suprasellar extension.

4.4.1.2. Pituitary Disorders

Tumors of the pituitary represent the most important as well as the most common etiology of galactorrhea. Although microadenomas (tumors less than 10 mm) are the most frequent etiology, macroadenomas secreting prolactin (chromophobe adenomas) and invasive macroadenomas are also associated with galactorrhea. In fact, so-called "nonsecretory" adenomas are associated with hyperprolactinemia in more than 50% of instances, even in the absence of galactorrhea. Cushing's disease and acromegaly are also associated with a significant incidence of concomitant hyperprolactinemia. One variety of hyperprolactinemia, called "functional" or "idiopathic," is characterized by hyperplasia of lactotrophs with no tumor demonstrable radiologically or during surgery. It is believed that all three conditions—hyperplasia, microadenoma, and macroadenoma—represent different stages of evolution in the spectrum of one disorder, often taking years to evolve.

4.4.1.3. Chest Wall Diseases

Trauma, herpes zoster, burns, etc. cause galactorrhea by stimulating the afferent arc in the reflex of lactation. Constant manipulation of the nipple or areola can lead to hyperprolactinemia even in nonsuckling subjects.

4.4.1.4. Miscellaneous Conditions

In this category are included diverse diseases with no common mechanism underlying the galactorrhea. The conditions in this category are primary hypothyroidism, hyperthyroidism, polycystic ovarian disease, head trauma, and precocious puberty.

4.4.1.5. Ectopic Prolactin Production

Nonendocrine tumors, in particular bronchogenic carcinoma, have been implicated in ectopic secretion of prolactin. This phenomenon, however, has been doubted by some.

4.4.2. Clinical Features

The clinical consequences of hyperprolactinemia are galactorrhea, amenorrhea, infertility, male hypogonadism, and, less frequently, osteopenia. Occasionally, in the case of a prolactin-secreting macroadenoma, the parasellar effects of the tumor may overshadow the effects of hyperprolactinemia.

4.4.2.1. Galactorrhea

Spontaneous galactorrhea or expression of milk on pressure on the nipples is the main complaint in 50–60% of patients with hyperprolactinemia. The level of prolactin does not correlate with the degree of galactorrhea. An exception to this is in males with galactorrhea, where the level of prolactin is impressively high (above 300 to 400 ng/dl).

4.4.2.2. Amenorrhea

Hyperprolactinemia constitutes a significant etiology (in some series as high as one-third of secondary amenorrhea. This underscores the need to screen all patients presenting with secondary amenorrhea for a high prolactin level in the serum. As with galactorrhea, there is no clear correlation between the degree of hyperprolactinemia and the menstrual irregularities. The mechanisms for amenorrhea are multifactorial. The chronic hyperprolactinemia impairs the gonadal responsiveness to gonadotropins, i.e., less secretion of estrogens in response to stimulation by pituitary FSH and LH. Consequently, in the classic setting, the hormonal profile of such patients is characterized by high prolactin, decreased 17β-estradiol, high LH, and high FSH. Other mechanisms for amenorrhea include destruction of the pituitary reserve by tumor and very rarely, impairment of the hypothalamic releasing factor, GnRH.

4.4.2.3. Infertility

The incidence of hyperprolactinemia as an etiology for infertility in an unselected population is probably no greater than 10%, but it represents an important cause because of its correctability. The reason for the infertility is anovulation; this is caused by inadequate estrogen synthesis resulting in failure to cause the LH surge, a prerequisite for ovulation.

4.4.2.4. Male Hypogonadism

Chronic hyperprolactinemia results in decreased testosterone production by the Leydig cells. As a consequence, decreased libido and impotence are frequent symptoms in males with chronic hyperprolactinemia. The mechanism for decreased testicular function is analogous to ovarian dysfunction caused by hyperprolactinemia. i.e., decreased responsiveness of Leydig cells to pituitary gonadotropins. Because of the reversible nature of the problem, it is important to screen all patients with male hypogonadism for a high prolactin level in the serum. Gynecomastia is not a feature of hyperprolactinemia *per se* unless complicated by concomitant hypogonadism.

4.4.2.5. Osteoporosis

The relationship between hyperprolactinemia and the development of osteoporosis is a well-noted one, but the mechanism has not been well elucidated. In part, the problem has been separating the effects of hypoestrogenemia from those of hyperprolactinemia in the development of osteoporosis. The patients prone to develop bone disease from hyperprolactinemia are older patients with longstanding hyperprolactinemia with especially high levels.

4.4.3. Diagnostic Studies

After a careful drug history is obtained and primary hypothyroidism is excluded, the only two tests required in a patient with galactorrhea are measurement of serum prolactin level and computerized tomography of the pituitary gland.

4.4.3.1. Serum Prolactin Level

To some extent, the degree of hyperprolactinemia correlates with the mass of lactotrophs. The normal level of prolactin in the serum of the nonpregnant, nonlactating female is 5 to 20 ng/dl. In patients with drug-induced hyperprolactinemia and in the "idiopathic" or "functional" variety, the levels range between 50 to 100 ng/dl. The prolactin level in patients with pituitary microadenoma range between 100 and 250 ng/dl. Levels in excess of 300 ng/dl usually are encountered with larger tumors. Highest levels of prolactin are encountered in patients harboring prolactin-secreting macroadenomas that have invaded above and sectioned the stalk.

Two practical points are worth noting. First, the pulsatile nature of prolactin release may lead to the missing of mild hyperprolactinemia. In such circumstances, obtaining three or four blood samples at 20-min intervals and measuring the serum prolactin in the pooled serum may provide diagnostic information. Second, the combination of amenorrhea and mild hyperprolactinemia may be indicative of pregnancy. Therefore, when in doubt, pregnancy should be ruled out before one obtains expensive computerized tomograms, which, incidentally, can be abnormal in pregnancy.

4.4.3.2. Computerized Tomography

High-resolution CT scans of the pituitary and suprasellar area have rendered routine skull films or polytomography obsolete in the evaluation of the hyperprolactinemic patient. An absolutely normal CT favors the diagnosis of "idiopathic" hyperprolactinemia (hyperplasia). Microadenomas (tumors under 10 mm) can be recognized by their unilateral position, especially postinfusion, in more than 90% of instances. When the CT scan is equivocal, a follow-up study is indicated in 6 months to a year. Macroadenomas (tumors >10 mm) can be readily recognized by computerized tomography. Similarly, suprasellar tumors and disorders involving the pituitary stalk lend themselves to excellent visualization by the CT study in appropriate views.

The evaluation of prolactin dynamics is hardly indicated in the patient with hyperprolactinemia and an abnormal CT study. It was once thought that in the patient with galactorrhea and a negative CT study, dynamic tests may permit separation between hyperplasia and CT-negative microadenoma. The plethora of tests devised for this purpose (TRH test, phenothiazine test, L-dopa test, L-dopa–carbidopa test, nomifensin test, etc.) are attestations to the fact that dynamic tests do not provide clear separation between the two conditions and hence are not clinically indicated.

4.4.4. Course and Prognosis

Most microadenomas are slow growing. The growth of microadenomas may be accentuated by estrogen excess. The slow growth and benign nature of these small tumors must be taken into consideration in formulating therapeutic options, especially when the hyperprolactinemia is mild and when the patient is not particularly bothered by symptoms.

4.4.5. Treatment

The three major alternatives that are available for the treatment of prolactinomas are surgery, radiotherapy, and medical therapy using dopamine agonists. Each of these modalities has some advantages and disadvantages; therefore, the identification of the single best therapy is difficult.

Transsphenoidal microsurgery has gained increasing popularity in the treatment of pituitary adenomas. The morbidity and mortality rate of this mode of surgery is very low, and the pituitary function is usually preserved following surgery. Correction of hyperprolactinemia as well as restoration of menstruation and fertility can be achieved in 50% to 90% of patients following microadenectomy. A high rate of success is usually seen in microadenomas with a modest degree of hyperprolactinemia, whereas the results are less satisfactory with tumors with very high levels of prolactin preoperatively. An important factor in determining the results of transsphenoidal microsurgery is the availability of a neurosurgeon with expertise. Even in the hands of experienced surgeons, recent data indicate that there is a high rate of delayed recurrences of hyperprolactinemia following "successful" surgery. The immediate postoperative plasma prolactin may be a predictive factor for delayed recurrences.

The role of radiotherapy in the treatment of prolactinomas is limited. The long period of time needed for normalization of prolactin level and the high incidence of hypopituitarism are the two major disadvantages. However, radiotherapy may be a useful adjunct to surgery in the treatment of macroadenomas, especially when complete cure is not achieved by surgery alone.

Bromocriptine has proved very effective in the treatment of prolactinomas. Normoprolactinemia can be reached in a high percentage of patients, and fertility is restored in 80% of patients. However, when bromocriptine is used to restore fertility two important issues are raised: the possible teratogenicity of the drug and the possible enlargement of pituitary tumors during pregnancy. Expansion of pituitary tumors resulting in field defects has been reported to occur during pregnancy. However, the risk of such a complication seems to be small for microadenomas (less than 1%) but significant for macroadenomas (approximately 10–15%). Because of this potential risk, many authorities recommend surgical treatment for women with macroprolactinomas when pregnancy is desired. As for the teratogenicity of the drug, surveillence of large numbers of patients who were given bromocriptine in the early weeks of pregnancy indicates no evidence for an increased risk of abortions or fetal malformations.

An important disadvantage of bromocriptine therapy is the need to continue the drug for a long period of time, perhaps life long. Although lasting remission after the discontinuation of bromocriptine has been reported, relapse of hyperprolactinemia with its clinical consequences usually occurs, as may reexpansion of the tumor, when the drug is discontinued. Therefore, the side effects associated with the long-term use of the drug and the economic factor should be considered when bromocriptine is chosen for the treatment of prolactinomas.

The choice of a particular modality of therapy in an individual patient should be based on several factors: (1) the desire for fertility, (2) the size of the tumor, (3) the presence of visual field defects, (4) the availability of surgical expertise, and (5) the economic factors. The recommendations given below may serve as general guidelines.

1. Macroadenomas with visual disturbances. The treatment for this group of patients should be surgical. Notwithstanding the reports in the literature attesting to a beneficial effect of bromocriptine in causing shrinkage of tumor mass, most authorities would agree that a surgical option is a wiser one. The choice of bromocriptine is tempered by the possible expansion of tumor during drug therapy, especially with the occurrence of pregnancy. The surgical approach for patients with macroadenomas is somewhat controversial. The success rate of transsphenoidal microsurgery in patients with invasive macroadenomas is only 25% in contrast to an 88% success rate for microadenomas. Therefore, many authorities recommend the transfrontal approach in the treatment of macroadenoma with significant extrasellar extension. In such patients, the role of drug therapy may be viewed as adjunctive to surgery.

2. Microadenomas. If the patient does not desire pregnancy and galactorrhea is not a distressing symptom, periodic follow-up without intervention is a reasonable choice. If fertility is desired, the treatment is either bromocriptine or transsphenoidal microsurgery. The choice between these two modalities largely depends on the availability of surgical expertise and the patient's preference. If bromocriptine is chosen, the drug should be discontinued when pregnancy occurs, and the patient should be followed closely for possible tumor expansion, although such an occurrence is rare with microprolactinomas.

3. Hyperprolactinemia with no demonstrable tumor by CT scan. This entity, referred to as idiopathic, functional, or hypothalamic galactorrhea, should be treated with bromocriptine if the patient desires pregnancy. Otherwise periodic follow-up studies with prolactin levels (and possibly CT scans) present a conservative option that can be offered to these patients.

5

Pituitary Hypofunction

5.1. Introduction

In this chapter the general aspects of hypopituitarism, as well as the specific syndromes that occur as a consequence of selective hormonal deficiencies will be discussed.

5.2. Hypopituitarism

Hypopituitarism occurs as a result of deficient secretion of one or more trophic hormones secreted by the pituitary gland. Panhypopituitarism or total deficiencies of all the hormones is a rare disorder. More often, pituitary failure is characterized by selective deficiency of one or more trophic hormones. The pituitary gland demonstrates an amazing ability to withstand the destructive effects of infiltrative or neoplastic processes, and hence clinically significant hypopituitarism does not ensue until more than 85% of the gland's reserve has been compromised. The clinical implications of this fact are threefold: first, the evolution of the clinical syndrome can be quite a slow process, indeed often taking years to evolve; second, partial deficiency of the trophic hormone(s) can be detected by sophisticated testing even in the absence of symptoms and third, even when only a single hormone is evidently affected (unitrophic) at the time of presentation, multiple trophic hormone deficiencies may develop later. This underscores the need for extended, even lifelong, follow-up of such patients. The traditional concept that gonadotropins and growth hormone are the earliest pituitary hormones to be lost, followed sequentially by TSH, ACTH, and prolactin, is observed more frequently when the pituitary reserve is compromised by tumor encroachment. However, the loss of hormone reserve can occur in any order.

5.2.1. Etiology

There are basically two major mechanisms that can cause pituitary hypofunction: loss of hormone reserve as a result of intrinsic pathology of the pituicytes (primary hypopituitarism) or loss of pituitary hormone reserve because of lack of the hypothalamic releasing factors that drive the gland to secrete (secondary hypopituitarism). The most common etiology of primary hypopituitarism is destruction of the pituicytes by tumor, vascular insufficiency, or infiltrative disorders; the most common cause for secondary hypopituitarism is developmental or acquired "stalk section," i.e., interruption of the hypothalamo–hypophyseal communication by pituitary tumors that extend above the sella or by suprasellar tumors that invade the stalk from above (Table 15).

It is essential that the multitude of causes of hypopituitarism be placed in perspective. In adults of both sexes, the most common cause for hypopituitarism is tumor of the pituitary gland, usually chromophobe adenoma. In females, Sheehan's syndrome and lymphocytic hypophysitis bear a temporal relationship to pregnancy. In children, the most common etiologies for hypopituitarism are developmental causes and craniopharyngioma. The rapid development of hypopituitarism (particularly ACTH deficiency) in patients of either sex, regardless of age, should always alert the physician to the possibility of pituitary apoplexy or rupture of an aneurysm of the cavernous portion of the internal carotid artery—catastrophic events characterized by extremely high mortality unless emergency decompression of the sella is carried out.

TABLE 15
Etiology of Hypopituitarism

Pituitary tumors	Usually chromophobe adenoma
Suprasellar tumors	Craniopharyngioma, meningioma, or dysgerminoma of the pineal gland
Vascular	Sheehan's syndrome, pituitary apoplexy
Lymphocytic hypophysitis	Restricted to females; often temporally related to pregnancy
Infiltrative disease	Metastatic disease (breast, GI tract, etc.); hemochromatosis
Granulomatous diseases	Sarcoidosis, Hand–Schuller–Christian disease, histiocytosis X, TB
Developmental	Congenital; usually affects growth; optic nerve abnormalities often present
Rare: postradiation or post-basilar-fracture of skull; maternal deprivation syndrome	Predominantly hypothalamic involvement

5.2.2. Clinical Features

The clinical features of hypopituitarism reflect the effects of the loss of various trophic hormones.

5.2.2.1. Constitutional Symptoms

The most common constitutional symptoms of hypopituitarism are tiredness, easy fatigability, and a general sense of ill health. These symptoms, which are invariably present when hypopituitarism becomes clinically significant, result from either ACTH deficiency (secondary hypoadrenalism) or TSH deficiency (secondary hypothyroidism). Changes in weight in either direction may occur, depending on the presence and relative degree of ACTH or TSH deficiency. When ACTH deficiency is significant, weight loss predominates; when TSH deficiency coexists, no change in weight or even a slight weight gain may be evident. However, since anorexia is present in most patients with hypopituitarism, weight loss is more frequently observed than weight gain. In extreme cases, the weight loss can be severe ("pituitary cachexia" or Simmond's syndrome). Depression and apathy are noted in more than one-third of patients.

5.2.2.2. Effects of ACTH Deficiency

These are most impressive and can be responsible for a strikingly dramatic presentation when adrenal crisis is precipitated by stress. In addition to easy fatigability, constant tiredness, anorexia, weight loss, and apathy, these patients are at constant risk for developing adrenal crisis. When hypothyroidism is associated with ACTH deficiency, the former, in a sense, is protective; i.e., the metabolic demands are so lowered by the presence of concomitant hypothyroidism (secondary to TSH deficiency) that these patients manage to get by at the basal state despite very little cortisol production. But when the system is stressed by infection or trauma, rapid decompensation occurs, and adrenal crisis develops. The presentation, severity, and clinical findings of adrenal crisis consequent to hypopituitarism are no different from those caused by primary adrenocortical failure. Although theoretically mineralocorticoid deficiency should not be a feature of chronic ACTH deficiency, it may occur, since ACTH plays a permissive role in the release of aldosterone by the zona glomerulosa in response to renin-mediated stimuli.

Several physical findings may be evident in the patient with ACTH deficiency. A low blood pressure and postural hypotension can be encountered in secondary adrenal insufficiency, although they are less common and less severe than in primary adrenocortical insufficiency. Lack of axillary hair, especially in females, is a striking indicator of loss of adrenal androgens; since ACTH and β-lipotropin share a common precursor peptide, ACTH deficiency is often associated with loss of the pigmentary hormone β-lipotropin. This may result in some generalized hypopigmentation. Occasionally, the loss of β-lipotropin can be so impressive as to give the skin an alabasterlike tone.

In summary, the effects of chronic ACTH deprivation include nonspecific but extremely important constitutional symptoms, hypotension, decreased skin pigmentation, loss of axillary hair (especially in females), and a heightened proclivity to decompensate into adrenal crisis during stress. This last aspect is the most crucial one to recognize, since untreated adrenal crisis is often fatal.

5.2.2.3. Effects of TSH Deficiency

The hypothyroidism that develops as a consequence of TSH deficiency is identical to primary thyroid failure. Characteristically, the thyroid gland is shrunken because of lack of TSH drive and hence not palpable. Hypothyroidism coupled with pallor (in the absence of significant anemia) may be a helpful clue to suggest hypopituitarism. It should be pointed out that lack of sexual hair, decreased libido, amenorrhea, and even hypotension can all be encountered in patients with primary hypothyroidism. Therefore, the above features, although often present in secondary hypothyroidism (hypopituitarism with TSH deficiency), are by no means pathognomonic for this entity. Pericardial effusions do occur in patients with pituitary hypothyroidism, but ascites is rare. The cutaneous, integumental, cardiorespiratory, hematologic, and metabolic consequences of hypothyroidism are the same regardless of whether the etiology is primary thyroidal or pituitary in origin.

5.2.2.4. Gonadotropin Deficiency

Deficiencies of LH or FSH are often the earliest markers to indicate the presence of hypopituitarism. *Decreased libido* in males and *oligomenorrhea, amenorrhea, or infertility* in the female are the most important symptoms. Atrophy of breasts or testes may be evident in longstanding cases.

5.2.2.5. Prolactin Deficiency

This becomes important only in the setting of the nursing mother in the postpartum period. The classic history of *inability to lactate* with amenorrhea following delivery is pathognomonic for postpartum pituitary necrosis of the Sheehan's type.

5.2.2.6. Growth Hormone Deficiency

Deficiency of growth hormone is a rare cause of *growth retardation* in children. In both adults and children, *hypoglycemia is an* important consequence of growth hormone failure. Characteristically, the hypoglycemia occurs during fasting and is particularly severe in the presence of concomitant ACTH deficiency.

5.2.2.7. Associated Features

Depending on the etiology of hypopituitarism, additional physical findings may be evident.

1. Headaches and visual field cuts is a patient with hypopituitarism are virtually diagnostic of pituitary tumor.
2. Diabetes insipidus (*polyuria, polydipsia*) in a patient with hypopituitarism signifies suprasellar disease caused by tumor (craniopharyngioma, dysgerminoma, etc.), metastatic disease (from breast, colon, etc.), or granulomatous disease (histiocytosis, Hand–Schuller–Christian disease, or sarcoidosis). It must be noted that the symptoms of diabetes insipidus are often masked by the concomitant presence of adrenocortical insufficiency. This is because in the absence of cortisol there is a marked reduction in the free water clearance by the renal tubule, imposing a nullifying effect on the lack of vasopressin (ADH). When the glucocorticoid deficiency is corrected by administering cortisol, the diabetes insipidus will become manifest, since now the renal tubules can excrete free water.
3. Galactorrhea, paradoxical as it may seem, may occur in association with hypopituitarism and is seen when hypopituitarism is secondary to stalk inhibition. When the pituitary stalk is interrupted (by a tumor), the result is loss of several hypothalamic factors that are trophic to secretion of ACTH, TSH, FSH, LH, and growth hormone. Therefore, with progressive loss of hypothalamic drive, deficiencies of any of the above hormones may develop. However, *pari passu* with loss of the trophic releasing factors, inhibition of the stalk also results in loss of the hypothalamic prolactin inhibitory factor (PIF). This leads to "escape" of the lactotrophs from the tonic negative influence of PIF, resulting in hyperprolactinemia and even in galactorrhea. Rarely, galactorrhea can occur in association with post-partum necrosis, when hypothalamic insult is coexistent with *partial* pituitary infarction.

The clinical features of hypopituitarism are summarized in Table 16.

5.2.3. Diagnostic Studies

Hypopituitarism should be suspected in any patient presenting with symptoms referable to failure of target glands, i.e., the thyroid, adrenal, gonads, or growth. There are three steps in the diagnostic work for hypopituitarism: (1) documentation of hypopituitarism by hormonal studies, (2) delineating whether the pituitary failure is "primary" (intrinsic pituitary disease) or "secondary" (to impaired synthesis, secretion, or transport of hypothalamic releasing factors), and (3) defining the etiology of hypopituitarism, with particular reference to anatomic causes.

TABLE 16
Clinical Consequences of Hypopituitarism

Hormone lost	Clinical consequence
ACTH	Constitutional symptoms: weight loss, tiredness, apathy; prone to adrenal crisis; postural hypotension; loss of axillary hair (esp. females)
β-Lipotropin	Generalized hypopigmentation
TSH	Secondary hypothyroidism, atrophied thyroid gland
Gonadotropin	Decreased libido, oligomenorrhea, amenorrhea, infertility
Prolactin	Inability to lactate
Growth hormone	Growth retardation; fasting hypoglycemia
Vasopressin	Polyuria, polydipsia

5.2.3.1. Documentation of Hypopituitarism by Hormonal Studies

This can be attained in one of the following two ways: (1) by simultaneous evaluation of the relationship between the target gland hormone and the trophic hormone of the pituitary or (2) by evaluating the reserve of each trophic hormone, employing appropriate provocative stimuli. The former is based on the negative feedback principle that when the target organ fails, the normal pituitary responds by secreting more of its trophic hormone. In essence, the demonstration of a low target-gland hormone (for example, T_4) and a nonelevated trophic hormone (pituitary TSH) implies impairment of TSH reserve. In the second method of testing, regardless of levels of basal hormone, the capacity of the pituitary gland to respond to trophic stimuli (thyrotropin-releasing hormone, hypoglycemia, or metyrapone) is evaluated. Both methods possess advantages as well as disadvantages.

The following general principles are applicable to the hormonal evaluation of pituitary function.

Measurement of a single basal sample of any pituitary hormone (without measuring the target gland hormone simultaneously) is absolutely useless for interpretation for two reasons. (1) The "normal" ranges for all the pituitary hormones at the basal state considerably overlap with the ranges seen in patients with hypopituitarism. (2) Further, the pulsatile nature of pituitary hormones is impressive enough to preclude making diagnostic conclusions based on a single sample drawn at an isolated period in time.

When both the target-gland hormone and the trophic hormone are clearly low, the diagnosis of hypopituitarism can readily be made.

When the target-gland hormone is low but the trophic hormone level is normal, pituitary dysfunction can be suspected but can not be established unless more detailed testing is undertaken.

When the target-gland hormone is low and the trophic hormone is elevated, pituitary dysfunction has been excluded.

From the above, it is evident that in the presence of a low target-gland hormone, the simultaneous demonstration of a low level of trophic hormone strongly supports hypopituitarism, whereas a clearly elevated level of trophic hormone excludes the diagnosis. Equivocal numbers mandate formal pituitary reserve testing with provocative stimuli to exclude or establish pituitary dysfunction.

Formal pituitary reserve testing involves evaluation of the response of each pituitary hormone to a specific provocative stimulus. Thus, the ability of TSH and prolactin to rise in response to intravenous TRH, the ability of ACTH and growth hormone to peak in response to hypoglycemia, and the ability of LH and FSH to respond to intravenous LH-RH are indicative of the pituitary reserve. Although these stimuli can be administered simultaneously, the test involves multiple samplings of six hormones at 30-min intervals for 2 to 3 hr, thus rendering the test expensive. The drawback is that physiologically, the definition of a "normal" response can be highly variable from person to person, and interpretation should take into consideration the multitude of factors that affect these responses in normal persons.

5.2.3.2. Distinguishing Primary from Secondary Hypopituitarism

The second step in the evaluation of hypopituitarism established by hormonal tests is to determine if the problem is primary or secondary. In general, distinction between primary and secondary hypopituitarism can be made by evaluating the response of the pituitary hormones to respective trophic stimuli. Patients with intrinsic pituitary disease show minimal or no response, whereas those with secondary hypopituitarism demonstrate a normal but delayed response. Also, patients with secondary hypopituitarism often demonstrate hyperprolactinemia.

5.2.3.3. Etiology

The third step is to determine the etiology of hypopituitarism. Since tumors represent the most important and most common etiology, the crucial test is imaging of the pituitary gland. Conventional X rays of the sella and polytomography have been replaced by the use of computerized tomography of the pituitary. However, the conventional skull X rays may sometimes provide clues to the underlying etiology of hypopituitarism. Thus, the double-floor sign (tumor), erosion of the clinoids (tumor), suprasellar calcification (craniopharyngioma), and asymmetric erosion by a calcified lesion (aneurysm) are important signs that can be detected by routine lateral skull films. Since hypopituitarism is caused only by the invasive macroadenomas, and since these are invariably visualized by CT imaging, a normal CT scan virtually excludes tumor as the etiology of hypopituitarism. Metastatic lesions as well as supra-hypophyseal lesions also lend themselves well to the resolution of comput-erized tomography. The possibility of a vascular etiology (postpartum necro-sis) should be considered when the history is suggestive. Lymphocytic hypophysitis and granulomatous diseases are rare and difficult to document. In essence, since the treatments of all "nontumorous" varieties of hypopitu-itarism are identical (i.e., replacement therapy), the major concern is to ex-clude tumors, and this can be done effectively by CT scans.

5.2.4. Treatment

The treatment of hypopituitarism should focus on the dual aspects of replacing the lost hormone(s) as well as correcting the etiologic factor such as tumor. When hypopituitarism is caused by a pituitary or suprasellar tumor, surgery is mandatory to prevent further pituitary destruction as well as to avoid serious complications such as visual loss and increased intracranial ten-sion.

When hypopituitarism is caused by nontumorous etiologies, the focus of therapy is on replacement of the deficient hormone(s). For example, TSH deficiency and the resultant secondary hypothyroidism readily can be cor-rected by the use of oral levothyroxine, 0.15 mg daily. Secondary adrenal failure form ACTH deficiency is treated by the use of oral hydrocortisone, 20 mg in the morning and 10 mg in the evening. With regard to replacement therapy with thyroxine and hydrocortisone, two facts should be stressed. First, when adrenal insufficiency coexists with hypothyroidism, thyroid replacement should be attempted only after building up the adrenal status. Vigorous thy-roid hormone replacement in a patient with undertreated adrenal insuffi-ciency imposes the unacceptable risk of precipitating adrenal crisis. The im-pact of such an error can be catastrophic. Second, patients with hypoadrenalism should be advised to double their replacement dose in the event of stress. Most importantly, these patients should wear identification tags to indicate the diagnosis and the need for intravenous steroids should the patient be found unconscious.

Gonadotropin deficiency and the resultant hypogonadism are best treated with testosterone or estrogen replacement therapy. The only exception to this is when fertility is desired, in which case therapy with human chorionic and human menopausal gonadotropins may be considered.

Growth hormone deficiency in the child should be treated with injections of growth hormone given once or twice a week under close supervision to monitor the response.

Replacement therapy with glucocorticoids and levothyroxine for hypo-pituitarism is life long. Therefore, when lifelong replacement therapy is being contemplated, establishing the correct diagnosis is crucial. The results of such therapy are extremely gratifying.

5.3. Sheehan's Syndrome

Sheehan's syndrome refers to the development of hypopituitarism as a consequence of pituitary necrosis in the immediate postpartum period (postpartum pituitary necrosis).

5.3.1. Etiology

The etiology of postpartum pituitary necrosis is vascular in nature. During the course of normal gestation, a gradual enlargement of the pituitary gland occurs secondary to the increased population and size of the lactotrophs. The increase in size is maximal during the third trimester, occasionally becoming significant enough to cause visual field defects. In addition, the vascularity of the gland is also considerably increased. The pituitary gland, under these circumstances, is quite vulnerable to ischemia, contrasting sharply to its customary resiliency. When a rapid or marked decline in systemic blood pressure occurs as a consequence of postpartum hemorrhage or obstetric shock, this is reflected as a drastic pressure drop in the portal blood flow to the hypophysis. The resultant arteriolar spasm and/or thrombosis leads to marked ischemia and consequently to extreme pituitary destruction. In severe cases, the entire population of cells within the pituitary can be wiped out. In some instances, diffuse intravascular coagulation of the hypothalamic portal blood vessels has been noted.

5.3.2. Clinical Features

The classic description of Sheehan's syndrome is the development of postpartum amenorrhea and inability to lactate following a difficult labor.

There are four important variations to this classic theme:

1. Although a history of bleeding, obstetric shock, or a difficult labor may be evident in most cases, approximately 5% of patients who develop Sheehan's syndrome in the postpartum period give no such history.
2. Although panhypopituitarism is the expected sequel to postpartum necrosis, this is not invariably so. Occasionally, selective unitrophic or bitrophic hormone deficiencies may be the only expression of hypopituitarism secondary to Sheehan's syndrome.
3. The causative pregnancy need not always be the last one. Occasionally, patients with postpartum necrosis have been known to become pregnant. This underscores the importance of obtaining a detailed obstetric history of each pregnancy in the past.
4. Rarely, hypothalamic dysfunction can coexist with pituitary damage caused by Sheehan's syndrome. This may result in the development of diabetes insipidus as a result of vasopressin deficiency. A seemingly

paradoxical effect of hypothalamic damage in Sheehan's syndrome is the occurrence of galactorrhea in this setting, coupled with pituitary failure. Such an outcome can be explained when hypothalamic damage (with loss of the prolactin inhibitory factor) is coupled with partial pituitary destruction (with survival of the densely populated lactotrophs).

5.3.3. Diagnostic Studies

The triad to establish the diagnosis of Sheehan's syndrome consists of (1) evidence of hypofunction of the pituitary (confirmed by reserve testing), (2) suggestive obstetric history of hemorrhage or hypotension in the immediate pre- or postpartum period, and (3) exclusion of tumor in the sellar or parasellar region by computerized tomography. In fact, the pituitary gland appears small and shrunken in computerized tomograms.

5.3.4. Treatment

The treatment is identical to that for all other forms of nontumorous hypopituitarism (see Section 5.2.5).

5.4. Hypopituitary Dwarfism

The pediatric definition of the term *dwarfism* is applied to children whose height is 4 standard deviations or more below the mean of their coevals. The term *hypopituitary dwarfism* indicates a pituitary etiology for the short stature.

Theoretically, growth hormone deficiency can be caused by one of the following mechanisms:

1. Decreased or absent production of growth hormone by the somatotrophs.
2. Production of biologically inactive growth hormone by the somatotrophs.
3. An inability of the normally produced growth hormone to generate somatomedin ("Laron dwarf").
4. Peripheral insensitivity to growth hormone (African pygmy).

The term hypopituitary dwarfism, in the strictest sense, should be restricted to growth failure secondary to deficient or absent growth hormone secretion by the pituitary gland.

5.4.1. Etiology

Growth hormone deficiency is rare and accounts for fewer than 10% of children with growth retardation. There are several etiologies for growth hormone deficiency in childhood:

1. Tumors (craniopharyngiomas and pituitary tumors) account for one-third of cases of growth hormone deficiency. These patients may, in addition, demonstrate failure of other trophic hormones of the pituitary.
2. Congenital maldevelopment of the pituitary or the somatotrophs is the next most common etiology. This entity is usually characterized by monotropic growth hormone deficiency.
3. Inflammation (meningitis, encephalitis) and trauma (perinatal trauma) account for a small number of cases.
4. Rarely, fibrotic disease (hypophyseal fibrosis) and granulomatous disease (Hand–Schuller–Christian) may underlie growth hormone deficiency.

5.4.2. Clinical Features

The five major facets of hypopituitary dwarfism are growth retardation, the presence of associated somatic abnormalities, concomitant endocrinopathies, psychological changes, and abnormalities in glucose metabolism.

5.4.2.1. Growth Retardation

The slow growth rate in children with hypopituitary dwarfism usually becomes apparent between the first and third year of life. The growth retardation is manifested much later (8–10 years of age) when the hyposomatotropism is secondary to tumors such as craniopharyngioma. Nearly all hypopituitary dwarfs are 3 to 4 S.D. below the mean height appropriate for age. The patient's skeletal proportions are often symmetrical and childish. There is a striking contrast between the childish body proportions and the prematurely aged appearance from fine wrinkling of the face.

5.4.2.2. Somatic Abnormalities

When hypopituitary dwarfism is secondary to a congenital etiology, several somatic abnormalities may be present. These include cleft palate, absent septum pellucidum, optic nerve dysplasia, and iris–dental dysplasia (Reiger's abnormality).

5.4.2.3. Concomitant Endocrinopathy

When hypopituitary dwarfism is secondary to tumors, loss of other trophic hormones may be evident. When TSH deficiency is associated with growth hormone deficiency, the growth retardation can be quite severe. Similarly, when gonadotropin deficiency is associated with growth hormone failure, the retardation is accentuated by loss of the pubertal growth spurt. It is a well-noted observation that the other trophic hormone deficiencies appear much later than growth hormone deficiency. The reason for this lag is not clear.

Diabetes insipidus secondary to loss of antidiuretic hormone (vasopressin) may be associated with growth hormone deficiency when suprasellar lesions (craniopharyngioma, Hand–Schuller–Christian disease, etc.) are etiologically related.

5.4.2.4. Psychiatric Changes

The intelligence level of hypopituitary dwarfs is normal. The psychiatric changes seen in patients with hypopituitary dwarfism are those shared by patients with dwarfism from any etiology. These include dependency, isolation, and a "desire to excel." The insecurities of a minority group, having to adjust to a culture where the notion "bigger is better" prevails as an unspoken code, are understandable. The tendency to treat such patients as children because of their size is a contributing factor for the development of dependency tendencies. The emergence of support systems for "little people" has considerably aided in the attainment of mental well-being for many a patient with dwarfism.

5.4.2.5. Changes Related to Abnormal Glucose Handling

Patients with monotropic growth hormone deficiency tend to demonstrate a tendency for fasting hypoglycemia. Defective gluconeogenesis (which is partly dependent on growth hormone) may account for the tendency towards fasting hypoglycemia. These patients tend to be insulinopenic and demonstrate hypersensitivity to exogenous insulin.

In contrast, some hypopituitary dwarfs demonstrate an impaired glucose tolerance and even diabetes. Notably, the diabetes is mild, and characteristically, the incidence of microangiopathic complications is considerably lower. (Indeed, this observation prompted the recommendation of hypophysectomy as a form of treatment in the late 1960s to prevent progression of diabetic microangiopathy.)

5.4.3. Diagnostic Studies

The three steps in the diagnostic evaluation of a patient with suspected growth hormone deficiency are (1) establishing the impairment in growth hormone reserve, (2) excluding intracranial tumors as the underlying etiology, and (3) evaluating the adequacy of other trophic hormones (TSH, FSH, LH, etc.) that may contribute to and aggravate the somatotropin deficiency.

Hormonal confirmation of growth hormone deficiency requires documentation of the lack of growth hormone response to two provocative stimuli. Hypoglycemia and oral L-dopa are used for this purpose. Failure of the growth hormone to exceed at least 7 to 10 ng/ml over the base line in response to both stimuli is indicative of impaired reserve. It should be noted that measurements of basal growth hormone level or somatomedin C level do not permit clear separation between normal and hypopituitary children.

After deficiency is established, the next step is to exclude intrasellar or suprasellar tumors as the etiology for the impaired pituitary reserve. Craniopharyngiomas and pituitary tumors account for nearly a third of all cases of hypopituitary dwarfism and can be demonstrated by computerized tomography of the sella and perisellar region. The sellar size is often reduced in patients with nontumorous hypopituitarism.

The third step in the evaluation of patients with hyposomatotropism is to exclude concomitant deficiency of TSH, LH, FSH, or ACTH. Pituitary hormone reserve testing should be performed periodically, since the development of trophic hormone deficiency can be a delayed occurrence.

Additional tests in the evaluation of patients with hypopituitary dwarfism include (1) measurement of somatomedin C response to an injection of growth hormone to ensure effectiveness of growth hormone therapy, (2) glucose tolerance test with measurement of blood glucose and immunoreactive insulin levels following an orally administered load of glucose to evaluate β-cell reserve, (3) ophthalmologic evaluation to exclude congenital defects in the iris or optic nerves as well as for visual fields when a tumor in the sellar or suprasellar area underlies the etiology of hypopituitary dwarfism, and (4) psychological evaluation to provide support when necessary.

5.4.4. Differential Diagnosis

As indicated earlier, growth hormone deficiency accounts for no more than 10% of children with growth retardation.

The causes of growth retardation are extensive, and important ones are listed in Table 17.

5.4.5. Treatment

The treatment of growth hormone deficiency is administration of human growth hormone extracted from cadavers.

The therapy is more effective when started at an earlier age, underscoring the need for early diagnosis. The dosage of growth hormone varies from patient to patient; calculating the dose based on body weight appears to be more efficacious than titrating a standard dose based on the response. The initial dose recommended is 0.06–0.10 units/kg i.m. three times a week. Therapy should be modified later depending on the response.

There are some important therapeutic aspects to be kept in mind in treating patients with hypopituitary dwarfism with human growth hormone. First, the therapeutic response to growth hormone gets blunted with concomitant glucocorticoid therapy, presumably because of peripheral antagonism. Should such therapy be indicated, the replacement maintenance dose should not exceed 10–15 mg hydrocortisone equivalent per square meter of body surface area (of course, this is not applicable when the patient is under stress). Second, concomitant thyroxine replacement may also blunt the effectiveness of growth hormone by causing epiphyseal fusion. Third, administration of

TABLE 17
Causes of Short Stature

Etiology	Comment
Constitutional	Often familial and corrects itself at puberty
Systemic disease	
Cardiac	Congenital heart disease
Renal	Chronic renal disease; Fanconi's
GI	Malabsorption syndromes
Pulmonary	Severe chronic lung disease
Hematologic	Sickle cell; Thalassemia major
Endocrine	
Pituitary dwarf	Monotropic hyposomatotropism
Laron dwarf	Failure to generate somatomedin
Peripheral resistance	African pygmies
Cushing's syndrome	Antigrowth effects of steroids
Hypothyroidism	Juvenile or cretinism
Precocious puberty, e.g., a-g syndrome	Epiphyseal closure triggered by sex steroids
Bartter's syndrome	Loss of K^+
Turner's syndrome	Genetically determined
Bone disease	
Rickets	Vitamin D deficiency (resistant variety)
Juvenile osteoporosis	
Achondroplasia	
Miscellaneous	
Emotional deprivation	
Metabolic diseases	

sex steroids, which also facilitate epiphyseal fusion, should be delayed until the maximal benefits of growth hormone therapy have been attained. Fourth, careful monitoring of bone age is needed, especially around puberty. Epiphyseal maturation would soon result in epiphyseal closure, a phenomenon that would render any further therapy with growth hormone useless.

The complications of therapy include the development of lipoatrophy or lipodystrophy at the injection sites and the development of glucose intolerance and even overt diabetes from the diabetogenic effects of somatotropin. Neutralizing antibodies to growth hormone, which develop in approximately 5% to 10% of patients, may blunt the effectiveness of therapy. In most patients, with careful attention to the above principles, eventual heights of 5 feet can be attained.

5.5. Kallmann's Syndrome

Kallmann's syndrome is a disorder characterized by hypogonadism and olfactory dysfunction (olfactogenital syndrome). The hypogonadism of Kallmann's syndrome is a classic example of hypogonadotropic hypogonadism;

i.e., it results from deficient or absent secretion of the pituitary gonadotropins FSH and LH. The olfactory dysfunction (anosmia or dysosmia) results from defective development of the olfactory lobe. The term Kallmann's syndrome, in a purist's sense, should be restricted to cases in which the dual components of the disorder are present. The term "isolated gonadotropin deficiency" is more apt when olfactory function is normal. The terms "male Kallmann's" and "female Kallmann's" are used to denote the occurrence of the syndrome in karyotypic males and females, respectively.

5.5.1. Etiology

The gonadotropin deficiency of Kallmann's syndrome is secondary to lack of hypothalamic decapeptide gonadotropin-releasing hormone (GnRH). This releasing factor is responsible for initiating pubertal events by stimulating the pituitary gonadotrophs to secrete and release FSH and LH. When the hypothalamus fails to secrete this peptide, there is failure of the central signals essential to set the stage for puberty. Thus, the disorder is an instance of puberty that failed to arrive. The exact mechanism(s) for failure to generate GnRH are not very clear. However, autopsy studies suggest a lack of development of the hypothalamic neurons that normally secrete the releasing factor. The concomitant presence of aplastic or hypoplastic olfactory lobes and the association with midline craniofacial abnormalities lend support to a congenital origin of the disorder. The hereditary nature of Kallmann's syndrome is supported by several studies that suggest an autosomal dominant pattern of inheritance with incomplete penetrance. The heterogeneous nature and partial expressions of this disorder are evidenced by the presence of anosmia in the eugonadal relatives of patients with fully expressed Kallmann's syndrome.

5.5.2. Clinical Features

The highlights of Kallmann's syndrome are the hypogonadism and olfactory dysfunction. In addition, several somatic features may be associated.

5.5.2.1. Hypogonadism

In males, delayed puberty or sexual infantilism are the important presenting features. When the gonadotropin deficiency is complete, the appearance of the patient is strikingly prepubertal. The youthful boyish appearance, accentuated by the near total lack of facial hair and very sparse pubic and axillary hair, is distinctive. The prepubertal phallic proportions, the nonrugous scrotum, and the soft, small testes are all indicative of lack of virilization. Gynecomastia is usually minimal or absent.

In females, primary amenorrhea and sexual infantilism are the presenting features. The degree of nonfeminization depends on the completeness of the gonadotropin deficiency. The physical findings are those common to all forms of prepubertal hypogonadism, i.e., poor development of breasts and external genitalia, presence of a shallow vagina, and a hypoplastic uterus. The skeletal proportions may be eunuchoidal (span greater than height) because of continued epiphyseal growth secondary to lack of sex steroids.

In both males and females, the hypogonadism can be of varying severity because of the heterogeneous nature of Kallmann's syndrome.

5.5.2.2. Olfactory Dysfunction

Disturbances in the perception of smell are more frequent in male Kallmann's syndrome. In mild cases, sophisticated olfactory testing may be required to detect the dysosmia.

5.5.2.3. Somatic Abnormalities

The somatic abnormalities that have been associated with the syndrome include cleft palate, harelip, craniofacial asymmetry, congenital deafness, and brachydactyly (short fourth metacarpal bone). These features are also more prevalent in male Kallmann's syndrome.

5.5.3. Diagnostic Studies

The hormonal hallmark of the Kallmann's syndrome is low levels of FSH and LH in the presence of low circulating sex steroids (testosterone or 17β-estradiol).

The diagnostic criteria for Kallmann's syndrome are (1) low or absent gonadotropins, (2) preservation of other pituitary hormones, i.e., normal reserve of TSH, ACTH, and growth hormone, and (3) a normal sella turcica, i.e., no evidence of tumor in the sellar or suprasellar area.

5.5.4. Differential Diagnosis

The combination of anosmia and hypogonadism unmistakably implies the diagnosis of Kallmann's syndrome. Isolated gonadotropin deficiency (without anosmia) clinically resembles other forms of prepubertal hypogonadism. In the female, the most important clinical differential diagnoses include Turner variants (without the Turner stigmata) and gonadal dysgenesis. Both of these conditions, however, are characterized by elevated LH and FSH levels. The differentiation between hypopituitarism (with intrinsic disease of the gonadotrophs) and Kallmann's syndrome can theoretically be made by the administration of exogenous synthetic LH-RH (luteinizing hormone-releasing hormone). In principle, there should be no LH or FSH response to LH-RH when the pituitary is intrinsically compromised, whereas the LH or FSH response is normal but delayed when the hypothalamus is at fault. In practice, however, the response patterns are seldom clear-cut enough to permit absolute delineation.

Male Kallmann's needs to be clinically differentiated from primary testicular failure (Klinefelter's syndrome), in which the LH and FSH levels are clearly elevated.

5.5.5. Treatment

The treatment of Kallmann's syndrome involves replacement therapy with gonadotropins or their releasing hormone.

Gonadotropin therapy using human chorionic gonadotropin (which possesses LH-like activity) and human menopausal gonadotropin (which contains FSH-like activity) can effectively induce stimulation of the testes or ovaries. The induction of puberty by this method is a slow but gratifying process. The weekly injections, the slow response, and the high cost of therapy are minor drawbacks considering the fact that such therapy offers the patient a chance at fertility. Most patients respond to therapy. However, some patients with male Kallmann's syndrome may, in addition to the central defect, possess a second defect at the testicular level. These patients may demonstrate a defect in testosterone synthesis and consequently not respond to gonadotropin administration.

The recent successes with therapeutic administration of LH-RH have added a new dimension in the treatment of Kallmann's syndrome. However, the availability of this form of therapy is limited. Considerable expertise is required to treat patients with LH-RH, since this therapy can be the proverbial double-edged sword. Given in very small doses in a pulsatile fashion, LH-RH stimulates the pituitary (agonist action). But given in large doses or on a constant, nonpulsatile basis, the same drug inhibits the pituitary release of gonadotropins. The best results are obtained when the drug is administered in small "pulses" delivered by a programmable insulin pump. The limitations and drawbacks of long-term pump therapy are obvious.

Treatment with androgens or estrogens can provide the desirable effect but minimize and even preclude fertility. Many patients prefer to use these agents to induce the necessary masculinization or feminization initially, switching to gonadotropin therapy when fertility is desired.

6

The Empty Sella Syndrome

6.1. Introduction

The term *empty sella syndrome* denotes the presence of an enlarged sella turcica containing a remodeled pituitary gland flattened against the posterior and inferior walls of the sella. The term "empty" is somewhat of a misnomer, since the sella is filled partially by the remodeled flat pituitary gland and partially by cerebrospinal fluid. The condition is a result of extension of the subarachnoid space into the sella as a result of incompleteness in the diaphragma sella. This weakness in the diaphragma sella, which is probably congenital, allows the extension of a small arachnoid diverticulum, filled with CSF, into the sella. The diverticulum enlarges slowly and gradually pushes the normal pituitary gland against the posterior and inferior wall. In chronic cases, the walls of the sella expand to accommodate the enlarged arachnoid diverticulum. The anatomic consequences of the empty sella syndrome are several (Table 18):

1. The enlarged sella caused by the empty sella syndrome is detected by routine skull films and is indistinguishable from other causes of sellar enlargement, particularly tumors. The distinction is very important because of the entirely different prognostic and therapeutic implications.
2. In severe cases, the floor of the sella can become eroded, rendering the resemblance to a tumor even closer.
3. Very rarely, the arachnoid diverticulum, after eroding the floor, may communicate with the sphenoid sinus, resulting in CSF rhinorrhea.
4. Rarely, when the weakness in the diaphragma sella is considerable, and when the intrasellar pressure is high because of the expanding arachnoid diverticulum, the optic chiasm, optic tract, and optic nerves may prolapse into the "empty" sella.

The term primary empty sella syndrome is used when the defect in the diaphragma sella is intrinsic, whereas the term secondary empty sella syn-

TABLE 18
Anatomic Consequences of a Defect in
Diaphragma Sella

Extension of arachnoid diverticulum through the diaphragm
Compression of the pituitary gland
Enlargement of the sellar walls
Thinning of sellar walls
Erosion of the sellar floor
Communication with sphenoid sinus inferiorly
Prolapse of optic tracts, optic nerves, or chiasm

drome indicates the development of the syndrome following surgery or radiation to the pituitary gland or after apoplexy in a preexisting tumor.

6.2. Clinical Features

Empty sella syndrome is approximately six times more frequently encountered in females; a direct correlation with multiparity and obesity has been suggested but not proven. Most patients with the primary empty sella syndrome are asymptomatic, and nearly all patients have normal pituitary function.

Occasional symptoms include nonspecific headaches and, rarely, visual field defects or CSF rhinorrhea. The last two symptoms are indicative of complications of the empty sella syndrome resulting in prolapsed optic tracts and communication with the sphenoid sinus, respectively.

6.3. Diagnostic Studies

6.3.1. Skull X Ray

Lateral X rays of the skull would demonstrate the enlargement of the walls of the sella turcica by the expanding arachnoid space. The empty sella syndrome may well represent the most common etiology for an enlarged sella. The appearance may mimic that of an enlarged sella secondary to a pituitary

TABLE 19
Radiologic Features of Empty Sella versus Tumor

Empty sella	Tumor
Tomography shows symmetric contours (globular shape)	Contours often asymmetric
Smoothly curved walls	Irregular walls
Erosion uncommon	Erosion often present

tumor. There are, however, some differences that may permit recognition (Table 19).

Occasionally, when the remodeling is asymmetric, and when erosion is present ("double floor"), the empty sella cannot be differentiated from a tumor by regular skull films or by hypocycloidal polytomography. Definitive distinction between the two can be made only by employing other tests.

6.3.2. Computerized Tomography

The fourth-generation CT scans have provided a noninvasive method to aid the diagnosis of empty sella syndrome. Although there is some difference of opinion as to the conclusiveness of the study, it is agreed that computerized tomography of the sellar region (axial and coronal views with metrizamide) should be carried out before resorting to invasive procedures such as pneumoencephalography. The attenuation density of the CSF can be traced from the suprasellar cistern down to the sella. Also, following injection of metrizamide, the pituitary stalk can be seen to extend far below its usual location, leading to the flattened gland in the posterior and inferior aspect of the sella.

6.3.3. Pneumoencephalography

This invasive procedure involving injection of air (and more recently metrizamide) into the cerebrospinal space is required only when computerized tomography has failed to demonstrate conclusively the empty sella. On lateral views, the demonstration of air (or metrizamide) entering into and filling the sella is absolutely confirmatory.

6.3.4. Endocrine Reserve Testing

Pituitary reserve testing is not indicated in the empty sella syndrome, since the hormonal reserve of the gland is usually not compromised. Subtle abnormalities may occasionally be detected by provocative testing, but seldom are these clinically significant. It should be remembered that, even though flattened (and pushed), the pituitary gland of the empty sella syndrome is not exempt from or immune to the diseases that affect the normal pituitary gland. This is especially so when microadenomas develop in the pituitary glands of patients with empty sella syndrome, resulting in hypersecretory syndromes. The diagnostic impact of such an occurrence is obvious, since the presentation would be characterized by hypersecretory syndromes, e.g., galactorrhea, acromegaly, Cushing's disease, and an enlarged sella turcica by routine X rays or polytomograms, suggesting a large tumor causing the hypersecretion. The documentation of the fact that the enlarged sella is caused by the empty sella syndrome and that the hypersecretory state results from a coexisting microadenoma originating in a flattened pituitary gland may be difficult, requiring sophisticated imaging techniques coupled with hormonal studies.

6.4. Differential Diagnosis

As indicated above, the major differential diagnosis of the empty sella syndrome is tumor of the pituitary gland. The use of computerized tomography and, rarely, pneumoencephalography aids in this important delineation.

6.5. Course and Complications

Uncomplicated primary empty sella syndrome has a benign course, most patients coming to attention merely on the basis of an abnormal skull X ray obtained serendipitously.

The three rare complications are CSF rhinorrhea, optic nerve prolapse, and increased intracranial tension. All three require surgical intervention.

6.6. Treatment

No treatment is required for uncomplicated primary empty sella syndrome. When complications occur, they should be treated by appropriate surgery. If present, CSF rhinorrhea is treated by transsphenoidal repair of the floor of the sella. Visual field defects, when caused by prolapse of the optic nerve, chiasm, or optic tract, are best treated by packing the empty sella (by muscle or bone chips) and pushing the visual tracts up to the original supradiaphragmatic position. Increased intracranial pressure would necessitate a shunt procedure.

7

Pituitary Tumors

7.1. Introduction

Pituitary tumors represent fewer than 5% of intracranial tumors, but the strategic location and the unusual syndromes associated with these tumors confer enormous significance. Although the neurosurgeon and the CT radiologist dominate the diagnostic arena of patients with pituitary tumors, the endocrinologic work-up of these patients assumes importance both pre- and postoperatively.

7.2. Classification

Pituitary tumors can be classified in several ways: according to histology (acidophilic, basophilic, chromophobe, according to size (microadenoma, macroadenoma, and invasive macroadenoma), according to electron microscopy (somatotroph adenoma, lactotroph adenoma, etc.), and according to their secretory activity (hypersecretory versus nonsecretory). The most common pituitary tumor is chromophobe adenoma, and the most common tumor of childhood is craniopharyngioma.

7.3. Clinical Features

The clinical presentation of pituitary tumors can be highlighted by parasellar symptoms, by hypersecretory syndromes, or by the development of hypopituitarism.

7.3.1. Parasellar Symptoms

Headaches and visual disturbances represent the two most common symptoms of pituitary tumors. Persistent headaches, most often caused by an in-

crease in the intrasellar pressure, should elicit a search for a pituitary neoplasm. The ophthalmologic symptoms are caused by pressure effects on the
optic chiasm and tract and may consist of a mild field cut (superior quadrantic
hemianopsia), a chiasmal effect (bitemporal hemianopsia), or severe optic tract
compression (optic atrophy and blindness).

7.3.2. The Hypersecretory Syndromes

The most common hypersecretory syndrome associated with pituitary
tumors is hyperprolactinemia, the most common cause of which is a pituitary
microadenoma (Section 4.4). Less commonly, acromegaly (Section 4.2) and
Cushing's disease (Section 4.3) may be encountered.

7.3.3. The Hypopituitary Syndromes

Tumors of the pituitary can cause hypopituitarism in one of two ways:
by encroaching on and destroying the normal tissue or by extending above
and disconnecting the pituitary from the stalk (tumorous stalk section). The
latter would result in loss of the hypothalamic trophic factors that travel via
the stalk. Tumor encroachment may result in loss of one, more than one, or
all pituitary hormones (panhypopituitarism). When partial hypopituitarism
develops as a consequence of tumors, the earliest hormones to be lost are
growth hormone and gonadotropins, followed by TSH, ACTH, and prolactin
(Section 5.2). The development of hypopituitarism secondary to pituitary
tumors is gradual except in the event of the catastrophic occurrence of apoplexy, which rapidly causes panhypopituitarism.

7.4. Diagnostic Studies

The four cornerstones in the diagnostic evaluation of pituitary tumors
are radiological, neuroradiological, endocrinologic, and ophthalmologic eval-
uations.

7.4.1. Radiological Studies

The emergence of high-resolution computerized tomography has rendered the use of lateral films and polytomography of the sella rather obsolete.
However, since asymptomatic pituitary tumors are often detected by seren-
dipity, when a skull film is obtained for unrelated reasons, it is essential to be
familiar with the appearance and size of a normal sella turcica on a plain
lateral skull film (Chapter 1). The causes for enlarged sella are several (Table
20).

Most of the other conditions that cause enlargement of the sella turcica
can be differentiated from pituitary tumor by the use of computerized tomography with infusion. In addition to establishing the presence of the pituitary tumor, the CT scan also can demonstrate suprasellar extension.

TABLE 20
Causes for Enlarged Sella

Pituitary tumors (chromophobe adenoma)
Suprasellar tumors (craniopharyngioma)
Empty sella syndrome
Aneurysm
Hypophysitis
Cysts
Metastases

7.4.2. Neuroradiological Studies

Since the advent of high-resolution CT scans, there has been a considerable decrease in the use of diagnostic pneumoencephalography in the evaluation of pituitary tumors. Carotid angiography, although not an absolute aid in diagnosis, provides information regarding the vascular supply of the region in the event of surgical intervention.

7.4.3. Endocrinologic Evaluation

The hormonal evaluation of patients with pituitary tumors focusses on two aspects: (1) the detection of hypersecretory syndromes involving prolactin, growth hormone, ACTH, and TSH or the subunits of glycoprotein hormones of the pituitary and (2) the determination of the presence and degree of compromise in pituitary function caused by tumor (Section 5.2.3).

Also, following surgical removal of the tumor, it is essential to evaluate the pituitary reserve for substitution therapy.

7.4.4. Ophthalmologic Evaluation

A properly performed perimetry to disclose the adequacy of visual fields is mandatory, even if the fields appear normal by confrontation tests.

7.5. Treatment

The optimal treatment for pituitary tumors depends on several factors such as size, rate of progression, the presence of perisellar invasion, and the presence of hyper- or hyposecretion of the pituitary hormones. The following general statements can be made.

Surgical intervention is clearly the choice of therapy in patients with invasive macroadenomas (especially with suprasellar extension). The documentation of visual field cuts that persist (or progress) is an indication for surgical intervention.

Noninvasive macroadenomas, i.e., those contained within the sella, probably should be removed since the outcome of untreated chromophobe adenoma is generally bad. In an asymptomatic patient with a noninvasive macroadenoma, the serial demonstration of progression (by CT) and or development of impaired reserve by hormone testing are convincing arguments to recommend surgical intervention. The route of entry (transsphenoidal versus transfrontal), the amount of normal tissue removed, and the complication rate of these types of surgery depend on the neurosurgical team and are beyond the scope (or control) of the endocrinologist.

The treatment of hypersecretory syndromes secondary to microadenomas has been discussed in Chapter 4.

The occurrence of clinical hypopituitarism in the presence of a pituitary tumor is an indication for surgical intervention.

Radiation to the pituitary gland as the primary mode of therapy for nonhypersecretory chromophobe adenomas is probably an inferior choice, since these tumors are not particularly radiosensitive. Radiation therapy as an adjunct to surgery is often used to prevent recurrence of the chromophobe adenoma.

Medical therapy for pituitary tumors is also, at best, adjunctive. Despite scattered reports of "tumor shrinkage" with bromocriptine used in extremely high doses, such therapy should be considered experimental for nonhypersecretory pituitary tumors.

8

The Neurohypophysis
The Regulatory Control and Actions of Vasopressin

8.1. Introduction

Vasopressin (Antidiuretic hormone, ADH) is the antidiuretic principle secreted by the supraoptic and paraventricular nuclei of the hypothalamus. Arginine vasopressin (AVP) is an octapeptide with a basic amine at the penultimate position of the side chain. The hypothalamus also secretes a polypeptide called neurophysin, which is believed to be a carrier protein involved in the intraneuronal transport of arginine vasopressin. Arginine vasopressin is transported through the pituitary stalk and is stored in the posterior pituitary. The median eminence of the hypothalamus represents a crucial location in this avenue of transport. Section of the pituitary stalk above the median eminence permanently disrupts the pathway, resulting in permanent loss of antidiuretic hormone.

8.2. Regulation of Vasopressin Release

The two major regulatory mechanisms for the synthesis and release of AVP are the osmotic and nonosmotic pathways.

The osmotic pathway is centered around the supraoptic and paraventricular nuclei of the hypothalamus. These two nuclei contain "osmoreceptors" that are exquisitely sensitive to even minor changes in the serum osmolarity. When there is an increase in plasma tonicity, the osmoreceptors "shrink" and trigger the release of AVP from the hypothalamic nuclei. Conversely, when there is a decrease in plasma tonicity, the osmoreceptors "swell" and in turn suppress the release of AVP. It is important to recognize that the osmoreceptors respond to hypertonicity only when hypernatremia contributes to the hypertonicity.

The plasma tonicity is maintained within the narrow range of 270–275 mOsm/kg. When the plasma tonicity increases (as in dehydrated states), the appropriate responses are stimulation of AVP release followed by antidiuresis, increased water reabsorption by the renal tubules, conservation of water, and restoration of plasma tonicity to normal. Physiologically, therefore, the urine is highly concentrated (800–1000 mOsm) during AVP release. Failure of AVP to be released in response to dehydration characterizes central diabetes insipidus (DI).

When the plasma tonicity decreases (as in hyponatremia), the appropriate responses are suppression of AVP followed by decreased water reabsorption by the renal tubules, resulting in increased free water clearance and eventual restoration of plasma tonicitiy to normal. Physiologically, therefore, the urine is maximally dilute (50–100 mOsm) during AVP suppression. Failure to physiologically suppress in response to hypotonicity, reflected as a less than maximally dilute urine, characterizes the syndrome of inappropriate ADH secretion (SIADH).

The osmoregulatory center is physiologically and anatomically closely related to the thirst center. Thus, hypertonicity of plasma (dehydration) increases thirst, resulting in increased consumption of water in an attempt to restore eutonicity. Conversely, hypotonicity of plasma decreases thirst in an attempt to avoid further dilution. Figure 5 illustrates the physiological responses to plasma hypertonicity, as with dehydration.

The nonosmotic factors involved in the mediation of the secretion and

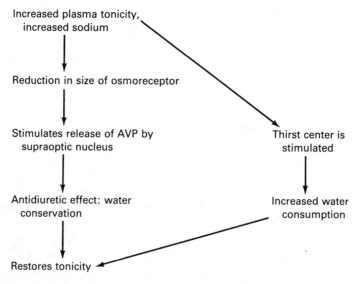

FIGURE 5. Physiological response to increased plasma tonicity.

TABLE 21
Chemical Factors That Affect AVP Release

Stimulate AVP release	Suppress AVP release
Nicotine	Alcohol
Analgesics	Diphenylhydantoin
Barbiturates	
Cyclophosphamide	
Vincristine	
Chlorpropamide [a]	
Clofibrate[a]	

[a]Also enhance peripheral action of AVP.

release of AVP include volume receptors in the left atrium, baroreceptors in the carotid sinus and the aortic arch, and hormonal and chemical factors.

The volume receptors in the wall of the left atrium are exquisitely sensitive to pressure changes within that cavity. The afferent impulses from the left atrium are conducted through the vagus nerve and are inhibitory to the release of AVP. Thus, an increase in the left atrial pressure distends the left atrial wall and stimulates these volume receptors with a consequent increase in the parasympathetic drive and suppression of AVP. This is the mechanism that underlies the polyuria of paroxysmal atrial tachycardia, a condition characterized by increased distension of the left atrium. Conversely, any decrease in the left atrial pressure results in suppression of parasympathetic drive and hence stimulates release of AVP. This is the mechanism that underlies the release of AVP (and SIADH) in patients receiving positive-pressure ventilatory assistance.

The baroreceptors in the aortic arch and carotid sinus are sensitive to changes in arterial blood pressure. A drop in the arterial blood pressure stimulates these receptors, resulting in the release of AVP. The afferent pathways for this reflex arc are the vagus and glossopharyngeal nerves. This is the mechanism whereby volume depletion and hypotension (from dehydration, hemorrhage, shock, etc.) result in an increased release of AVP in an attempt to replete volume by water conservation. This mechanism is also the reason that precludes diagnosis of SIADH in the presence of volume depletion, a condition expected to elicit an appropriate increase in the synthesis and release of AVP.

Hormonal factors, particularly catecholamines and angiotensin II, can modify the release of AVP from the hypothalamus. The well-recognized suppression of AVP in response to pain, fear, or stress belongs in this category.

Chemical factors play an important role in drug-induced AVP release and suppression. Drugs and chemicals should be carefully excluded while patients with disorders of vasopressin secretion are evaluated. Table 21 illustrates the variety of drugs capable of affecting vasopressin release.

Hormonal and chemical stimuli do not play a dominant role in the day-to-day physiology of AVP control. The two most important stimuli for the release of AVP are hypertonicity of plasma (increased sodium) and hypotension (from volume depletion). Of these two, the more sensitive is the osmotic stimulus. A 1% to 2% change in osmolarity will stimulate AVP release, whereas a 5% to 10% change in blood volume is necessary to cause the same effect. Although the osmotic pathway is more sensitive, the baroreceptor pathway elicits a more potent response in terms of AVP release. Once stimulated by the nonosmotic pathway, the response of AVP occurs in a geometric manner, perhaps accounting for the greater response. Usually, the osmoreceptor and the baroreceptor pathways work in concert.

8.3. Action of Vasopressin

The action of vasopressin is to increase the permeability of the distal convoluted tubule and the collecting ducts to water. Thus, AVP is a hormone that promotes urinary concentration. The concept of the countercurrent system is used to illustrate the process of urine concentration. The renal medullary interstitium is an extremely important structure that, along with AVP, regulates this process. The countercurrent system is visualized as resembling a fluid stream bent back on itself like a hairpin, with fluid flowing in opposite directions but very close to each other. This system is buried in the substance of the renal medullary interstitium, which provides the tonicity needed for the functioning of this countercurrent system. Another anatomic fact that has enormous significance is that the proximal and distal convoluted tubules are in the cortex of the kidney, whereas the Henle's loop with both its limbs and the collecting tubules are in the medullary interstitium (Figure 6).

The glomerular filtrate is isosmotic to the plasma with an osmolality of 280 to 300 mOsm/kg. The proximal tubule neither concentrates nor dilutes the urine, but performs the phenomenal task of reabsorbing almost 120 liters of filtrate per day. It delivers 40 liters of isotonic filtrate to the descending limb of the loop of Henle. The loop of Henle is closely intertwined with blood vessels of the vasa recta, an important anatomic consideration for the events of the countercurrent system that subsequently take place.

Two facts govern the events occurring at the descending limb of the loop of Henle: first, the descending limb is freely permeable to water, and second, the adjoining medulla is relatively concentrated. Therefore, as the filtrate moves down along this limb, it becomes progressively concentrated, because the water exits from the descending limb into the concentrated medulla. Maximal concentrations are reached at the hairpin bend.

The concentrated filtrate reaches the ascending limb. This structure actively removes sodium from the tubule into the medullar interstitium but is impermeable to back diffusion of water; i.e., sodium leaves the ascending limb into the interstitium to increase its solute content without a simultaneous efflux of water. As the dilute filtrate moves up, it reaches the distal convuluted tubule with an osmolarity around 100 mOsm.

The events described thus far are independent of AVP. The role of AVP

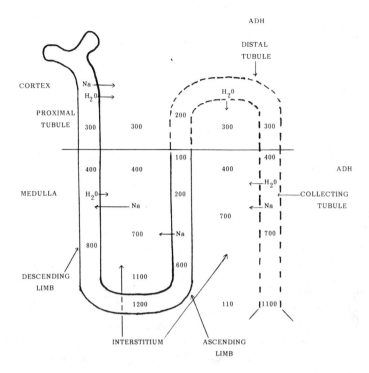

FIGURE 6.   The descending limb of the loop of Henle is freely permeable to water, whereas the adjoining medulla is relatively concentrated. Hence, the filtrate progressively becomes concentrated. In the ascending limb, sodium is removed from the tubule without a simultaneous efflux of water. Thus, the filtrate reaching the distal tubule has an osmolarity of 100 mOsm. Vasopressin increases water permeability at the distal and collecting tubules.

becomes manifest at the distal and collecting tubules. If the urine needs to be concentrated, AVP is released and acts on the distal and collecting tubules to reabsorb water and concentrate the urine. Vasopressin increases water permeability by opening membrane pores. After the hypotonic fluid reaches the distal tubule, a large fraction of water is reabsorbed under the influence of AVP, resulting in isosmotic fluid being delivered to the cortical interstitium (about 300 mOsm).

The filtrate, thus rendered isosmotic, reaches the collecting tubule. This structure is buried in the medullary interstitium. Under the influence of vasopressin, water reabsorption continues, resulting in progressively increased amounts of fluid leaving the collecting tubules. This process continues until the filtrate reaches equilibrium with the medullary interstitium. The final urine, therefore, can be, even at the height of AVP action, only similar to the concentration of the medullary interstitium and never can exceed it. At the height of vasopressin action, urinary concentrations of 1000–1200 mOsm/kg can be attained. When AVP is totally absent, the final urine osmolarity ranges between 50 to 100 mOsm. Even in the absence of AVP, dehydration alone can result in a urinary concentration around 300 mOsm, an accomplishment entirely achieved by the hypertonic medullary interstitium.

In general terms then, the medullary countercurrent system forms the basis for excreting urine of widely variable concentrations, but it is AVP that modulates the fine tuning. If water homeostasis demands a concentrated urine, AVP is released and can concentrate the final urine. If, on the other hand, the homeostasis requires a dilute urine, AVP is suppressed, and the final urine remains hypoosmolar.

The water-reabsorbing action of AVP on the distal and collecting tubules is achieved by an increase in the number and size of pores in the luminal membrane. Vasopressin binds to specific receptors located on the contraluminal surface of the tubular epithelial cells. Following its binding to membrane receptors, vasopressin activates adenylate cyclase, which effects the conversion of ATP to cyclic AMP. This in turn stimulates intracellular protein kinases that express the hormonal effect of AVP. The peripheral effect of AVP on the renal collecting tubules can be potentiated by chlorpropamide and inhibited or impaired by lithium carbonate, demeclotetracycline, hypercalcemia, hypokalemia, and a hypotonic medullary interstitium.

The disorder that results from insufficient or ineffective AVP is diabetes insipidus. The disorder resulting from excess and inappropriate secretion of AVP is called the syndrome of inappropriate ADH secretion (SIADH). These two sets of disorders are discussed in the next two chapters.

9

Diabetes Insipidus

9.1. Introduction

Diabetes insipidus (DI) is a condition characterized by the passing of large quantities of extremely dilute urine. The basic defect in diabetes insipidus is the inability of the renal tubules to concentrate the urine. When the defect is caused by partial or complete absence of vasopressin, the term *central diabetes insipidus* is used to denote the disorder; when the defect results from resistance of the renal tubules to vasopressin, the condition is called *nephrogenic diabetes insipidus*. Regardless of the mechanism, the consequences and clinical features are the same.

9.2. Etiology

9.2.1. Central Diabetes Insipidus

The most common form of central DI is idiopathic, accounting for 50% to 60% of all such cases. Idiopathic central diabetes insipidus is inherited as an autosomal dominant and less frequently as an X-linked trait. The exact reason for the development of central DI is not clear, but pathological examination of the brain of some patients with the disorder reveals a striking depletion of Nissl granules in the supraoptic and paraventricular hypothalamic nuclei. Central DI is extremely heterogeneous in presentation, with a spectrum ranging from severe disease presenting in childhood to mild disease manifesting for the first time in adulthood.

Although idiopathic central DI is the most common form of spontaneous central DI, the most frequently encountered cause for central DI is trauma, especially surgical trauma. Transient DI is extremely common following pituitary surgery because of removal of the neurohypophysis. Permanent DI develops only when the pituitary stalk is damaged above the median eminence.

Next to the idiopathic and surgical etiologies, tumors constitute an im-

TABLE 22
Etiology of Central Diabetes Insipidus

Idiopathic
Pituitary surgery
Suprasellar tumor
  Craniopharyngioma
  Meningioma
  Dysgerminoma
  Hamartoma
Metastastic malignancy
  Breast
  Colorectal cancer
Sarcoidosis
Hand–Schuller–Christian disease (histiocytosis X)
Vascular
  Sheehan's apoplexy
  Wegener's granulomatosis
Infections
  Encephalitis
  Rarely, basal meningitis
Traumatic
  Basal skull fracture

portant etiology for central DI. Diabetes insipidus is often the earliest and indeed the only manifestation of a suprasellar tumor such as craniopharyngioma. Less commonly, metastases (from the breast or colon) can present with central DI. The rare causes for central DI are outlined in Table 22.

9.2.2. Nephrogenic Diabetes Insipidus

Nephrogenic DI, characterized by target organ resistance to the action of vasopressin, can be congenital or acquired.

TABLE 23
Etiology of Nephrogenic
Diabetes Insipidus

Congenital
  X-linked
Acquired
  Hypercalcemia
  Hypokalemia
  Drugs: lithium carbonate, demeclocycline
  Chronic renal disease
  Sickle cell disease
  Amyloidosis
  Multiple myeloma
  Sjogren's syndrome

Congenital nephrogenic DI, is predominantly seen in boys and is inherited as an X-linked disorder. (It is believed that the gene for nephrogenic DI was introduced into the North American continent by the Ulster clan from Scotland, who landed in 1761 in Halifax, Nova Scotia, aboard the carrier "The Hopewell.") The disorder is a consequence of failure to generate cyclic AMP in the renal tubular cell in response to vasopressin.

The most frequent causes for acquired nephrogenic DI are metabolic abnormalities (hypokalemia, hypercalcemia) and drugs that inhibit the action on vasopressin (lithium, demeclocycline). Table 23 outlines the varied etiologies of nephrogenic DI.

9.3. Clinical Features

The two salient symptoms of any form of diabetes insipidus are polyuria and polydipsia. The physical examination is usually negative; the presence of associated features depends on the underlying etiology.

9.3.1. Polyuria

In complete DI, the urine output can exceed 10 liters a day. The onset is acute in central idiopathic DI, patients often being able to recall the exact day the polyuria started. Nocturia is invariably present. The severity of the polyuria poses restrictions on the patient's lifestyle, often to a frustrating degree. The description of the urine is often characteristic: pale, dilute, water-like urine.

9.3.2. Polydipsia

Increased thirst invariably accompanies the polyuria of diabetes insipidus as a compensatory mechanism to balance the fluid losses in the urine. The only situation in which thirst may be absent is when central DI is caused by a suprasellar tumor that has also encroached on and destroyed the thirst center in the hypothalamus. Such a combination is obviously disastrous, since such patients rapidly become dehydrated.

9.3.3. Associated Features

These depend on the underlying etiology and are mostly encountered when the diabetes insipidus is of central origin.

1. Signs of chiasmal compression are indicative of a suprasellar tumor causing DI.
2. Optic atrophy or papilledema with central DI points toward increased intracranial tension, usually secondary to tumors that obstruct the flow of CSF.

3. The demonstration of the "Parinaud's sign," impairment of upward gaze, in a patient with DI is highly suggestive of a pinealoma (dysgerminoma).

4. The combination of DI and precocious puberty again suggests a suprasellar tumor as the etiology for both.

5. The development of DI in a patient with a past or present history of breast cancer or colorectal cancer is indicative of metastatic disease to the median eminence of the hypothalamus.

6. The features of clinical hypopituitarism in a patient with diabetes insipidus suggest a suprasellar tumor extending inferiorly or an intrasellar tumor extending upwards.

It should be realized that the development of hypoadrenalism tends to "mask" or improve the diabetes insipidus. This is because of the marked decrease in free water clearance that develops secondary to glucocorticoid deficiency. On replacement with glucocorticoids, the polyuria of DI becomes apparent and is "unmasked."

9.4. Diagnostic Studies

The standard test used in the distinction of the various types of diabetes insipidus is the water deprivation test. The assay for vasopressin, at best, only assumes an adjunctive role in the diagnosis. Additional tests are employed depending on whether the DI is central or nephrogenic in origin.

9.4.1. The Water Deprivation Test

The principle of this test is to evaluate the release of vasopressin, the antidiuretic hormone, in response to a potent physiological stimulus such as rendering the plasma hypertonic by dehydration. The test, usually performed in the morning, begins by the obtaining of the basal parameters: weight, blood pressure, pulse rate, urine output, and serum and urine osmolarity. Water is withheld, and the response of the urine osmolarity and urine output is evaluated on an hourly basis. The serum osmolarity should be measured at the beginning and at the end of the test. As the water deprivation proceeds, the patient with true DI becomes desperate for water and will obtain water by any means unless closely supervised. The endpoint of fluid deprivation can be any of the following occurrences:

1. When three consecutive urine samples are nearly identical (less than 30 mOsm difference).

2. When the patient shows clinical evidence of volume depletion.

3. When there is a loss in body weight exceeding 3–5% of the weight at the start of the study.

The second part of the water deprivation test involves evaluating the urinary concentrating ability following the injection of 5 units of aqueous vasopressin.

The normal subject, following water deprivation, shows a rapid increase in urinary osmolarity, reaching isosmotic levels within hours. By 4 to 6 hr, the urinary osmolarity reaches 800–1000 mOsm with a prompt drop in the urine flow. These effects result from the physiological release of vasopressin in response to dehydration. After maximal concentration has been attained, as demonstrated by a plateau in the urine osmolarity, further injection of aqueous vasopressin fails to significantly increase the urinary concentration.

The patient with complete central DI responds in a characteristic manner to water deprivation: to begin with, these patients start with a very low urinary osmolarity (50–100 mOsm) and hardly attain an isosmotic range by dehydration; however, following aqueous vasopressin administration there is a dramatic increase in the urinary osmolarity, often exceeding 800 to 1000 mOsm.

The patient with nephrogenic DI behaves similarly to the patient with central DI during the first part of the test; however, there is a characteristic failure to respond to vasopressin during the second part of the test, highlighting the target organ resistance of the renal tubules to vasopressin.

Partial central DI is characterized by a slow, steady, but inadequate increase in the urinary osmolarity. In fact, the endpoint in these patients takes a frustratingly long time to be reached. Following the administration of aqueous vasopressin, there is an increase in the urine osmolarity by 25% or more over

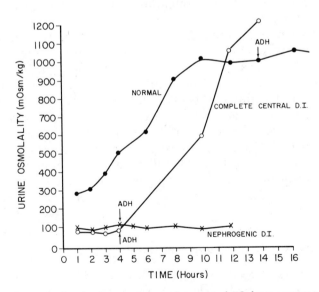

FIGURE 7. The water deprivation test in complete central DI demonstrates no urinary concentration with water deprivation but normal concentration following ADH. The water deprivation test in nephrogenic DI resembles complete central DI during the first part of the test. However, the disease is characterized by failure to respond to ADH administration.

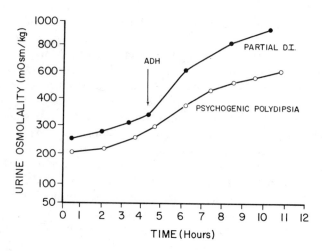

FIGURE 8. The results of the water deprivation test in patients with partial DI may resemble those of patients with psychogenic polydipsia (see text).

the base line. This contrasts sharply with the normal individual, who attains maximal concentration with dehydration, following which vasopressin injection causes little if any change.

Patients with psychogenic polydipsia, a disorder characterized by compulsive water drinking, can be regarded as having two separate problems. First, because of chronic water ingestion, there is suppression of endogenous vasopressin; therefore, there is sluggishness in responding to water deprivation, and the first part of the test resembles partial central DI. Second, the renal medullary interstitium of these patients has been rendered hypotonic ("dilute") as a result of chronic water inbibing; therefore, there is impairment even in responding to exogenous aqueous vasopressin. Thus, the second part of the test demonstrates an element of vasopressin resistance. The patient with psychogenic polydipsia starts with a urine osmolarity of 200 to 300 mOsm and then shows a gradual but inadequate concentrating ability, reaching a plateau between 400 and 600 mOsm. Up to this point the results of the study resemble partial DI. However, following exogenous vasopressin, the increase in urine osmolarity is less than 20% of the base line, indicating inability to concentrate adequately despite vasopressin administration. Figures 7 and 8 illustrate the responses of urine osmolarity to water deprivation in various disease states.

9.4.2. Plasma Arginine Vasopressin Levels

Measurement of AVP levels performed in conjunction with the water deprivation test can provide a clear separation among normals, patients with central DI, and those with nephrogenic DI. More importantly, the assay provides a means to differentiate patients with partial DI, from those with psychogenic polydipsia.

9.4.3. Topographical Tests

If central DI is diagnosed, the single most crucial test is evaluation of the suprasellar and sellar area by computerized tomography. Exclusion of tumors is a prerequisite for the diagnosis of idiopathic DI. A bone survey to detect lytic lesion may be essential if Hand–Schuller–Christian disease is suspected.

9.5. Differential Diagnosis

Diabetes insipidus needs to be distinguished from other polyuric states; the important ones include solute diuresis from hyperglycemia (diabetes mellitus), hypercalcemia, chronic renal interstitial or renal tubular disease, bilateral hydronephrosis, hypokalemia, the diuretic phase of acute renal failure, and, most importantly, excessive administration of intravenous fluids containing solute. This situation is particularly common in postoperative patients; the increased output seen in these patients may merely reflect the excessive fluids administered. "Weaning" the fluids, in these situations, is attended by a corresponding decline in urine output.

Psychogenic polydipsia, or compulsive water drinking, is caused by an underlying psychiatric problem. These patients consume enormous quantities of water for "self-satisfaction." (The author knew of a memorable case in which the patient would "quench" her thirst by stuffing a fully open garden hose in her mouth!) The diagnostic studies in patients with compulsive water drinking can mimic partial DI to a remarkable extent. One clue may be derived by the serum osmolarity and serum sodium; mild decrements in the serum osmolarity and serum sodium may be observed in patients with psychogenic polydipsia. Assay of vasopressin in the plasma during the water deprivation test may help in distinguishing the condition from true DI.

9.6. Complications

The most dangerous complication of complete DI is the development of volume depletion and dehydration. This occurs when access to water is denied, as when the patient is unconscious.

Bladder distension and even hydronephrosis can complicate severe disease.

9.7. Treatment

The treatment for acute DI with dehydration is liberal fluid replacement coupled with the use of a short-acting vasopressin preparation such as aqueous vasopressin.

For chronic DI, where the symptoms are distressing and interfere with the patient's life style, replacement therapy with 1-desamino-8-D-arginine vasopressin (dDAVP) or with a long-acting preparation such as pitressin tannate in oil is indicated. Of the two, dDAVP is superior for a variety of reasons. First, the drug can be conveniently administered intranasally twice a day. Second, the drug is highly potent; doses as small as 2.5 μg twice a day provide effective relief from polyuria. Third, the drug has a relatively longer duration of action, permitting b.i.d. dosage. Fourth, side effects such as vasoconstriction, hypotension, and, particularly, water intoxication are seldom encountered with dDAVP. Finally, the development of resistance to the drug with continued use is rare with dDAVP. Thus, therapy with dDAVP is a most effective, convenient, and safe modality. The only drawback is the expense, since the drug is costly.

Pitressin tannate in oil is a long-acting vasopressin preparation. However, its duration and potency are unpredictable, especially with long-term treatment. The particular danger with long-term use is the vasoconstrictive effect on arteries, especially the coronaries. Other undesirable effects include water intoxication and the development of resistance to the drug. A practical point that should be remembered is that the "hormone" is contained in a brown speck at the bottom of the ampule and needs to be gently hand warmed prior to injection. (If this is not done properly, the patient would be injecting peanut oil, which obviously does not possess any antidiuretic properties.)

Patients with partial central DI may be tried on chlorpropamide, which has dual actions. It can potentiate the release of vasopressin from the hypothalamus when the deficiency is partial and also augment the peripheral action of vasopressin on the renal tubules by enhancing receptor sensitivity. The drug does not work in the complete form of central DI or in nephrogenic DI.

Treatment of nephrogenic DI is extremely difficult. Paradoxically, the use of hydrochlorothiazide with a reduction in glomerular filtration rate improves the polyuria of nephrogenic diabetes insipidus.

10

Syndrome of Inappropriate ADH Secretion

10.1. Introduction

The syndrome of inappropriate ADH secretion (SIADH) represents one of the most frequent metabolic disorders encountered in hospitalized patients. The diverse diseases that cause this syndrome, the clinical features, and the criteria for establishing the diagnosis, as well as the therapeutic options for this disorder constitute this chapter.

10.2. Definition

The syndrome of inappropriate ADH secretion is defined as a metabolic disorder characterized by continued secretion of antidiuretic hormone (arginine vasopressin) despite hypotonicity.

10.3. Pathophysiology

The excess AVP in SIADH can be secreted by either the hypothalamus or an ectopic source. Regardless of the source, the pathophysiology of SIADH is identical. The effects of excess secretion of AVP are dual: decreased free water clearance because of increased reabsorption of water by the distal and collecting tubules and hypotonicity of the plasma as a result of dilution. The hallmark of SIADH is nonsuppressible AVP secretion despite hypotonicity of plasma. This is in contrast to the normal subject, where prompt suppression of AVP is the response to hypotonicity. With the continuous secretion of AVP, dilutional hyponatremia occurs, analogous to water intoxication. This hyponatremia is compounded by natriurisis, a paradox, in light of the fact that the serum Na^+ is already low. Table 24 contrasts the physiological response to hypotonicity in normals and in the patient with SIADH. The specific mechanisms underlying the pathophysiology of each facet of SIADH are discussed in Section 10.6.

10.4. Etiology

There are several disorders that are etiologically related to the development of SIADH. Despite the variety of disorders that cause SIADH, the majority of cases result from malignant disease or infectious disease of the CNS or lungs. Table 25 illustrates the numerous etiologies of SIADH. When no etiology for SIADH is discerned, the diagnosis of idiopathic SIADH can be made, a disorder especially prevalent in older patients.

TABLE 24
Response to Hypotonic Plasma in the Normal State and in SIADH

Normal	SIADH
Hypotonic plasma	Hyponatremia/hypotonic plasma
Prompt suppression of vasopressin (ADH)	Failure of vasopression suppression (or increased vasopressin levels)
Prompt suppression of water reabsorption in distal and collecting tubule	Continuous water reabsorption at the distal and collecting tubule
Dilution of urine due to increased water excretion	Urine relatively concentrated
Conservation of solute	Continuous natriuresis
Excretion of dilute urine	Excretion of less than maximally dilute urine
Restoration of plasma osmolality to normal	Persistance of low plasma osmolality

TABLE 25
Etiology of SIADH

Malignancy
  Bronchogenic carcinoma
  Pancreatic carcinoma
  GI neoplasms
  Hodgkin's and non-Hodgkin's lymphoma
  Thymoma
Nonmalignant pulmonary disease
  Tuberculosis
  Bacterial and viral pneumonia
  Lung abscess
  Empyema
  Fungal diseases
CNS disease
  Head injury
  Subarachnoid and subdural hemorrhage
  Meningitis, encephalitis
  Brain abscess
Drug induced
  Chlorpropamide
  Carbamazepine
  Clofibrate
  Vincristine
  Cyclophosphamide
  Tricyclic antidepressant
Idiopathic
Miscellaneous
  Acute psychosis
  Acute intermittent porphyria
  Positive-pressure ventilatory assistance

10.5. Clinical Features

The features of SIADH result from the effects of hyponatremia. The clinical features of SIADH evolve slowly and are characterized by fatigue, muscle weakness, and dizziness. As the disorder progresses, muscle twitching, alteration in behavior, and drowsiness supervene. When the serum sodium declines below 120 mEq/liter, stupor, convulsions, and coma occur. The development of metabolic encephalopathy depends on the severity of the hyponatremia as well as the rapidity with which the syndrome evolved. Edema or dehydration are characteristically absent.

10.6. Diagnostic Studies

The criteria for the diagnosis of SIADH are (1) hypotonicity of plasma, (2) hyponatremia, (3) less than maximally dilute urine, (4) natriuresis despite hyponatremia, and (5) the exclusion of hepatic, renal, thyroid, and adrenal dysfunction.

The hypotonic plasma and the hyponatremia are a consequence of dilution from excessive water reabsorption by the distal and collecting tubules as well as from urinary losses of sodium secondary to natriuresis. The exact mechanism for the sodium loss in SIADH is not clear, but it is probably a result of extracellular fluid (ECF) volume expansion. As a consequence, there is suppression of renin and aldosterone, which leads to decreased proximal tubular reabsorption of sodium and an increase in the filtered sodium. Severe salt restriction corrects the urinary sodium loss by stimulating renin and aldosterone with a resultant increase in sodium reabsorption.

The demonstration of a less than maximally dilute urine in the presence of a hypotonic plasma constitutes one of the most important criteria for the diagnosis. The reasons for this phenomenon are the continuous water reabsorption at the distal and collecting tubules and the continuous natriuresis, both of which are conducive to excretion of a concentrated urine. In general, the patient with SIADH demonstrates a urine osmolarity greater than the plasma osmolarity. It should be emphasized that the urine/plasma osmolarity greater than 1 is valid only when the patient has a hypotonic plasma. For example, any normal individual who has been deprived of water overnight will have a urine/plasma osmolarity greater than 1. The serum osmolarity in these normal subjects is not low.

Occasionally, a severely solute-restricted patient with SIADH may demonstrate a urine osmolarity below the plasma osmolarity, but the inappropriateness, i.e., the less than maximally dilute nature, will be evident. For instance, a severely salt-restricted patient with SIADH may have a plasma osmolarity of 250 mOsm and a simultaneous urine osmolarity of 200 mOsm. Even though below the plasma, the urine osmolarity in this situation is higher than one would expect for the degree of hypotonicity of the plasma. In normal situations, a plasma tonicity of 250 mOsm is associated with a very dilute urine, not exceeding 100 mOsm. Thus, in comparing the urine and plasma osmolarities in the diagnosis of SIADH, the question is not whether the urine osmolarity is greater than that of the plasma but whether the urine is less than maximally dilute. This criterion, however, is shared by several other situations (see Section 10.7). Continued natriuresis despite hyponatremia is a result of expansion of ECF and suppression of the renin–aldosterone system.

The exclusion of hepatic, cardiac, renal, and adrenal dysfunction as well as volume depletion is an essential criterion for the diagnosis of SIADH. Several conditions are characterized by dilutional hyponatremia, decreased free water clearance, and production of a less than maximally dilute urine in the presence of a hypotonic plasma. Cirrhosis, nephrotic syndrome, congestive failure, and volume depletion are all characterized by a reduction in "effective circulating blood volume." A decrease in renal flow or GFR is associated with production of urine more concentrated than the plasma even in the absence of AVP. The sequence for this occurrence is as follows:

1. A decrease in the effective circulating blood volume results in a decreased GFR.
2. The decrease in GFR stimulates the renin–angiotensin–aldosterone system.
3. This results in increased proximal tubular reabsorption of sodium.
4. Therefore, there is a reduced delivery of filtrate to the diluting segment of the nephron, i.e., the ascending limb of the loop of Henle.
5. The diluting process in this region depends on movement of sodium from the ascending limb into the medullary interstitium, thereby rendering the fluid progressively more dilute.
6. Since the ascending limb is impermeable to back diffusion of water, a decreased delivery of filtrate to the diluting segments will result in impairment of the diluting ability.
7. The decreased filtrate is conducive to a decreased flow rate through the distal tubule and collecting ducts, an area somewhat permeable to back diffusion of water into the medullary interstitium.
8. Most importantly, the decrease in the effective circulating blood volume stimulates the baroreceptors with the appropriate release of AVP.
9. The AVP further compounds the events at the collecting tubules, resulting in further concentration of urine. The net result is the production of a less than maximally dilute urine.

Thus, the diagnosis of SIADH can not be made in the presence of conditions that reduce the effective circulating blood volume. The two reasons that preclude the diagnosis of SIADH under these circumstances are:

1. These conditions can produce an identical abnormality in the handling of water by the renal tubules.
2. These conditions elicit an appropriate response in AVP release mediated by the nonosmotic pathways of AVP release. The importance of excluding adrenal or thyroid function is discussed in Section 10.7.

Based on the foregoing, the following tests would be required when the diagnosis of SIADH needs to be established:

1. BUN and creatinine.
2. Liver profile.
3. Thyroid function tests.
4. Serum cortisol and, when indicated, rapid ACTH stimulation test.

10.7. Differential Diagnosis

As indicated earlier, the combination of hyponatremia, natriuresis, and the production of a less than maximally dilute urine in the presence of a hypotonic plasma is not unique for SIADH. Volume depletion, ascites, nephrotic syndrome, hepatic failure, renal disease, and congestive cardiac failure are some common situations in which such a combination is frequently encountered. These can be excluded on the basis of clinical examination and routine laboratory tests. Three situations are particularly relevant in the differential diagnosis of SIADH from the endocrine standpoint: these are Addison's disease, hypothyroidism, and the "sick-call syndrome." All three can present with a metabolic picture identical to SIADH.

Adrenocortical failure is associated with decreased free water clearance and an inability to maximally dilute the urine. These abnormalities are caused by salt and water depletion and a decrease in the GFR; this results in increased reabsorption of water in the proximal tubule (vasopressin independent), reducing the delivery of filtrate to the diluting segments of the nephron. Since both SIADH and adrenocortical failure present with hyponatremia, and since tuberculosis and lung cancer frequently exist in the background of both diseases, the distinction is important in clinical practice. Three findings permit delineation: first, the patient with adrenocortical failure is often volume depleted and dehydrated; second, hyperkalemia is present in more than two-thirds of patients with adrenal insufficiency; third, the low serum cortisol levels may help in suggesting adrenocortical failure. When in doubt, evaluation of adrenal reserve by the administration of ACTH should be performed to exclude Addison's disease.

The hyponatremia and the decreased free water clearance of myxedema are multifactorial; decreased GFR, resetting of the osmoreceptors, relative glucocorticoid deficiency, and decreased clearance of vasopressin may all be contributory.

The hyponatremia of the "sick-cell syndrome" is observed in the chronically debilitated patient. The mechanism is presumably a result of shift in sodium ions from the extracellular to the intracellular compartment in contrast to dilutional hyponatremia, which is characterized by defective water excretion. The pathophysiology underlying the sick-cell syndrome is unclear, but it may be related to loss of organic intracellular osmoles (products of cellular metabolism) as a consequence of cachexia or malnutrition. Alternatively, the condition may be caused by resetting of osmostats as a result of chronic disease, since the majority of such patients are able to excrete a dilute urine following a water-loading test.

10.8.   Treatment

The cornerstone for the treatment of SIADH is fluid restriction, usually limited to 600–800 ml/day. With this intake, the patient should soon develop negative fluid balance because of the continued insensible losses; the serum sodium gradually increases as the water intoxication is treated by simple water restriction. A good indication that the water restriction is working is to demonstrate weight loss. As the weight decreases, the plasma osmolarity and the serum sodium rise. This treatment usually increases the serum osmolarity to normal within 7 to 10 days.

Demeclocycline is a useful adjunct to fluid restriction. This drug interferes with the action of vasopressin at the level of the distal and collecting tubules. The drug blocks the action of vasopressin regardless of whether it is secreted by the hypothalamus or secreted ectopically by a tumor. In most patients, the electrolyte abnormality is restored to normal within 5 to 14 days. Demeclocycline is given in doses of 900 to 1200 mg/day. The occasional side effects include the occurrence of renal failure and bacterial superinfection. In general, the side effects are minimal, and the drug can be used safely, provided there is adequate follow-up and monitoring of renal function.

The use of hypertonic saline may be considered when the serum sodium is below 115 mEq/liter. The rapid correction of hyponatremia may result in the development of central pontine myelinolysis, a serious complication.

Selected Readings

Anderson, R. J., Chung, H., Kluge, R., *et al.*: Hyponatremia: A prospective analysis of its epidemiology, and the pathogenetic role of vasopressin, *Ann. Intern. Med.* **102**:164, 1985.

Antunes, J. L., Housepian, E. M., Frantz, A. G., *et al.*: Prolactin secreting pituitary tumors, *Ann. Neurol.* **2**:148, 1977.

Archer, D. R.: Physiology of prolactin, *Clin. Obstet. Gynecol.* **23**:325, 1980.

Aron, D. C., Tyrrell, J. B., Fitzgerald, P. A., *et al.*: Cushing's syndrome: Problems in diagnosis, *Medicine* **60**:25, 1981.

Asa, S. L., Bilbao, J. M., Kovacs, K., *et al.*: Lymphocytic hypophysitis of pregnancy resulting in hypopituitarism, *Ann. Intern. Med.* **95**:166, 1981.

Bartter, F. C., and Schwartz, W. B.: The syndrome of inappropriate secretion of antidiuretic hormone, *Am. J. Med.* **42**:790, 1967.

Berl, T., Anderson, R. J., McDonald, K. M., *et al.*: Clinical disorders or water metabolism, *Kidney Int.* **10**:117, 1976.

Besser, G. M., Wass, J. A. H., Thorner, M. O., *et al.*: Bromocriptine in the medical management of acromegaly, *Adv. Biochem.* **23**:191, 1980.

Bowers, C. Y., Freisen, H. G., Hwang, P., *et al.*: Prolactin and thyrotropin release in man by synthetic pyroglutamyl-histidyl-prolinamide, *Biochem. Biophys. Res. Commun.* **45**:1033, 1971.

Brown, M. R., and Fisher, L. A.: Brain peptides as intracellular messengers. Implications for medicine, *J.A.M.A.* **251**:1310, 1984.

Chrousos, G. P., Schulte, H. M., Oldfield, E. H., *et al.*: The corticotropin-releasing factor stimulation test. An aid in the evaluation of patients with Cushing's syndrome, *N. Engl. J. Med.* **310**:662, 1984.

Clemmons, D. R., Van Wyke, J. J., Ridgway, E. C., *et al.*: Evaluation of acromegaly by measurement of somatomedine-C. *N. Engl. J. Med.* **301**:1138, 1979.

Cook, D. M., Kendall, J. W., and Jordon, R.: Cushing's syndrome, current concepts of diagnosis and therapy, *West. J. Med.* **132**:111, 1980.

DiChiro, G., and Nelson, K. B.: The volume of the sella turcica, *Am. J. Roentgenol. Rad. Ther. Nucl. Med.* **87**:989, 1962.

Eastman, R. C., Gorden, P., Roth, J., *et al.*: Conventional supervoltage irradiation is an effective treatment for acromegaly. *J. Clin. Endocrinol. Metab.* **48**:931, 1979.

Faglia, G., Beck-Peccoz, P., Ferrari, C., *et al.*: Plasma growth hormone response to TRH in patients with active acromegaly, *J. Clin. Endocrinol. Metabl.* **36**:1259, 1973.

Findling, J. W., Aron, D. C., Tyrrell, J. B., *et al.*: Selective venous sampling for ACTH in Cushing's syndrome. Differentiation between Cushing's disease and ectopic ACTH syndrome, *Ann. Intern. Med.* **94**:647, 1981.

Fitzgerald, P. A., Aron, D. C., Findling, J. W., *et al.*: Cushing's disease: Transient secondary insufficiency after selective removal of pituitary microadenomas; evidence for a pituitary origin, *J. Clin. Endocrinol. Metab.* **54:**413, 1982.

Foley, T. P., Owings, J., Hayford, J. T., *et al.*: Serum thyrotropin responses to synthetic TRH in normal children and hypopituitary patients: A new test to distinguish primary releasing hormone deficiency from primary pituitary hormone deficiency, *J. Clin. Invest.* **51:**431, 1972.

Frantz, A. G., and Rabkin, M. T.: Human growth hormone. Clinical measurement of response to hypoglycemia and suppression by corticosteroids, *N. Engl. J. Med.* **271:**1375, 1964.

Frey, H. M.: Spontaneous pituitary destruction in diabetes mellitus, *J. Clin. Endocrinol. Metab.* **19:**1642, 1959.

Goldfine, I. D., Lawrence, A. M.: Hypopituitarism in acromegaly, *Arch. Intern. Med.* **130:**720, 1972.

Goldstein, C. S., Braunstein, S., and Goldfarb, S.: Idiopathic syndrome of inappropriate antidiuretic hormone secretion possibly related to advance age, *Ann. Intern. Med.* **99:**185, 1983.

Hardy, J.: Transsphenoidal surgery of hypersecreting pituitary tumors, in Kohler, P. O., and Ross, G. T. (eds.): *Diagnosis and Treatment of Pituitary Tumors.* Amsterdam, Excerpta Medica, 1973.

Jacobs, L. S., Snyder, P. J., Utiger, R. D., *et al.*: Prolactin response to TRH in normal subjects, *J. Clin. Endocrinol. Metab.* **36:**1069, 1973.

Kleinberg, D., Noel, G., and Frantz, A.: Galactorrhea—a study of 235 cases, including 48 with pituitary tumors, *N. Engl. J. Med.* **296:**589, 1977.

Kreiger, D. T.: Endorphins and enkephalins, *D Mo* **28:**3, 1982.

Lawrence, A. M.: Hypothalamic hypopituitarism after pituitary apoplexy in acromegaly, *Arch. Intern. Med.* **137:**1134, 1977.

Lawrence, A. M., Goldfine, I. D., Kirsteins, L., *et al.*: Growth hormone dynamics in acromegaly, *J. Clin. Endocrinol. Metab.* **31:**239, 1970.

Liddle, G. W., and Givens, J. R.: The ectopic ACTH syndrome, *Cancer Res.* **25:**1057, 1965.

Lin, T., and Tucci, J. R.: Provocative tests of growth hormone release. A comparison of results with seven stimuli, *Ann. Intern. Med.* **80:**464, 1974.

Lindholm, J., Riishede, J., Vestergaard, S., *et al.*: No effect of bromocriptine in acromegaly a controlled trial, *N. Engl. J. Med.* **304:**1450, 1981.

Loh, Y. P., and Loriaux, L. L.: Adrenocorticotropic hormone, β lipotropin, and endorphin related peptides in health and disease, *J.A.M.A.* **247:**1033, 1982.

Luton, J. P., Mahoudeau, J. A., Bouchard, P. H., *et al.*: Treatment of Cushing's disease by 0,p'DDD, *N. Engl. J. Med.* **300:**459, 1979.

McGuffin, W. L., Sherman, B., Roth, J., *et al.*: Acromegaly and cardiovascular disorders. A prospective study, *Ann. Intern. Med.* **81:**11, 1974.

Merker, E., and Futterweit, W.: Postpartum amenorrhea, diabetes insipidus and galactorrhea, *Am. J. Med.* **56:**554, 1974.

Mortimer, C. H., Besser, G. M., McNeilly, A. S., *et al.*: Interaction between secretion of the gonadotrophins, prolactin, growth hormone, thyrotrophin and corticosteroids in man: The effects of LH/FSH-RH, TRH and hypoglycemia, alone and in combination, *Clin. Endocrinol.* **2:**317, 1973.

Moses, A. M., and Notman, D. D.: Diabetes insipidus and SIADH, *Adv. Intern. Med.* **27:**73, 1982.

Noell, K. T.: Prolactin and other hormone-producing pituitary tumors: Radiation therapy, *Clin. Obstet. Gynecol.* **23:**441, 1980.

Orth, D. N., and Liddle, G. W.: Results of treatment in 108 patients with Cushing's syndrome, *N. Engl. J. Med.* **285:**243, 1971.

Pearson, O. H., Arafah, B., Brodkey, J., *et al.*: Management of acromegaly, *Ann. Intern. Med.* **95:**225, 1981.

Quigley, M. M., and Haney, A. F.: Evaluation of hyperprolactinemia: Clinical profiles, *Clin. Obstet. Gynecol.* **23:**337, 1980.

Randall, R. V.: Empty sella syndrome, *Compr. Ther.* **10:**57, 1984.

Reichlin, S.: Somatostatin, *N. Engl. J. Med.* **309:**1495, 1983.

Savage, D. D., Henry, W. L., Eastman, R. C., *et al.:* Echocardiographic assessment of cardiac anatomy and function in acromegalic patients, *Am. J. Med.* **67:**823, 1979.

Schuster, L. D., Bantle, J. P., Oppenheimer, J. H., *et al.:* Acromegaly—reassessment of the long term therapeutic effectiveness of transsphenoidal pituitary surgery, *Ann. Intern. Med.* **95:**172, 1981.

Sheehan, H. L.: Post partum necrosis of anterior pituitary, *J. Pathol. Bacteriol.* **45:**189, 1937.

Singer, P. A., Mestman, J. H., Manning, P. R., *et al.:* Hypothalamic hypothyroidism secondary to Sheehan's Syndrome, *West. J. Med.* **120:**416, 1974.

Synder, P., and Utiger, R. D.: Response to thyrotropin releasing hormone in normal man, *J. Clin. Endocrinol. Metab.* **34:**380, 1972.

Spark, R. F., Baker, R., Bienfang, D. C., *et al.:* Bromocriptine reduces pituitary tumor size and hypersecretion. Requiem for pituitary surgery, *J.A.M.A.* **247:**311, 1982.

Swanson, H. A., and du Boulay, G.: Borderline variants of the normal pituitary fossa, *Br. J. Radiol.* **48:**366, 1975.

Teramato, A.: Immunohistochemical studies on the functioning pituitary adenomas, *Brain Nerve* **32:**1163, 1980.

Urbanic, R. C., and George, J. M.: Cushing's disease—18 years experience, *Medicine* **60:**14, 1981.

Vaughn, T. C., and Hammond, C. B.: Prolactin-producing pituitary tumors: Medical therapy, *Clin. Obstet. Gynecol.* **23:**403, 1980.

Wise, J., Morris, M. A., and Handwerger, S.: Measurement of prolactin, *Clin. Obstet. Gynecol.* **23:**315, 1980.

Woolf, P. D., and Schalch, D.: Hypopituitarism secondary to hypothalamic deficiency, *Ann. Intern. Med.* **78:**88, 1973.

Zerbe, R. L., and Robertson, G. L.: A comparison of plasma vasopressin measurements with a standard indirect test in the differential diagnosis of polyuria, *N. Engl. J. Med.* **305:**1539, 1981.

II

The Thyroid Gland

11

The Anatomy of the Thyroid Gland

The thyroid gland consists of two lobes, a right and left, connected by an isthmus. The upper margin of the isthmus lies just below the cricoid cartilage. The lobes, which measure 4 cm in length and 2 to 2.5 cm in width and thickness, lie alongside the lateral aspects of the lower half of the thyroid cartilage. The entire gland, including the isthmus, is enveloped by connective tissue that is continuous with the thyrocervical fascia. Thus, the thyroid is affixed to the anterior and lateral surface of the trachea and, hence, moves with deglutition. The normal gland weighs approximately 20 g.

The anatomic relations of the thyroid gland includes several important structures. Anteriorly, the thyroid lobes are separated from the subcutaneous tissues of the neck by the thin, ribbonlike infrahyoid muscles. Posteriorly, the lobes are related to the trachea. The recurrent laryngeal nerves lie in the groove between the lobes and the trachea. The parathyroid glands also form an important posterior relationship, normally situated as two pairs, one on each side, on or beneath the posterior surface of each lobe in the upper and lower poles. Laterally, the three important structures are the carotid sheath (containing the carotid vessels), the sternocleidomastoid muscles, and the cervical lymph nodes.

Embryologically, the thyroid gland is derived from the epithelium in the pharyngeal floor, originating as a diverticulum. This diverticulum gradually elongates and moves caudally, the primitive elongated stalk being present as the thyroglossal duct. At the diverticulum develops, it assumes a bilobar butterfly shape, fusing with the ventral aspect of the fourth pharyngeal pouch. The thyroglossal duct involutes by the second month, and its adult representation is a dimple called the foramen cecum at the base of the tongue.

Four variants of thyroid development are noteworthy. The right lobe of the thyroid gland is usually slightly larger than the left; this difference is magnified during diffuse enlargement, the right lobe showing a tendency to enlarge more than the left. Another variant is the pyramidal lobe, a fingerlike structure directed upward, originating from the isthmus and located slightly left of the midline. An important embryological variant is hemiagenesis of a lobe, resulting in total absence of one lobe. Rarely, the thyroid gland may be entirely absent, with a lingual thyroid representing the remnant.

The thyroid gland is highly vascular, the blood flow averaging 5 ml per minute per gram of tissue. The arterial supply is derived from the superior thyroid arteries (branches of external carotids) and the inferior thyroid arteries (branches of subclavian arteries). The highly vascular thyroid gland becomes even more so during diffuse hyperfunction of the gland, resulting in the familiar bruits heard—and occasionally even felt—on the thyroid lobes.

Physiology
The Secretion, Regulatory Control, and Actions of the Thyroid Hormones

The two principal hormones secreted by the thyroid gland are thyroxine (T_4) and triiodothyronine (T_3). Both hormones are synthesized by the thyroid gland from iodine. The first step in thyroid hormonogenesis is *trapping*. The thyroid cells are extremely effective in trapping iodine from the plasma against a concentration gradient, since the concentrations of iodine in the plasma are extremely low (0.1 to 1 µg/dl). The trapped iodine is immediately oxidized. Unless oxidized, the iodine cannot be incorporated into tyrosyl residues, a process called *organification*. The trapped, oxidized iodine undergoes organification instantaneously by a number of enzymes, in particular, the peroxidases. The tyrosyl is provided by thyroglobulin, a large-molecular-weight protein contained within the colloid. The process of iodination of thyroglobulin results in the formation of monoiodotyrosine (MIT). A series of coupling reactions results in the formation of diiodotyrosine (DIT) and tetraiodothyronine (T_4). Similarly, coupling of one DIT with one MIT results in the formation of triiodothyronine (T_3).

After synthesis, the next step is secretion. The iodination of thyroglobulin and the formation of all the iodoproteins including T_4 and T_3 occur at the apical border of the cell, with exocytosis into the colloid. When secretion and release are activated, the thyroglobulin actually undergoes phagocytosis, with the formation of a "colloid droplet." The colloid droplet, which makes it way from the apical to the basal border of the cell, combines with lysosomal enzymes with proteolytic properties. As a result of proteolysis, T_4 and T_3 are cleaved from thyroglobulin and released from the basal border of the cell into the circulation. The deiodinase enzymes that are present in the colloid remove iodine from T_4 as well as MIT and DIT in order to conserve and recycle iodine.

The thyroid hormones circulate in blood as both bound and free hormones: Approximately 99.5% of thyroxine is bound to plasma proteins; less than 0.5% is free. It is this free moiety that is biologically active, enters the target cells, and regulates the pituitary secretion of TSH. Yet the radioimmunoassay for T_4 measures only the bound T_4, which is biologically inactive and subject to alterations in the proteins to which it is bound. The major protein that carries T_4 is thyroxine-binding globulin (TBG). To a lesser extent, T_4 is bound to thyroxine-binding prealbumin (TBPA) and albumin. The TBG, the predominant carrier protein of T_4 (and T_3), is an inter-α-globulin and is synthesized by the liver. There is an equilibrium between the free and bound fractions of T_4, and generally, in the absence of abnormalities in TBG or other binding proteins, the bound thyroxine correlates well with the free fraction. The following equation typifies the relationship between the free and bound fractions:

Free hormone is proportional to TBG-bound T_4/unoccupied TBG

The factors that affect TBG (and therefore affect T_4) and the correction factors employed are discussed in Chapter 13.

The major metabolic fate of T_4 is peripheral deiodination to T_3. The T_4-to-T_3 conversion primarily occurs at the liver and kidney. Loss of one iodine at the distal ring results in the formation of T_3 (3,5,3′), with three to four times the metabolic potency of T_4. Approximately 80% of the T_3 in the circulation is derived in this manner. Several factors inhibit the peripheral conversion of T_4 to T_3. These include renal or hepatic disease, severe acute or chronic illness, and a variety of drugs such as propylthiouracil (PTU), glucocorticoids, propranolol, and iopanoic acid. The most common setting is severe illness, and the low T_3 seen in this entity is referred to as the "sick euthyroid syndrome." When the T_4-to-T_3 conversion is impaired, regardless of the cause, the thyroxine in the blood is converted instead into reverse T_3 (3,3′,5′), a metabolically inert isomer formed by monodeiodination of T_4 at the proximal ring.

The regulation of thyroid function by pituitary TSH is discussed in Chapter 2. In summary, TSH stimulates all aspects of thyroid function and is mediated by the cyclic AMP system. Autoregulatory mechanisms mediated by iodine can modify the effect of TSH on the thyroid to some extent. The negative feedback effect of the thyroid hormones on TSH secretion and release is discussed in Chapter 2.

The action of thyroid hormones is mediated by binding of these hormones to nuclear proteins. The affinity of the nuclear receptors to T_3 is greater than to T_4. After binding to nuclear receptors, the thyroid hormones alter DNA transcription with a subsequent increase in messenger RNA formation and eventual protein synthesis. The three major effects of thyroid hormones are increased protein synthesis (anabolic), uncoupling of oxidative phosphoryl (catabolic) resulting in increased oxygen consumption by tissues, and increased ion transport across membranes (calorigenic).

13

Testing Thyroid Function

13.1. Introduction

The commonly used thyroid function tests can be divided into three categories: blood tests that assess the functional status of the thyroid gland (T_4, T_3R, T_3RIA, TSH), tests that dynamically evaluate the pituitary–thyroid axis (TRH test, cytomal suppression test), and *in vivo* isotopic tests (radioiodine uptake tests, thyroid scan, etc.). In addition, several adjunctive tests (thyroglobulin, antithyroid antibodies, human thyroid stimulators, free hormones, etc.) can be utilized when indicated.

13.2. Tests to Assess the Functional Status

The diverse clinical indications that require screening for adequacy of thyroid function are outlined in Table 25. The indications, utility, and physiological bases for abnormalities in each of the tests form the subject of this chapter.

13.2.1. Serum Thyroxine

A sensitive radioimmunoassay is available for the measurement of thyroxine, and has replaced the older method of measurement by column. The T_4 radioimmunoassay measures the thyroxine bound to the carrier proteins, particularly TBG (thyroxine-binding globulin). Thus, other than thyroid dysfunction, the most significant factor that alters the measurement of T_4 by radioimmunoassay is a change in the binding proteins (see Table 28).

In addition to alterations in TBG, abnormal carrier proteins in the plasma (bisalbumin) as well as the presence of circulating "inhibitors" that prevent the binding of T_4 to TBG can also affect the measurement of thyroxine in

TABLE 25
Indications to Screen for Thyroid Function

Overt or suspected hyper- or hypofunction
Cardiac disease
  Arrythmia
"Refractory" cardiac failure
  Coronary heart disease
  Pericardial effusion
Unexplained weight loss (or gain)
Unexplained diarrhea or constipation
Menometrorrhagia, amenorrhea
Thyromegaly
Proptosis
Growth retardation
Mental retardation
Unexplained fatigue, cramps, etc.
Anxiety or psychiatric syndromes
Unexplained hypercalcemia

the plasma. The various causes for elevated and decreased T_4 are outlined in Table 26. An abnormal serum thyroxine level should always be interpreted along with the results of the T_3R uptake test in order to correct for alteration in the TBG level, a major parameter that affects the measurement of the bound hormone.

The normal range of thyroxine in most laboratories is 4–11 µg/dl; with the exception of patients with T_3 toxicosis (hyperthyroidism caused by preferential hypersecretion of triiodothyronine but not thyroxine), hyperthyroidism can be established with ease by the measurement of serum levels of thyroxine. A single sample of blood is usually adequate for diagnostic purposes, since the hormone shows negligible fluctuation throughout the day. Thus, the sensitivity of the test to document hyperthyroidism is excellent. As far as the diagnostic specificity, the only common reasons for a false-positive ele-

TABLE 26
Causes for Elevated and Decreased Thyroxine

Increased T_4	Decreased T_4
Hyperthyroidism	Hypothyroidism
Increased TBG	Decreased TBG
Familial hyperthyroxinemia (caused by abnormal albumin)	
Peripheral resistance to thyroid hormone	Acromegaly, Cushing's disease
Drugs: amiodarone, heparin, thyroxine	Drugs: salicylate, diphenylhydantoin, cytomel, thionamides
Rarely, in severely ill patients	Severe illness
Antibodies to T_4 (depending on method)	Antibodies to T_4 (depending on method)

vation of T_4 in the euthyroid state are quantitative or qualitative abnormalities in TBG. This can be corrected for by performing the T_3 resin uptake test.

13.2.2. The T_3 Resin Uptake Test

The T_3 resin uptake test (T_3R, T_3RU) is a simple and effective *in vitro* test to determine the TBG binding capacity. The test is based on the following principles. First, the thyroxine-binding capacity of TBG in the plasma is never completely saturated. Second, when a measured amount of radiolabeled T_3 is incubated with the patient's plasma, the hot T_3 occupies sites available on the TBG. Third, the number of sites available on the TBG for exogenous labeled T_3 to bind depends on the number of sites that are already occupied by endogenous thyroxine as well as on the absolute amount of TBG that is present in the patient's plasma. Fourth, the amount of radiolabeled T_3 that is not picked up by the TBG following incubation is competitively picked by a nonspecific resin. This amount is expressed as the percentage of the radiolabeled T_3 taken-up by the resin and, in the normal euthyroid person, represents 25% to 35% of the radiolabeled amount. Thus, under normal circumstances, 65% to 75% of radiolabeled T_3 binds with the TBG.

When the patient's TBG is increased, as, for example, in the pregnant state, a greater proportion of labeled T_3 binds to the patient's TBG because of the dramatic increase in the availability of binding sites. As a consequence, less labeled T_3 is available to be taken up by the resin, and hence, the T_3R uptake is decreased. The measured T_4 under this circumstance is increased, reflecting the greatly enhanced carrying capacity of the plasma TBG.

When the patient's TBG is decreased, as, for example, in hypoproteinemic states, only a small amount of radiolabeled T_3 can be bound to the TBG because of the greatly diminished availability of binding sites. As a consequence, a large proportion of the T_3 would be taken up by the resin, and hence the T_3R uptake is increased. The measured T_4 under this circumstance is decreased, reflecting the greatly diminished carrying capacity of the plasma TBG.

In the truly hyperthyroid patient, the TBG sites are already occupied to accommodate the increased quantities of hormone produced by the hyperactive thyroid gland. Therefore, when exogenous labeled T_3 is added to the patient's plasma, fewer sites are available on the TBG molecule to bind the labeled T_3. As a result, more is available to be picked up by the resin, and hence the T_3R uptake is increased. The T_4 in this circumstance would also be elevated, reflecting the increased production of the hormone.

In the truly hypothyroid patient, the TBG sites are relatively unoccupied by the endogenous hormone as a result of suboptimal production by the thyroid gland. Therefore, when exogenous labeled T_3 is added to the patient's plasma, a greater proportion of the hot T_3 binds to TBG to occupy empty sites. As a result, less is available to be picked up by the resin, and hence the T_3R uptake is decreased. The measured T_4 in this circumstance would also be decreased, reflecting the diminished production of hormone by the thyroid.

TABLE 27
T$_4$ and T$_3$ Resin Uptake Test
Results in Different Conditions

Condition	T$_4$	T$_3$R
Increased TBG	↑	↓
Decreased TBG	↓	↑
Hyperthyroidism	↑	↓
Hypothyrodism	↓	↑

From the foregoing discussion it should be evident that when changes in TBG affect the measurement of T$_4$, the alteration in the T$_3$R uptake test is in the opposite direction, whereas when true disease (hyper or hypo) affects the measurement of T$_4$, the alteration in the T$_3$R uptake test is in the same direction (see Table 27).

Quantitative as well as qualitative alterations in thyroxine-binding gluobin may be encountered in several physiological and pathological states. The more frequent causes of alterations in TBG are outlined in Table 28.

The requirement in interpreting the T$_4$ level is that the T$_4$ level should always be evaluated in light of the T$_3$R uptake test. Several mathematical derivations have been devised for reporting results of these two tests (free thyroxine index T_7, etc.). The most widely employed derivation, the free thyroxine index (FTI), can be calculated by multiplying the T$_4$ by the T$_3$R uptake and dividing the product by 30, which is the mean value of T$_3$R uptake in normals. The purpose of this derivation is to express the T$_4$ corrected for abnormalities in TBG binding. In euthyroid patients with abnormalities in T$_4$ exclusively caused by alterations in the TBG, the FTI would be in the normal range (4–12) in most instances. However, it should be realized that with a marked increase or decrease in TBG (at extremes), the FTI may not be completely reliable for interpretation. It is in these circumstances that measurement of the free, biologically active moiety of the hormone would be indicated to evaluate the metabolic state of the patient.

TABLE 28
Conditions That Affect TBG

TBG increase	TBG decrease
Pregnancy	Chronic liver disease
Oral contraceptive	Nephrotic syndrome
Acute hepatitis	Chronic renal failure
Congenital	Acromegaly
	Hypercortisolism
	Congenital
	Drugs (competition for sites): salicylates, diphenylhydantoin

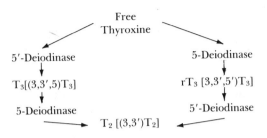

FIGURE 9. Conversion of T_4 to T_3.

13.2.3. Triiodothyronine

The T_3RIA measures the concentration of the circulating triiodothyronine level in the plasma (and should not be confused with the T_3 resin uptake). The predominant source (80%) of the circulating T_3 is peripheral deiodination of T_4 to T_3. Approximately 20% of circulating T_3 is from direct glandular secretion of this hormone. Triiodothyronine is two to four times more potent than thyroxine in terms of its calorigenic potential. The peripheral deiodination of T_4 can occur in all tissues but is most strikingly evident in hepatic tissue. The deiodination of T_4 to T_3 and the subsequent degradation of T_3 are outlined in Figure 9. The enzyme 5'-deiodinase is ubiquitous in all tissues and converts T_4 into T_3. When this enzyme is impaired or absent, free T_4 is converted to reverse T_3 by the enzyme 5-deiodinase. Reverse T_3 is not biologically active.

The indications to obtain serum T_3 levels include the following clinical settings:

1. When thyrotoxicosis is suspected but the T_4 levels are normal, to establish the diagnosis of T_3 hyperthyroidism (or T_3 toxicosis). This entity probably accounts for approximately 5% of all hyperthyroidism. It occurs preponderantly in certain settings such as hyperthyroidism occurring in areas of endemic iodine deficiency, hyperthyroidism developing in autonomously functioning thyroid nodules, (Plummer's disease), and in patients with recurrent hyperthyroidism following surgery or radioactive iodine.
2. When compensated euthyroidism is suspected following surgery or radioactive iodine therapy for Graves' hyperthyroidism. These are instances wherein euthyroidism is maintained despite a low serum thyroxine level at the expense of an elevated TSH secretion and a preferential production of T_3 by the compromised gland.
3. When factitious hyperthyroidism is suspected secondary to abuse of large amounts of exogenous preparations containing triiodothyronine such as *levo*-triiodothyronine (Cytomel).

The normal range of T_3 measured by radioimmunoassay is 80–180 ng/dl. The causes for an elevated and decreased serum triiodothyronine level are outlined in Table 29.

TABLE 29
Causes for Elevated and Decreased T₃ in the Circulation

Elevated T₃ RIA	Decreased T₃ RIA
Hyperthyroidism	Hypothyroidism
T₃ toxicosis	Drugs that interfere with peripheral conversion of T₄ to T₃
	Propylthiouracil (not tapazole)
"Factitious"	Glucocorticoids
hyperthyroidism	Iopanoic acid
with T₃	Amiadarone
Peripheral	Sick euthyroid syndrome
resistance	

13.2.4. Thyrotropin

The indications for and utility of the TSH assay are discussed in Chapter 2.

13.3. Tests to Assess the Pituitary–Thyroid Axis

The T_3 suppression test and TRH stimulation test both essentially evaluate the same phenomenon but in different ways. The T_3 suppression test evaluates the suppressibility of TSH (and, consequently, the radioactive iodine uptake by the thyroid gland) by exogenous administration of *levo*-triiodothyronine, whereas the TRH test evaluates the response of TSH to the exogenous administration of TRH, a response that is modified by the level of circulating thyroid hormones.

13.3.1. Suppression Test

This test is based on the principle that the exogenous administration of T_3 to normal subjects is associated with a prompt decrease in basal TSH level. The mechanisms that underlie the negative feedback effect of thyroid hormones are outlined in Chapter 2.

The test is performed by administering 25 μg of *levo*-triiodothyronine (Cytomel) three times a day orally for 7 days. The parameter compared is the 24-hr radioactive iodine uptake before and after the administration of L-triiodothyronine. In the normal individual, administration of exogenous T_3 is attended by a decline in the 24-hr radioactive iodine uptake by 50% or more compared to the pretest base line. This decrease reflects the suppression of the pituitary thyrotroph in response to exogenous T_3. Thus, the normal individual demonstrates suppressible thyroid function. Nonsuppressibility to exogenous T_3 administration is said to exist when the 24-hr radioactive iodine fails to decline (by 50% of the base line) following the drug. Nonsuppressible thyroid function is encountered in the following circumstances:

1. Graves' hyperthyroidism. Virtually all patients with untreated Graves' hyperthyroidism demonstrate nonsuppressibility for two reasons. First, the TSH is already maximally suppressed because of increased circulating thyroid hormones, and, second, the thyroid gland in this entity is driven by stimulators other than TSH.
2. Approximately 50% to 65% of patients with euthyroid Graves' disease may demonstrate nonsuppressible radioactive iodine uptake. The seeming paradox of nonsuppressibility despite normal levels of thyroid hormones may reflect a change in the thyroid hormone level compared to the patient's basal level—although the level is in the "normal" range, a slight increase is perceived by the thyrotroph as significant—or an alteration in the sensitivity of the hypothalamic–pituitary–thyroid axis resulting in decreased sensitivity of the thyrotroph to TRH.
3. Occasionally a patient with Hashimoto's thyroiditis may demonstrate nonsuppressibility.
4. Nonsuppressibility can be a localized phenomenon within a portion of the thyroid gland, as seen in patients with autonomous functioning ("hot") thyroid nodules.

The indications for performing the T_3 suppression test have considerably declined in the past decade because the widespread application of the TRH test. The only indication in which the T_3 suppression test has not been usurped by the TRH test is in the evaluation of autonomous ("hot") nodules (Table 30).

TABLE 30
The T_3 Suppression Test

	T_3 suppression test	Alternate test
Indications	To establish thyroid autonomy, i.e., Graves' hyperthyroidism, when the clinical and lab data are equivocal	TRH test
	To establish Gravesian ophthalmopathy as the cause of proptosis	Ultrasonography of the orbit is superior
	To delineate "responders" from "nonresponders" in patients on thiocarbamide therapy for Graves' hyperthyroidism	Thyroid-stimulating immunoglobulins
	In evaluating hyperfunctioning nodules	None
Disadvantages	Cost	$60.00 for TRH
	Cardiotoxic potential	test, which has no
	Time consuming	adverse effect
Diagnosis of nonsuppression	Graves' hyperthyroidism or euthyroid Graves' disease	Diagnosis of nonresponsive TSH to TRH is diverse
False positive	Almost none	

The T_3 suppression test should not be performed in patients who are clearly thyrotoxic or in those with underlying cardiac disease (in particular, angina or cardiac arrythmias).

13.3.2. The Thyrotropin-Releasing Hormone Test

The principle, interpretation, indications, and clinical utility of this test, which evaluates the TSH response to exogenous administration of TRH, are outlined in Chapter 2.

13.4. The *in Vivo* Isotopic Tests

The two most frequently employed *in vivo* isotopic tests are the radioactive iodine uptake study and the thyroid scan.

13.4.1. Radioactive Iodine Uptake

This test estimates the percentage of radioactivity in the thyroid 24 hr after the administration of radioactive iodine orally. Radioactive iodine uptake is a reflection of trapping, organification, and release. Radioactive iodine uptake by the thyroid gland is not a sensitive test to establish the diagnosis of hyper- or hypothyroidism, since the functional state of the thyroid gland is evaluated best by the measurement of hormone levels. This is especially so for hypothyroidism, since the lower limits of the normal 24-hr radioiodine uptake considerably overlap with the range encountered in hypothyroid patients.

TABLE 31
Hyperthyroidism and ^{131}I Uptake

Hyperthyroidism with ↑ 24-hr ^{131}I uptake
  Graves' hyperthyroidism
  Plummer's disease (toxic adenoma or toxic MNG)
  Molar thyrotoxicosis
  TSH secreting pituitary adenoma
Hyperthyroidism with normal uptake
  Grave's hyperthyroidism with rapid biological turnover
  Toxic adenoma
  Grave's hyperthyroidism associated with iodine contamination or treated with
    thiocarbamides
  Hashitoxicosis
Hyperthyroidism with a low uptake
  Subacute thyroiditis
  Silent thyroiditis (lymphocytic thyroiditis with spontaneously resolving hyperthyroidism)
  Factitious hyperthyroidism
  Jod–Basedow phenomenon
  Hyperthyroidism in ectopic tissue (struma ovarii)
  Functioning metastases of differentiated thyroid carcinoma

The test is performed simply by administering a tracer dose of radioactive iodine and following this by a repeat count over the gland 24 hr later. This count is expressed as the percentage of the original tracer dose administered.

The three common indications to perform a 24-hr radioactive iodine study are:

1. To assist in the etiologic diagnosis of hyperthyroidism. This is the single most important indication for obtaining the radioactive iodine uptake. In hyperthyroid patients without the Graves' stigmata, especially when the duration of disease has been short, the radioiodine uptake study considerably aids in the exclusion of the thyroidites that cause transient hyperthyroidism, an important therapeutic concern. Hyperthyroid patients with subacute and silent thyroiditis demonstrate low uptakes, whereas patients with hyperthyroidism secondary to Graves' disease demonstrate an elevated radioactive iodine uptake (Table 31).
2. To assist in the calculation of the therapeutic dose of ^{131}I for treatment of hyperthyroid Graves' disease. The dose of ^{131}I administered to treat such patients is directly proportional to the gland size and inversely proportional to the 24-hr radioactive iodine uptake, i.e., the lower the uptake, the higher the calculated dose.
3. In performing the T_3 suppression test. As indicated above, the parameter that is evaluated to define suppressibility to exogenous tri-iodothyronine is the 24-hr ^{131}I uptake before and after the oral administration of T_3 for 7 days. Suppressibility is defined as a decline in the post-T_3 radioactive iodine uptake by at least 50% compared to the base line.

13.4.2. The Thyroid Scan

The thyroid scan is an imaging method to visualize the thyroid. The most important indication to obtain a thyroid scan is in the evaluation of thyroid nodules. The utility of the thyroid scan is in the evaluation of thyroid nodules. The utility of the thyroid scan in evaluation of hyperfunctional and nonfunctional nodules is discussed in Chapter 17.

14

Thyroid Hyperfunction

14.1. Introduction

The terms hyperthyroidism and thyrotoxicosis are interchangeably used to denote increased production (or release) of thyroid hormones. In the next section of this chapter, the etiology and clinical features of hyperthyroidism in general are reviewed. In the following section Graves' disease is separately discussed. The final section of the chapter deals with hyperthyroidism secondary to the autonomously functioning thyroid nodule.

14.2. Hyperthyroidism

14.2.1. Etiology

There are several etiologic conditions that can result in increased production of thyroid hormones (Table 32). *Graves' hyperthyroidism* is the most frequent etiology, accounting for nearly 60–70% of hyperthyroidism, and is caused by autonomous hyperfunction of the entire thyroid gland. *Plummer's disease* is the development of hyperthyroidism in autonomously functioning single or in multiple thyroid nodules.

In contrast to the hyperthyroidism of Graves' and Plummer's diseases, which represent sustained hypersecretion, the following four conditions are characterized by transient hyperthyroidism: subacute thyroiditis, silent thyroiditis, hashitoxicosis, and Jod–Basedow phenomenon. *Subacute thyroiditis* is an inflammatory condition of the thyroid believed to be of viral etiology. The clinical hallmark here is pain. *Silent (painless) thyroiditis,* a condition associated with pregnancy and the puerperium, is believed to be autoimmune in nature but distinctly different from Hashimoto's lymphocytic thyroiditis. *Hashitoxicosis* represents a uniquely schizoid instance in which both Hashimoto's and Graves'

TABLE 32
Etiology of Hyperthyroidism

Condition	Characteristics	Diagnostic feature
Graves' disease	Diffuse thyromegaly, chronic symptoms, Graves' stigmata may be present	Elevated radioactive iodine uptake
Plummer's disease	Single or multiple nodules	Autonomous function of nodules
Subacute thyroiditis	Pain, mild to modest thyromegaly, symptoms mild	Low radioactive iodine uptake
Silent thyroiditis	Related to pregnancy; painless thyromegaly	Low radioactive iodine uptake
Hashitoxicosis	Mild symptoms, brief duration; rapid progression to hypothyroidism	Normal radioactive iodine uptake; strong antimicrosomal antibodies
Jod–Basedow (iodine induced)	Nodule(s) present; history of exposure to iodine; transient hyperthyroidism	Low radioactive iodine uptake
Thyrotoxicosis factitia	No thyroid enlargement	Low radioactive iodine uptake
Molar thyrotoxicosis	Mild hyperthyroidism; pregnancy evident	Markedly elevated HCG
Thyrotroph adenoma	Often associated with other hypersecretory states	Abnormal CT of sella; elevated TSH

diseases cohabit the same gland with eventual dominance of the Hashimoto's thyroiditis.

The term *Jod–Basedow phenomenon* refers to iodine-induced hyperthyroidism, historically occurring when iodine is introduced in areas of endemic iodine deficiency. In areas where iodine is plentiful, the phenomenon is observed following the administration of iodinated contrast material to patients with nodular disease of the thyroid. The importance of grouping these four entities together is to underscore two characteristics shared by all these entities: the self-limited, transient nature of hyperthyroidism and the unelevated radioactive iodine uptakes by the thyroid gland.

Factitious hyperthyroidism (thyrotoxicosis factitia) is a not infrequent cause of hyperthyroidism and can be secondary to the abuse of thyroxine or triiodothyronine. The condition should be suspected in the absence of thyromegaly coupled with extremely low radioactive iodine uptakes.

Rare causes of hyperthyroidism need to be mentioned only for the sake of completion. Functional metastases to the bones from a well-differentiated thyroid carcinoma should become rare with the application of justifiably aggressive maneuvers to treat the primary carcinoma. Rarely, hyperthyroidism can result from localized thyroid carcinoma of both differentiated and undifferentiated varieties. *Molar thyrotoxicosis* is a result of thyroid stimulation by molar thyrotropin, a variety of placental TSH secreted in large quantities by hydatidiform moles (molar pregnancy) or choriocarcinoma. Asian and Oriental women are particularly at high risk for the development of molar pregnancy and molar hyperthyroidism. *Struma ovarii* also represents a rare cause of hyperthyroidism, resulting from hyperfunctioning ectopic thyroid tissue in an ovary that usually harbors a solid tumor (teratoma). In this instance it is not the hormone that is being ectopically produced; rather, it is ectopic thyroid tissue that synthesizes excessive quantities of the hormone. Finally, there is the rare pituitary tumor that secretes TSH and causes secondary hyperthyroidism; TSH-induced hyperthyroidism is usually seen in conjunction with other hypersecretory states such as acromegaly. Patients with Albrights' syndrome (polyostotic fibrous dysplasia) are also prone to develop such a phenomenon.

From the foregoing discussion, it may appear that the etiologic spectrum of hyperthyroidism is extensive. In clinical practice, the etiology of hyperthyroidism can be easily arrived at by five basic observations (Table 32).

1. Evidence for Graves' stigmata (infiltrative ophthalmopathy or infiltrative dermopathy).
2. Presence or absence of thyromegaly (lack of thyromegaly suggests factitious hyperthyroidism; rarely, Graves' hyperthyroidism can occur in the absence of thyromegaly, especially in older individuals).
3. Diffuse thyromegaly versus nodular thyromegaly (diffuse thyromegaly is seen in hyperthyroidism associated with Graves' disease, whereas nodular thyromegaly is encountered in Plummer's disease).
4. Chronicity of symptoms and degree of hyperthyroidism.
5. The radioactive iodine uptake study (Table 31 in Chapter 13).

14.2.2. Clinical Features

Regardless of etiology, the clinical consequences of hyperthyroidism are the same. Chronic and sustained hypersecretion of thyroid hormones results in a multisystem disorder with protean manifestations. When the onset of hyperthyroidism is recent and the disease mild, the physical findings may not be impressive. But in chronic hyperthyroidism, the clinical picture is striking enough to permit instant recognition. However, all findings may not be present in all patients.

14.2.2.1. Symptoms

Several symptoms of hyperthyroidism are shared by other diseases as well. Table 33 outlines the diversity of symptoms encountered in hyperthyroidism as well as the differential diagnosis of each symptom.

TABLE 33
Symptoms of Hyperthyroidism

Symptom	Differential diagnosis
Weight loss despite hyperphagia	Diabetes mellitus, malabsorption
Heat intolerance	Any hypermetabolic state (Luft's syndrome, pheo, carcinoid, etc.)
Increased diaphoresis	Chronic infections (TB) acromegaly, hypermetabolic states, congestive failure
Increased nervousness	Anxiety neurosis, islet cell tumor, pheochromocytoma
Hair loss	Hypothyroidism
Weakness of shoulders or thighs ("giving out after using")	Any proximal myopathy
Palpitations	Anxiety, pheochromocytoma, cardiac arrhythmias
Dyspnea on exertion	Cardiac failure
Increased bowel movements or diarrhea	GI disturbance
Increased generalized pigmentation	Addison's disease (especially when combined with weight loss, weakness, and diarrhea)
Swelling in the neck	Thyromegaly from any cause
Oligomenorrhea or amenorrhea	Gynecological disorder

14.2.2.2. Signs

The skin of hyperthyroid patients is soft, smooth (velvety), warm (vaso-dilated), and moist. Generalized hyperpigmentation may be evident. When Graves' disease underlies the etiology, vitiligo may be seen (4–6%), as may infiltrative dermopathy in the pretibial region (pretibial myxedema). The hair is often thin and brittle with alopecia, usually localized but occasionally resulting in severe hair hair loss and even baldness. The nails reveal onycholysis (Plummer's nails). The nail is lifted from the nailbed as a result of subungual accumulation of dirt, resulting in the replacement of the normal convex dirt line by an irregular concave, jagged line.

The cardiovascular signs of hyperthyroidism are extremely important and include several features. Tachycardia and an increase in the sleeping pulse rate are quite common in hyperthyroid patients. With progressive disease, there is the development of high-output failure characterized by cardiomegaly and a wide pulse pressure. It should be remembered that an S_3 or S_4 and a wide variety of functional murmurs, both systolic and diastolic, may be encountered in hyperthyroid patients even in the absence of cardiac failure. Among these murmurs, the Lerman–Means murmur is particularly prevalent and consists of an ejection systolic murmur with a harsh scratching quality heard at the pulmonic area. The presence of a mitral click indicating mitral valve prolapse points to Graves' disease as the underlying etiology because there is a striking prevalence of "floppy" mitral valve in patients with Graves' hyperthyroidism. Although supraventricular arrhythmias (atrial fibrillation or flutter) are the most common arrhythmias seen in hyperthyroidism, rarely conduction disturbances (first-degree A–V block) may highlight the course. Finally, coronary heart disease (angina pectoris or myocardial infarction) can be associated with or even caused by hyperthyroid heart disease.

The gastrointestinal manifestations of hyperthyroidism include hyperdefecation or diarrhea when the disease is severe. Vague abdominal pain is not uncommon. The GI manifestations may predominate in elderly patients with hyperthyroidism. The presentation of these older patients with weight loss, weakness, vague abdominal pain, anorexia, and a paucity of other thyrotoxic symptoms often leads to a search for GI neoplasm ("masked" hyperthyroidism, which in reality is "missed" hyperthyroidism, since the diagnosis should be considered in anyone with weight loss). Regarding hepatic involvement in hyperthyroidism, mild elevation of transaminases and alkaline phosphatase is frequent. Hepatomegaly and jaundice, when present, indicate severe hyperthyroidism. Hypoalbuminemia from rapid catabolism of albumin can be quite severe, giving rise to edema and occasionally even anassrca. The constellation of these features may result in mistaken diagnosis of primary liver disease.

The muscle involvement of hyperthyroidism is of five types: thyrotoxic myopathy, thyrotoxic periodic paralysis, bulbar myopathy, coexistent myasthenia gravis, and external ophthalmoplegia. Of these, thyrotoxic myopathy is the most prevalent form of muscle disease and is characterized by involvement of the proximal muscles—shoulder and pelvic girdle muscles. Inability to keep the arms raised above the shoulders and difficulty in sustaining the raised straight leg are characteristic. The myopathy can become so severe that practically any group of voluntary muscles may be involved, rendering the patient considerably disabled, even bedridden. Distal muscle involvement can be rarely encountered.

Thyrotoxic period paralysis resembles the familial periodic type in the sudden onset of profound muscle weakness. The patient often falls to the floor and cannot arise. This entity is more prevalent in Oriental and perhaps Hispanic patients with hyperthyroid Graves' disease and is more common in males. The episodes tend to occur after a meal, and the serum potassium during such episodes may be normal, high, or low. The duration of these episodes can be quite variable, lasting from minutes to several hours. The third form of myopathy, bulbar myopathy, is a potentially fatal one, affecting older patients with severe thyrotoxic myopathy. In this variety, the involuntary muscles controlling deglutition and respiration are involved. Dysphagia and nasal regurgitation of fluids are harbingers of the development of the more serious respiratory failure. These were once considered uniformly fatal, but the use of heavy-dose propranolol has lowered mortality. The fourth muscle disease, myasthenia gravis, is associated with Graves' hyperthyroidism at an incidence of 2–4%. The occurrence of ptosis, dysphonia, or dysphagia in a patient with Graves' hyperthyroidism should involve the suspicion of concomitant myasthenia. Finally, external ophthalmoplegia is involvement of eye muscles and is discussed under Graves' hyperthyroidism (Section 14.3). It should be noted that severe muscle disease of any variety is usually seen in conjunction with Graves' hyperthyroidism, since this entity represents the prototype for chronic and sustained hypersecretion.

The neurological manifestations of hyperthyroidism include tremors, hyperactive DTRs, and, rarely in children, chorea and other involuntary extrapyramidal movements.

The psychiatric changes in hyperthyroidism range from anxiety or nervousness to paranoid ideation, psychosis, and even suicidal tendencies. The psychiatric manifestations are intensified during thyroid crisis.

The skeletal changes of hyperthyroidism occur as a consequence of increased bone turnover. Mild hypercalcemia occurs in one-fourth of hyperthyroid patients. Osteoporosis and fractures occur in elderly females with chronic hyperthyrodism.

There are two situations of hyperthyroidism that require special recognition. Since detection is of paramount importance, the first is apathetic hyperthyroidism, a very atypical hyperthyroid state and hence easy to miss; the second is thyroid storm, which is potentially fatal.

Apathetic hyperthyroidism is characterized by the triad of apathy ("flat affect"), paucity of typical hyperthyroid symptoms ("oligosymptomatic"), and biochemical hyperthyroidism occurring in an elderly patient. The following features are often present in varying combinations:

1. The patient is usually elderly and withdrawn, with chronic "depression."
2. Anorexia (rather than hyperphagia) and weight loss are consistent symptoms.
3. GI disturbances—vague abdominal pain and constipation—are frequent.
4. Cardiac disease is usually present and is often mistakenly ascribed to atherosclerotic heart disease.
5. Varying degrees of myopathy are evident, in extreme cases rendering the patient bedridden.
6. Thyromegaly is minimal and may even be absent.
7. Ptosis (rather than the stare) may complicate the picture, giving a myxedematous look.

Apathetic hyperthyroidism is entirely curable with extraordinarily gratifying results. Unfortunately, the diagnosis is often missed since the psychiatric, behavioral, cardiac, and musculoskeletal manifestations of this disease are incorrectly attributed to senility or dementia.

Thyroid storm, on the other hand, is difficult to miss if the condition is kept in mind. The triad to lead to suspicion of thyroid storm consists of an actually ill hyperthyroid patient with tachycardia (>120) and a fever ($>100°F$). Thyroid storm is regarded as a breakdown in the body's tolerance to chronic excess of thyroidal hormones. Therefore, features of chronic hyperthyroidism are generally evident. Thyroid storm is often ushered in with GI symptoms such as nausea, vomiting, anorexia, abdominal pain, and diarrhea. The classic appearance of the desperately ill patient, often agitated, tremulous, and even delirious with fever, dehydration, and tachycardia is unmistakable. Cardiac tachyarrhythmias or even congestive failure can and often do complicate the picture.

Thyroid crisis is often precipitated by an infection. Less frequent causes for exacerbation include surgery, ^{131}I therapy, withdrawal of iodine or thionamide therapy, and thyroid hormone overdose.

The treatment of thyroid storm is outlined in Table 34.

From the foregoing description, it should be apparent that hyperthyroidism is a multisystem disorder with the brunt of systemic effects falling on the cardiac and muscular systems. The severity of the systemic effects of hyperthyroidism are directly related to the chronicity of the disease, and the prototype for sustained, chronic hypersecretion of thyroidal hormones is Graves' disease, which is reviewed in the following section.

14.3. Graves' Disease

Graves' disease is an autoimmune disease characterized by a triumvirite consisting of thyroid dysfunction, infiltrative ophthalmopathy, and infiltrative dermopathy. These three components may be temporally separated in terms of their occurrence in a given patient, and the expression may not even be complete in several instances. The thyroid dysfunction takes the form of hyperthyroidism (hyperthyroid Graves' disease) but less commonly can be expressed as diffuse thyromegaly in a euthyroid person (euthyroid Graves' disease). The gravesian ophthalmopathy can occur concurrently with the hyperthyroid state, may precede it, or may occur in an absolutely euthyroid person (euthyroid Graves' disease). Infiltrative dermopathy, the rarest gravesian manifestation, can occur concurrently with the hyperthyroid state but more commonly occurs years after treatment for hyperthyroidism. Widely diverse as these three manifestations are, the single common link present in most, if not all, gravesian patients is nonsuppressible thyroid function.

TABLE 34
Treatment of Thyroid Storm

General supportive measures
    Hydration
    Reduction of fever (ice blankets, antipyretics)
    Oxygen
    Treatment of precipitating factor(s)
Specific measures
    Stable iodine (to block hormone release)
    Thionamide (to block hormone synthesis)
    Propranolol (to block peripheral effects)
    Dexamethasone (to block T_4 to T_3 conversion)

14.3.1. Etiology

Although Graves' disease is categorized as an autoimmune disorder, the exact mechanisms that underlie the pathophysiology remain enigmatic. The "antigen," in this instance, is the TSH receptor on the membrane of the thyroid follicle cell. The autoantibodies are collectively referred to as "thyroid-stimulating immunoglobulins (TSI)," a generic term to indicate a variety of γ-globulins that circulate in the blood of patients with Graves' disease. These antibodies are unique in two ways. First, they represent one of the few known instances in which antibodies stimulate function (in contrast to most situations, where autoantibodies are destructive in nature), and second, these antibodies depose TSH from its role as the thyroid stimulator. Thus, thyroid regulation in Graves' disease is controlled by a group of IgG immunoglobulins that not only stimulate the gland but do so too well, resulting in hyperfunction. These thyroid-stimulating immunoglobulins are secreted by the B lymphocytes. The reason for these "humoral" antibodies to be secreted by the B lymphocytes may have to do with the T lymphocytes. It is believed that an underlying defect in cell-mediated immunity results in random appearance of a forbidden clone of helper T cells; this abnormal clone of T cells, located in abundance within the thyroid tissue, interacts with the normal thyroid cell membrane and initiates the production of TSI by the B lymphocyte. It is believed that the abnormal T lymphocyte becomes sensitized to the thyroid membrane containing the TSH receptor as a result of a defect in immune surveillance (Table 35).

The "gravesian diathesis" appears to be an inherited one. Such predisposition is supported by several lines of evidence: the strong familial aggregation of Graves' disease, the strong concordance of the disease in monozy-

---

TABLE 35
The Pathogenesis of Graves' Hyperthyroidism

Genetic predisposition (HLA type)
  + Defective cell-mediated immunity
      ↓
Dysfunction of specific suppressor T lymphocytes
      ↓
Survival of forbidden clone of helper T lymphocytes
      ↓
Interaction with thyroid cell membrane
      ↓
Stimulation of B lymphocytes
      ↓
Production of TSI
  LATS
  LATS-P
  TDA (TSH displacing)
  TAC (adenylate cyclase stimulating)

gotic twins, and the high prevalence of HLA-B8 tissue type in Caucasians with Graves' disease.

14.3.2. Clinical Features

The three aspects of Graves' disease are the hyperthyroidism, the ophthalmopathy, and the dermopathy.

14.3.2.1. Hyperthyroidism

The consortium of signs and symptoms resulting from hyperthyroidism is discussed in Section 14.2.2. The thyromegaly of Graves' hyperthyroidism is diffuse, often variably enlarged, can be asymmetric, and rarely can be absent. In children with Graves' hyperthyroidism, lymphadenopathy and splenomegaly may be present. In young males with Graves' hyperthyroidism, gynecomastia may be present. "Gravesian stigmata," i.e., ophthalmopathy or dermopathy, are evident in a third of patients.

14.3.2.2. Ophthalmopathy

In approximately 35% to 40% of patients with Graves' hyperthyroidism, some degree of infiltrative ophthalmopathy is usually evident clinically. As indicated above, ophthalmopathy may never develop in some, but in others it may antedate the occurrence of hyperthyroidism by months to years. Rarely, ophthalmopathy may be the one and only manifestation, with preservation of entirely normal thyroid function.

The abridged staging of opthalmopathy as recommended by the American Thyroid Association is outlined in Table 36 and can be remembered by the catchy mnemonic "NO SPECS."

From a clinical standpoint, distinction must be made between noninfiltrative and infiltrative eye changes. The stare, the lid retraction, and lid lag

TABLE 36
Staging of Gravesian Ophthalmopathy

Class	Description
0	No signs, no symptoms
1	Only signs (upper lid retraction, stare lid lag, proptosis >22 mm); no symptoms
2	Soft tissue involvement (above with symptoms: lachrymation, congestion)
3	Proptosis 22 mm
4	Extraocular muscle involvement
5	Corneal involvement
6	Sight loss: optic nerve involvement

are noninfiltrative eye signs and can be caused by any hyperthyroid state regardless of etiology. The infiltrative eye signs, i.e., proptosis, external ophthalmoplegia, and optic neuritis, are unique for Graves' disease and represent infiltration of the retrobulbar and peribulbar tissue by mucopolysaccharides and lymphocytes with intense fibrous tissue proliferation.

The degree of proptosis should be measured carefully by the Hertel's exophthalmometer to record progression. The upper limits for normal eyes are 20 mm for Caucasians and 21 mm for blacks. Proptosis greater than 25 mm is referred to as malignant exophthalmos because of its potential for keratitis and visual loss. Extraocular muscle weakness or even paralysis (external ophthalmoplegia) is a serious complication resulting in troublesome diplopia and difficulty in reading. The fundus should be examined carefully and the visual acuity carefully tested to detect optic nerve involvement. The four ophthalmic features that require medical intervention with steroid therapy are malignant exophthalmos, progressive ophthalmopathy, external ophthalmoplegia, and optic neuritis.

When the ophthalmopathy is unilateral and occurs in the euthyroid person, the distinction from orbital tumor is the most obvious and important one to make. This distinction can be made by the use of orbital ultrasonography or computerized tomography of the orbit. Patients with gravesian ophthalmopathy demonstrate changes in the lateral rectus muscle bilaterally even when the proptosis is unilateral. A CT of the orbits outlines unilateral tumors accurately.

14.3.2.3. Infiltrative Dermopathy

The third component of Graves' disease is the least frequently encountered one. The term "pretibial myxedema" is in a sense a misnomer and is obsolete. Although the changes are most frequently and consistently seen in the pretibial area, infiltrative dermopathy can occur anywhere. The change consists of thickening of the skin (and subcutaneous region) as a result of an infiltrative phenomenon. The violaceous pigmented, leathery skin with coarse hair and little pitting is classical. Less frequently, infiltrative dermopathy may resemble erythema nodosum. Rarely, the appearance may simulate venous stasis of legs with pitting edema and discoloration but only minimal thickening. Pain is notably absent in all forms of infiltrative dermopathy. Infiltrative dermopathy can, in its severe form, extend and progress relentlessly, causing ulceration, infection, and gross disfiguration.

14.3.3. Diagnostic Studies

The laboratory studies in patients with Graves' hyperthyroidism can be categorized into hormonal studies, isotopic studies, and nonendocrine routine tests.

14.3.3.1. Hormonal Studies

The diagnosis of hyperthyroidism can easily be established by measurement of circulating thyroxine (T_4) and the T_3 resin uptake (T_3RU). The calculated free thyroxine index (FTI) would be elevated. These two simple tests are the only ones needed in most cases. The indications to obtain circulating levels of T_3, TSH, free hormones, TSI, or to perform a TRH study or a T_3 suppression test are outlined below.

Measurement of the T_3 level in the serum is indicated only when T_3 toxicosis is suspected. These are patients presenting with the clinical picture of hyperthyroidism but with a normal T_4. In such instances, selective hypersecretion of T_3 should be excluded by measuring the serum levels of T_3. No diagnostic purpose would be served by measuring the serum level of triiodothyronine in hyperthyroid patients with a clearly elevated T_4, since the T_3 would be expected to be elevated as a consequence of the increased substrate, T_4. The three clinical situations with a proclivity for development of T_3 toxicosis are toxic nodules, recurrent hyperthyroidism following surgery or radioactive iodine, and hyperthyroidism occurring areas endemic for iodine deficiency.

There is no indication to measure the circulating TSH level in patients with Graves' hyperthyroidism since it would be suppressed. The difference in "suppressed" versus "low normal" ranges is not significant enough to permit diagnosis of Graves' hyperthyroidism on the basis of a basal TSH level.

The role of measurement of free T_4 (and free T_3) levels for establishing the diagnosis of hyperthyroidism is limited to situations in which a quantitative or qualitative abnormality of TBG clouds the interpretation of the T_4 and T_3RU.

The clinical indication to measure thyroid-stimulating immunoglobulin is when pregnancy is complicated by Graves' hyperthyroidism. These immunoglobulins can be transferred across the placenta to the fetus, resulting in stimulation of the fetal thyroid. Extremely high titers of TSI predispose the fetus to a higher risk of developing neonatal hyperthyroidism.

The TRH study is employed for diagnostic purposes when the circulating thyroid hormone levels are borderline but hyperthyroidism is suspected on clinical grounds. In such a setting, failure of TSH to rise following intravenous TRH is diagnostic of hyperthyroidism. The other causes for a blunted or absent TSH response are malnutrition, old age, chronic illness, anorexia nervosa, hypopituitarism, Cushing's acromegaly, and euthyroid Graves' disease.

The T_3 suppression test for the diagnosis of hyperthyroidism has been superseded by the TRH test (Section 3.3).

14.3.3.2. Isotopic Studies

The 24-hr radioactive iodine uptake is elevated in Graves' hyperthyroidism. Occasionally, the uptake may be "normal" because of an extremely rapid biological turnover of the isotope by the very hyperthyroid gland. In such an instance, an early uptake study (4- or 6-hr uptake) will demonstrate the elevated uptake.

The scintiscan in Graves' hyperthyroidism will demonstrate the diffuse enlargement with uniform uptake of radionuclide.

14.3.3.3. "Routine" Nonendocrine Tests

The abnormalities that may be present in the "routine" tests are outlined in Table 37.

14.3.4. Treatment

The options for the treatment of Graves' hyperthyroidism revolve around the trinity of radioactive iodine ($Na^{131}I$), antithyroid drug therapy (thionamides), and surgery (subtotal thyroidectomy). Each of these modalities has one major drawback: with radioactive iodine the chances for eventually developing hypothyroidism is extremely high; with thionamide therapy the chance of eventually enjoying a permanent remission is disappointingly low; and with subtotal thyroidectomy, the mortality (anesthetic death) and morbidity (damage to the recurrent laryngeal nerve or the parathyroids), no matter how low, constitute risks that are not acceptable when alternative therapies are available. If one accepts the inevitability of eventual hypothyroidism—and indeed some of it may reflect the natural history of Graves' disease regardless of the form of therapy employed—and if one also accepts the premise that detected hypothyroidism is an easier disease to treat than recurrent or unremitting hyperthyroidism, then radioactive iodine therapy emerges as the safest, surest, most effective, least costly, and indeed best form of treatment for Graves' hyperthyroidism. Yet, there are selected indications for which one form of therapy may be more suitable than the others. Hence, it is necessary to focus on each form of therapy.

TABLE 37
Nonendocrine Tests in Graves' Hyperthyroidism

Test	Abnormality
CBC	Anemia (normochromic, normocytic); neutropenia with relative lymphocytosis
Calcium	Mild hypercalcemia
Liver function	Elevated SGOT, SGPT; elevated alkaline phosphatase; hypoalbuminemia
Lipids	Low cholesterol, low triglycerides
Glucose	Abnormal GTT (glucose intolerance)
EKG	Sinus tachycardia
Chest X ray	Cardiomegaly; widened mediastinum in children (from thymic enlargement)

14.3.4.1. Thionamides

The mode of action, dose, indications, contraindications, adverse effects, and drawbacks of thionamide therapy are outlined in Table 38. The major advantage of thionamide therapy, no permanent damage to the thyroid, has to be weighed against its greatest drawback, an extremely disappointing rate of achieving permanent euthyroidism after a prolonged course of the drug. When patient compliance is assured, the efficacy of thionamides in restoration of euthyroidism has never been questioned. In fact, given the right dose, ranging from 300 to as much as 1500 mg a day of PTU, practically any patient can be rendered euthyroid with thionamides. The realistic factor that limits the usage of thionamides is that even after an 18-month course, the rate of relapse following discontinuation of PTU is extremely high, in some series approaching 70–80%. Thus, at best, no more than a third of patients placed on PTU respond gratifyingly with a long-term remission following a protracted course of the drug. Attempts at identifying these responders early in the course of therapy, e.g., 6 months after initiating thionamide therapy, have not been consistently successful. The use of the TRH test, the T_3 suppression test, the circulating level of TSI, and the HLA type have all been used for this purpose but without a consistently significant prognostic value.

Although thionamide therapy may fall short of expectations in "curing" Graves' hyperthyroidism, this form of therapy enjoys an unparalleled repu-

TABLE 38
Key Facts Regarding Thionamides

Generic names	Propylthiouracil (PTU) Methimazole
Mode of action	Block organification Block coupling Block peripheral conversion of T_4 to T_3 (only PTU) ? immunologic effect on T lymphocytes
Dose	Starting dose: PTU 100–150 mg t.i.d.; methimazole 30 to 45 mg a day (single dose)

Indications	Adjunctive
	  In preparation for surgery
	  In treatment of storm
	  After [131]I
	Definitive
	  During pregnancy
	  In children, adolescents

Contraindications	Past history of agranulocytosis to thionamide or sulfa drugs Severe liver disease
Adverse effects	Skin rash, itching Bone marrow depression (less than 0.5%) Hepatotoxicity (rare)
Drawbacks	Compliance Extremely low permanent remission rate

tation as adjunctive therapy for hyperthyroidism. The three situations that are noteworthy for the use of thionamides are in the preparation of the hyperthyroid patient for subtotal thyroidectomy, in the pregnant hyperthyroid patient, and in the treatment of moderate or severe hyperthyroidism while waiting for the ^{131}I therapy to take full effect.

14.3.4.2. [131]I Therapy

Radioiodine therapy (using ^{131}I) is an ablative form of therapy. Following an avid uptake by the hyperthyroid gland, the ^{131}I emits high-energy radiation with a long path length. As a result, the distally placed nucleus at the base of the thyroid follicle cell and its replicative and biosynthetic machinery are exposed to the irradiation effects of ^{131}I and are destroyed gradually.

The safety of ^{131}I therapy is a matter of record. It is noncarcinogenic (the incidence of thyroid cancer following ^{131}I is lower than that in patients treated with surgery or thionamides); ^{131}I therapy is nonleukemogenic (the incidence of leukemia is slightly higher in Graves' patients as a whole); ^{131}I therapy is nonmutagenic (the gonadal radiation to the ovaries following ^{131}I therapy for Graves' hyperthyroidism is approximately 1 rad, equivalent to that obtained with a barium enema or an excretory urogram). Finally, the effects of ^{131}I are nonsystemic (therefore, patients do not suffer the adverse effects of radiation sickness such as nausea, vomiting, hair loss, and skin changes).

As a result of such an impeccable safety record encompassing over 40 years of experience, radioiodine is becoming the safest, surest, and least expensive method for treating Graves' hyperthyroidism. Most patients are rendered euthyroid in 2 to 6 months following [131]I. The age limit for administering ^{131}I has gradually declined in the past decades. Since an increase in the incidence of thyroid nodules has been noted when ^{131}I is used in children and adolescents, many thyroidologists reserve this form of therapy for patients over 20 or 25 years of age. However, it should be point out that many reputable centers administer ^{131}I even to children with Graves' hyperthyroidism.

The absolute contraindication for the use of ^{131}I is pregnancy: [131]I crosses the placenta and will irradiate the fetal thyroid, which is capable of trapping iodine by the 12th week. The teratogenic effect to the developing embryo is also a concern. The relative contraindications for the use of ^{131}I are few. Very large glands (>100 g) are less likely to respond to [131]I. The coexistence of a thyroid nodule in a young person with Graves' hyperthyroidism is a situation in which the patient's interests are best served by surgery. And finally, the patient who is obsessed with the fear of ^{131}I despite assurance is probably best treated by other modalities. As indicated earlier, young age is not considered to be an absolute contraindication by many.

Radioactive iodine is administered orally in a single sitting. The immediate adverse effects are practically none. Thyroiditis and precipitation of thyroid storm are only seen when very large doses of ^{131}I are given to very toxic patients on the verge of decompensation. The rare adverse effect, obviously, is the development of permanent hypothyroidism. It has become apparent over the years that permanent hypothyroidism following ^{131}I is inevitable. Reduction of the dose is attended with a lower cure rate and a higher recurrence rate. Although various centers provide different figures, the experience at Cook County Hospital, encompassing nearly 1000 patients, is as follows: the incidence of permanent hypothyroidism following ^{131}I is 30% in the first year, 50% by the fifth year, and nearly 70% by the tenth year. The incidence is probably universal by the 20th year. Thus, the acceptance of an easily treatable disease as a "trade-off" seems justifiable.

14.3.4.3. Subtotal Thyroidectomy

The safety of ^{131}I, even in younger patients, has resulted in a decline in recommending subtotal thyroidectomy for the treatment of Graves' hyperthyroidism. The indications for considering subtotal thyroidectomy are the following:

1. In children and adolescents who are "PTU failures" and in whom the use of ^{131}I is considered unsafe by patient, parent, or physician.
2. In the young hyperthyroid patient with a coexistent solitary thyroid nodule.
3. In the hyperthyroid patient with extremely large glands (>100 g), especially those causing pressure symptoms.

The patient who undergoes subtotal thyroidectomy for Graves' hyperthyroidism should be meticulously prepared for such surgery. Absolute rendition of euthyroidism, both clinically and biochemically, with the use of thionamides is a prerequisite. A week prior to surgery the patient should be "Lugolized," to decrease the vascularity and "firm up" the gland.

The immediate risks relate to anesthesia, bleeding, infection, and damage to the recurrent laryngeal nerve or the parathyroid glands. Some of these are preventable, but some, such as anesthetic complications, are not. The late complications relate to the development of hypothyroidism and recurrence of hyperthyroidism. Although the incidence of permanent hypothyroidism in the early years after surgery is far lower than after ^{131}I, the gap narrows significantly in the later years. The incidence of recurrent hyperthyroidism following successful surgery is approximately 13%, whereas the rate of recurrence following successful ablation with ^{131}I is negligible.

Thus, for all the above reasons, surgery is being recommended less frequently for the treatment of Graves' hyperthyroidism. But the same cannot be said for its role in treatment of Plummer's disease, which is discussed in the next section.

14.4. Plummer's Disease

Plummer's disease refers to the development of hyperthyroidism in an autonomously functioning solitary nodule. Less commonly, a similar phenomenon can occur in a multinodular goiter.

Autonomously functioning thyroid nodules (AFTN) probably account for fewer than 10% of all thyroid nodules. The appearance of the AFTN is classic on a radionuclide scan (Figure 10). The palpable nodule characteristically concentrates increased amounts of isotope, while the paranodular tissue demonstrates little or no isotopic concentration. The AFTN also characteristically demonstrates nondependence on TSH for growth and function. The "autonomously" functioning nodule does not suppress in response to oral administration of T_3 (Figure 11) and does not intensify in response to injections of bovine TSH (Figure 12), whereas the dormant, suppressed paranodular tissue "lights up" in response to TSH administration (Figure 12).

The natural history of the AFTN is highly variable. Some remain as such for years showing no change, some regress and become "less autonomous," and some begin to produce excess amounts of hormones. It is the last category that evolves into Plummer's disease. The incidence of the development of hyperthyroidism is much more common (18%) than previously supposed (5%). Two risk factors that merit mention are the age of the patient and the size of the nodule. The incidence of hyperthyroidism in patients over 60 harboring AFTN is two- to threefold greater than that in younger age groups. Similarly, toxicity tends to occur much more commonly in nodules larger than 3 cm.

The differences between Graves' disease and Plummer's disease are outlined in Table 39. Clinically, these patients are older, the palpatory findings reveal a solitary nodule, the cardiovascular effects of hyperthyroidism are severe, and infiltrative ophthalmopathy is not part of the disease. Biochemically, T_3 toxicosis is particularly prevalent, underscoring the need to obtain the T_3 level in the serum when screening for hyperthyroidism. Isotopic studies reveal, at best, only normal or minimally elevated ^{131}I uptake.

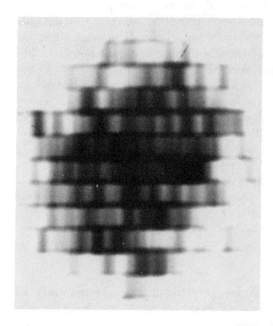

FIGURE 10. Patient with 3-cm nodule palpable on the left lobe of the thyroid gland. Thyroid scan demonstrates isotopic concentration limited to the palpable nodule with no visualization of paranodular tissue.

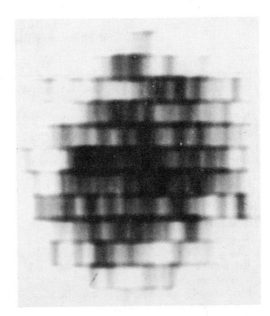

FIGURE 11. The autonomously functioning thyroid nodule fails to suppress in response to exogenous administration of triiodothyronine.

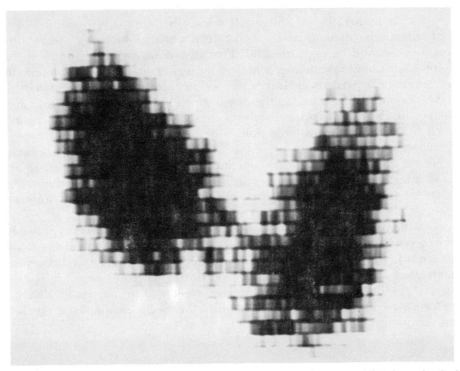

FIGURE 12. Administration of exogenous TSH "lights up" the paranodular tissue that had been suppressed by the AFTN.

TABLE 39
Graves' and Plummer's Diseases: A Comparison

Feature	Graves'	Plummer's
Age	Any age, predominantly below 50	Over 50
Thyroid gland	Diffusely enlarged	Nodule, usually single
Eyes	Infiltrative ophthalmopathy often present	Infiltrative ophthalmopathy never seen
Cardiovascular complication	May be present	Very often evident
T_3 toxicosis	Rare	Very frequent
Jod–Basedow	Rare	Common
24-hr RAIU	Elevated	Often normal
Treatment		
Response to ^{131}I	Usually excellent	Less responsive
Dose	5–12 mCi	Larger doses (15–25 mCi)
Release of preformed hormone	Negligible	Significant
Incidence of permanent hypothyroidism	30 to 100%	Low, since dormant paranodular tissue does not trap ^{131}I

The best therapy for Plummer's disease is rather controversial. When ^{131}I therapy is contemplated for the treatment of Plummer's disease, the following should be kept in mind. First, the doses required to ablate the hyperfunctioning nodule are considerably higher than those employed for treatment of hyperthyroid Graves' disease because of their relatively low uptake. Second, the response to therapy is much less gratifying, resulting in a higher incidence of treatment failures compared to Graves' disease treated with ^{131}I. Third, when a large dose is delivered to a small mass of hyperfunctioning tissue, there is the possibility of release of preformed hormone from the nodule. This, in an older individual, can precipitate cardiac arrhythmias, angina, or even a myocardial infarction. Fourth, the incidence of past ^{131}I hypothyroidism is much lower in this disease, since the dormant paranodular tissue fails to pick up isotope.

In the younger patient (<40) with Plummer's disease, surgery is probably the choice of therapy, since large doses of ^{131}I are required, and the possibility of requiring retreatment is real. In the older patient, the choice between a high dose of ^{131}I and surgery is an individual one, and there are strong supporters for either modality. As for the problem of "prophylactic" ablation of a euthyroid AFTN in a high-risk patient, there is no unanimity of opinion on the matter.

15

Thyroid Hypofunction

15.1. Introduction

Hypothyroidism is a common disorder. The incidence of subclinical hypothyroidism in the general population, derived from population surveys, ranges from 2% to 9%.

15.2. Etiology

Hypothyroidism is usually classified as primary, secondary, and tertiary hypothyroidism based on the level at which the problem originates. The fourth, and recent, addition to this conventional classification is hypothyroidism resulting from complete peripheral resistance (target organ insensitivity) to thyroidal hormones.

Primary hypothyroidism represents the most common variety of hypothyroidism and is caused by intrinsic thyroid disease. The prototype diseases representing this group are the spontaneous hypothyroidism of Hashimoto's thyroiditis (Section 16.5) and postablative hypothyroidism following radioactive iodine or surgery for Graves' hyperthyroidism.

Secondary hypothyroidism (pituitary hypothyroidism, thyroprivic hypothyroidism) is a consequence of TSH deficiency, the single most important cause of which is tumor of the pituitary gland. In this form of hypothyroidism, the thyroid gland stops functioning because of loss of its trophic stimulus from the pituitary.

Tertiary hypothyroidism is caused by lack of the hypothalamic peptide thyrotropin-releasing hormone (TRH). This may be congenital or may result from a suprasellar tumor such as craniopharyngioma.

The rare syndrome of complete resistance of peripheral tissues to thyroidal hormone occurs from an inability of T_4 and T_3 to bind to their respective nuclear receptors in the target cells or from a lack of these receptors.

TABLE 40
Etiology of Hypothyroidism

Primary hypothyroidism	Secondary hypothyroidism	Tertiary	Peripheral resistance
Hashimoto's disease	Tumors of the pituitary	Congenital lack of TRH	Lack of nuclear receptor
Postablative therapy for Graves' hyperthyroidism	Seehan's	Suprasellar tumors (craniopharyngioma, etc.)	Failure of T_4, T_3 to bind to receptors
Postablative Rx for thyroid cancer	Nontumorous isolated TSH deficiency		?Postreceptor defects
Lingual thyroid	Apoplexy		
Congenital athyrotic cretinism	After surgery or radiation to the pituitary		
Riedel's thyroiditis			
"Burnt out" Graves'			
Goitrogenic drugs			
Congenital dyshormonogenesis			
Chronic endemic iodine deficiency			
Infiltrative diseases of the thyroid			

The common and not so common causes of hypothyroidism are outlined in Table 40.

15.3. Clinical Features

Many symptoms of hypothyroidism are vague, notoriously nonspecific, and can be encountered in *euthyroid* individuals with a spectrum of disorders such as anemia, depression, and plain obesity (Table 41). The early stage of the disease is characterized by a plethora of symptoms in the absence of any objective physical findings. Therefore, it is essential to consider screening for hypothyroidism in patients with any of the symptoms listed in Table 41. Since hypothyroidism occurs much more frequently in females, the tendency to minimize the importance of these symptoms is to be deplored.

The obviousness of the physical findings of hypothyroidism is directly related to the duration and severity of the hypothyroid state (Table 42). These findings can be subtle enough to be missed by the untrained eye or can be striking enough to permit instant recognition of myxedema. The term myx-

TABLE 41
Symptoms of Hypothyroidism

Tiredness	Increased somnolence
Lack of energy	Muscle weakness
"Bloated" feeling	Constipation
Weight gain	Cold intolerance
Headaches	Chest discomfort
Muscle cramps	Dry skin
Decreased libido	Hair loss
Psychiatric changes (depression)	

edema is indicative of severe chronic, untreated hypothyroidism characterized by accumulation of mucoproteinaceous material in various body spaces, particularly in the subcutaneous tissue, resulting in edema.

The early signs of hypothyroidism are reflected in the skin, which is characteristically dry, cold (vasoconstricted), and often scaly. The combination of hypothyroid symptoms and the skin changes is the most frequent presentation that is encountered. As the hypothyroidism progresses, the severity of symptoms increases, and other changes become obvious. The dry skin continues to become drier, thick, and coarse, and changes in the hair become evident. These consist of changes in the texture, resulting in coarse brittle hair that falls off easily on brushing. The alopecia is usually localized but rarely can become severe and more generalized. Loss of hair in the outer third of eyebrows can be striking in some patients. Varying degrees of periorbital puffiness is usually present. At this stage most patients demonstrate mild sinus bradycardia and a clear delay in the relaxation phase of the deep tendon reflexes (DTR), particularly impressive over the Achilles tendon. Thus,

TABLE 42
Signs of Hypothyroidism

Mild hypothyroidism
Mostly symptoms
Dry skin
Moderate hypothyroidism
Dry, scaly, cold skin
Sinus bradycardia
Delay in the relaxation phase of DTR
Periorbital puffiness
Hair loss
Severe hypothyroidism
All of the above
Multisystem involvement

the four important changes of hypothyroidism are to be found in the skin, hair, pulse rate, and DTR. The presence of thyromegaly in the hypothyroid patient strongly indicates primary thyroid disease as the etiology, but an absence of such enlargement is consistent with both primary and pituitary disease.

Progressive severe hypothyroidism gradually evolves into myxedema. The changes in the skin are accentuated by desquamation and extreme dryness. A characteristic lemon-yellow tinge is imparted to the skin as a result of hypercarotenemia. The puffy face, the coarse brittle hair, the hoarse, low-pitched voice, and the inappropriate affect ("myxedema madness") are unmistakable. Dependent edema and accumulation of protein-rich transudates in the pleural, pericardial, and even the peritoneal cavity can result in mistaken diagnoses of pleuropulmonary, cardiac, or hepatic disorders. Myxedematous patients are at high risk for developing myxedema coma, a lethal complication.

Severe hypothyroidism affects practically every organ system. The effects of chronic hypothyroidism on the cardiovascular, respiratory, gastrointestinal, neuromuscular, reproductive, and hematopoietic systems highlight the importance of thyroid hormones in the normal functioning of these organ systems.

15.3.1. Cardiovascular

The three facets of hypothyroid heart disease are cardiomyopathy, pericardial effusion, and coronary atherosclerosis. The cardiac muscle dysfunction in hypothyroidism is characterized by abnormal hemodynamic parameters such as a decrease in cardiac output, stroke volume, and left ventricular ejection fraction. It is important to recognize that even asymptomatic patients with subclinical hypothyroidism may demonstrate abnormal myocardial contractile function. With protracted hypothyroidism, congestive failure may develop. Hypothyroidism should be suspected as the cause of congestive cardiac failure when the edema is disproportional to dyspnea and pulmonary congestion, when there is lack of significant tachycardia, and in the presence of exquisite sensitivity to digintoxication. The characteristic electrocardiographic changes include short-amplitude QRS complexes, sinus bradycardia, nonspecific ST,T changes, and intraventricular conduction defects. The addition of even small doses of *levo*-thyroxine results in a salubrious diuretic response. The mild hypertension observed in hypothyroid persons does not require specific treatment.

Although pericardial effusion occurs more commonly in primary hypothyroidism, more frequently in severe disease, and seldom results in hemodynamic compromise, these effusions have been described in patients with pituitary hypothyroidism or mild disease and can rarely result in cardiac tamponade. The pericardial effusion characteristically demonstrates slow resolution after initiation of *levo*-thyroxine therapy.

The primary hypothyroid state strongly favors the development of coronary atherosclerosis as a consequence of the increased cholesterol and triglyceride level as well as the accumulation of mucopolysaccharides in the intima of small blood vessels. The incidence of *symptomatic* coronary heart disease is low in relation to the high prevalence of coronary atherosclerosis in autopsy studies and is probably a reflection of the decreased myocardial oxygen consumption seen in this disease. Unfortunately, when myocardial oxygen consumption is raised with *levo*-thyroxine therapy, the symptoms appear, leading to angina or even acute myocardial infarction.

15.3.2. Respiratory

The most important effect of hypothyroidism is on the respiratory center, which is rendered relatively sluggish to hypoxia and hypercarbia. This sluggishness, in its extreme form, is exemplified in myxedema coma, where CO_2 retention as a result of respiratory hypoventilation dominates the picture. This central effect is aggravated by the decreased "bellows action" of the thorax in myxedematous patients.

15.3.3. Gastrointestinal

Severe hypothyroidism affects intestinal motility, resulting in paralytic ileus and even intestinal obstruction. Myxedema should be recognized as a rare cause of adynamic ileus, since surgical intervention will prove catastrophic for these patients. Rarely, myxedema can result in malabsorption syndrome. Ascites is also a rare manifestation of myxedema and is almost always seen in *primary* myxedema.

15.3.4. Neuromuscular

The two common neurological features of hypothyroidism are abnormal stretch reflexes and entrapment neuropathies; less commonly, a cerebellar syndrome and myxedema coma can complicate the picture of hypothyroidism.

The characteristic neurological sign of hypothyroidism is the "pseudo myotonic" reflex, i.e., the delayed relaxation phase. This finding, although quite frequently encountered in hypothyroidism, is not unique for this disease. Diverse disease states such as diabetic neuropathy, hypoalbuminemia, and pernicious anemia may be associated with a delay in the relaxation of DTRs. Carpal tunnel syndrome and entrapment neuropathies occur in approximately a third of hypothyroid patients.

The cerebellar syndrome associated with myxedema is characterized by ataxia and other cerebellar signs, mimicking a cerebellar tumor. The condition responds favorably to *levo*-thyroxine therapy. Myxedema coma is the penultimate manifestation of chronic untreated hypothyroidism. Obtundation, hypoventilation, hypothermia, and hypotension dominate the clinical picture. Myxedema coma is often precipitated by infection or the use of sedatives. Even with aggressive therapy, myxedema coma carries an extremely high mortality rate.

The muscle disease of hypothyroidism is of two forms: a biochemical syndrome and a clinical syndrome. The biochemical syndrome is extremely common in hypothyroid patients and consists of elevated muscle enzymes (CPK, aldolase) in the absence of any myopathic symptoms or signs. The clinical syndrome of hypothyroid myopathy is particularly common in children and young adults and is characterized by the bizarre combination of subjective and objective weakness in muscles that appear hypertrophied (Hoffmann's syndrome). Cramps, stiffness, and weakness dominate the symptomatology of patients with the Hoffmann's type of hypothyroid myopathy. Both the biochemical and clinical forms of hypothyroid myopathy respond excellently to *levo*-thyroxine therapy.

15.3.5. Reproductive System

Oligomenorrhea and anovulation in females and impotence in males can be secondary to hypothyroidism. Menorrhagia is the most frequent menstrual abnormality seen in hypothyroid women. A rare manifestation of hypothyroidism in prepubertal girls is the syndrome of precocious puberty. This syndrome is characterized by the constellation of primary hypothyroidism, breast enlargement, galactorrhea, hypertrophy of labia minora, and occasionally menstruation. The causative mechanism of this syndrome, somehow related to prolactin excess, is still unclear. The institution of therapy with *levo*-thyroxine results in gradual amelioration of all features.

15.3.6. Hematopoietic

Anemia is an extremely common finding in hypothyroidism. Microcytic anemia is often secondary to menorrhagia, and normocytic normochromic anemia results from poor erythropoiesis. The association between pernicious anemia and autoimmune thyroiditis is a frequent one; therefore, the association of macrocytic indices should occasion the screening for pernicious anemia with B_{12} levels. In patients with myxedema, intestinal malabsorption of iron, folic acid, and B_{12} further complicates the hematopoietic picture.

Table 43 illustrates the protean manifestations of chronic untreated hypothyroidism.

In addition to the well-recognized multisystem involvement of chronic hypothyroidism, there are three important metabolic alterations associated with this disorder.

1. The tendency to develop fasting hypoglycemia is a reflection of impaired gluconeogenesis and glycogenolysis.
2. The hyponatremia and hypotonicity of plasma with a less than maximally dilute urine can mimic the syndrome of inappropriate ADH secretion.

TABLE 43
The Multisystem Involvement of Hypothyroidism

System	Manifestation
General constitutional	Fatigue, lethargy, memory lapses, headaches, muscle aches, cold intolerance, depression, exercise intolerance
Hematologic	Anemia Microcytic: Fe deficiency from poor absorbtion or blood loss Normocytic Macrocytic: folate or B_{12} deficiency
Cardiovascular	"Hypothyroid heart," congestive failure Pericardial effusion Bradycardia, hypertension Coronary heart disease
Respiratory	Decreased ventilatory drive, sluggish respiratory center, impaired bellows action of lungs, tendency to retain CO_2
Gastrointestinal	Atrophic gastritis Malabsorption Constipation Myxedema ileus
Musculoskeletal	Asymptomatic CPK ↑ Hoffman's syndrome (triad of increased muscle stiffness and weakness and marked elevation of CPK)
Neurological	Pseudomyotonic stretch reflexes Mental changes Myxedema coma Cerebellar ataxia Associated subacute combined degeneration Carpal tunnel syndrome
Renal	Decreased free water clearance Tendency to water intoxication SIADH-like state with hypoatremia, hypotonic plasma, less than maximally dilute urine and natriurisis
Joints	Arthralgias Hyperuricemia; attacks of gout in the genetically predisposed SLE and Hashimoto's
Reproductive	Decreased libido Menorrhagia, oligomenorrhea, amenorrhea Primary amenorrhea Sexual infantilism Precocious puberty Galactorrhea

3. Finally, the perturbations of lipid metabolism in hypothyroidism are noteworthy. Practically every variety of dyslipoproteinemia has been described in association with the hypothyroid state. Although elevated cholesterol (and β-lipoproteins) is the most impressive abnormality, patients with hypothyroidism may demonstrate elevated triglycerides, reflecting increases in VLDL, chylomicrons, and even the intermediate LDL.

15.4. Diagnostic Studies

15.4.1. Hormonal Determinations

The only tests required in the initial evaluation of hypothyroidism are T_4, T_3R, and a serum TSH. The serum *thyroxine* is reasonably reflective of the degree of hypothyroidism (in the absence of significant TBG deficiency), and the TSH assay will permit differentiation of primary hypothyroidism from hypothalamic pituitary etiologies; an elevated TSH in the presence of a low serum thyroxine is diagnostic of primary hypothyroidism, whereas a low or even normal TSH in the presence of low thyroid hormones is suggestive of pituitary–hypothalamic dysfunction.

Measurement of serum triiodothyronine (T_3) levels in the serum is not indicated, since this would be expected to be low when the substrate (T_4) is low. Measurement of free hormones is also not indicated unless a concomitant abnormality in TBG is suspected. The most frequent diagnostic consideration that enters the differential diagnosis of true hypothyroidism is the "sick euthyroid syndrome," which is characterized by an extremely low serum triiodothyronine level and often may also be associated with a low serum thyroxine, the hormonal profile thus resembling hypothyroidism. The measurement of reverse T_3 in the circulation permits distinction between the two conditions; the reverse T_3 is elevated in the sick euthyroid syndrome because of a preferential increase in the peripheral deiodination of T_4 into reverse T_3, an inactive isomer of T_3; in true hypothyroidism, both T_3 and reverse T_3 are low because of inherently impaired production of T_4.

15.4.2. Antithyroid Antibodies

Measurement of antithyroglobulin or antimicrosomal antibodies is indicated in patients with primary hypothyroidism to document an autoimmune etiology.

15.4.3. Skull X Ray and CT Scans of Sella

These are indicated only in the hypothyroid patient with low TSH levels to exclude a pituitary neoplasm causing TSH deficiency and hypothyroidism. It must be recognized that, rarely, chronic primary hypothyroidism may also be associated with enlargement of the pituitary gland or the sella. This is secondary to hyperplasia of thyrotrophs in response to chronic hypothyroxinemia and hypotriiodothyroninemia.

15.5. Course and Prognosis

The syndrome of hypothyroidism that evolves from thyroid hormone deficiency completely regresses following institution of replacement therapy with *levo*-thyroxine with a gratifying response to treatment. Therapy is life long. The penultimate expression of chronic severe untreated hypothyroidism is myxedema coma. As a consequence of protracted deficiency of thyroid hormones, the metabolic machinery of all tissues comes to a crashing halt. The exact cellular basis for myxedema coma is unclear, but it is felt that chronic deficiency of thyroid hormones depletes the red cells of their 2,3-DPG content; this results in a shift in the oxygen dissociation curve of the hemoglobin unfavorable to oxygen delivery to tissues. The CNS is the tissue that is most severly affected by this tissue anoxia, leading to depression of higher functions and eventually the cardiac center, temperature centers, and respiratory center of the brain. The result is coma, hypotension, hypothermia, and hypoventilation in the myxedematous patient. Even with early recognition and aggressive treatment, myxedema coma carries an extremely high mortality rate, which ranges between 50% and 60%. Therefore, the emphasis is on preventing the occurrence of myxedema by early detection and institution of treatment.

15.6. Treatment

Replacement therapy for hypothyroidism is by the oral administration of *levo*-thyropine. Before initiating *levo*-thyroxine therapy, it is essential to evaluate three·important aspects of the patient's illness:

1. The presence of concomitant adrenal insufficiency.
2. The presence of underlying coronary heart disease.
3. The severity of the hypothyroidism.

Each of the above aspects has an important bearing on therapy.

If concurrent adrenal insufficiency is missed and the patient is started on *levo*-thyroxine, the results can be disastrous, with precipitation of adrenal crisis following the increase in metabolism. Both pituitary and primary hypothyroidism can be associated with adrenal insufficiency, in the former instance by the concomitant deficiencies of TSH and ACTH and in the latter situation by the combination of autoimmune thyroiditis and autoimmune adrenalitis. When adrenal and thyroid failure occur concurrently, replacement thyroxine therapy should be deferred until glucocorticoid therapy has been initiated.

The presence of underlying coronary heart disease poses a formidable therapeutic challenge in the treatment of hypothyroidism because of the high risk of precipitating overt myocardial infarctions with *levo*-thyroxine replacement. In such patients, therapy should be started with extremely low (25-μg) doses of *levo*-thyroxine with cautious stepwise (25-μg) increments every 2 to 3 weeks providing there are no chest pains or cardiographic abnormalities. In many instances *levo*-thyroxine therapy becomes a balancing act of titration therapy, most patients never achieving the full replacement level and hence mildly undertreated by necessity.

The more severe the hypothyroidism, the more gradual must be the replacement with *levo*-thyroxine. The starting dose in a myxedematous patient should not exceed 50 μg of *levo*-thyroxine.

The maintenance dose of *levo*-thyroxine is 150 μg for most patients. Older patients require a lower maintenance dose. The optimal maintenance dose should be based on the clinical response, the serum thyroxine, and in the case of primary hypothyroidism, on the serum TSH level. The dose of levo-thyroxine that maintains the serum TSH in the normal range (below 5 μU) is the optimal dose. Of course, the TSH level is not a parameter to follow when the hypothyroidism is secondary to TSH deficiency. Also, the measurement of TSH does not aid in determining "overmedication," since the degree of suppression does not permit distinction between adequate and overtreatment. That distinction is best made on clinical grounds and on the basis of serum level of thyroid hormones.

Therapy for hypothyroidism is life long, and this should be made clear to the patient. The dose of replacement thyroxine may fluctuate during the lifelong course of these patients. Since different commercial preparations possess variability in the bioavailability of the hormone, these patients are best maintained on the same brand of preparation throughout.

16

The Thyroidites

16.1. Introduction

Acute or pyogenic thyroiditis is rare. This chapter focuses on the four varieties of nonacute thyroiditis: subacute thyroiditis, silent thyroiditis, Hashitoxicosis, and Hashimoto's thyroiditis. The first three conditions are characterized by the development of transient hyperthyroidism and hence are often referred to as "hyperthyroidites." The fourth condition, Hashimoto's thyroiditis, represents the most common etiology of spontaneous hypothyroidism in adults as well as in children.

16.2. Subacute Thyroiditis

Subacute thyroiditis, also referred to as de Quervain's thyroiditis, was once thought to be rare but is being recognized with increasing frequency. According to some estimates, this entity constitutes approximately 15% of all newly diagnosed cases of hyperthyroidism.

16.2.1. Etiology

Subacute thyroiditis is believed to be secondary to a viral infection. The biopsy of the affected gland demonstrates a classical appearance characterized by infiltration of the edematous follicle with chronic inflammatory cells and giant cells, forming granulomas ("granulomatous thyroiditis"). Attempts to positively link this syndrome with Coxsackie viruses have not been entirely successful.

16.2.2. Clinical Features

In the classic case, subacute thyroiditis evolves in four phases: the hyperthyroid phase, the transition phase, the hypothyroid phase, and the recovery phase. These phases often evolve with rapidity, and the patient may seek help during any of these phases, resulting in a presentation not as clear-cut and compartmentalized as the clinical description that follows.

16.2.2.1. The Hyperthyroid Phase

The two hallmarks of this phase are painful thyromegaly and self-limited hyperthyroidism. The pain in the region of the neck can be extremely severe, radiating to the jaw or the ears. Some degree of dysphagia is invariably present. The thyromegaly can be diffuse or localized and limited to only one lobe. Tenderness to palpation is a characteristic sign evident in more than 90% of patients. In some instances the thyromegaly is unimpressive and easily missed. The patient often admits to antecedent sore throat or upper respiratory infection and experiences significant constitutional symptoms such as low-grade fever and malaise. The constellation of fever, malaise, neck pain, and dysphagia often leads to the mistaken diagnosis of pharyngitis, esophagitis, tonsillitis, cervical lymphadenitis, or even cellulitis of the neck.

The hyperthyroidism of subacute thyroiditis results from release of the preformed hormones from the inflamed gland into the circulation. The two features of this type of hyperthyroidism are its mildness and self-limited nature (2–6 weeks). The most common symptoms experienced by these patients include nervousness, palpitations, mild weight loss, and hyperdefecation. The hyperthyroidism lasts only as long as the inflamed gland keeps releasing the preformed hormones into the circulation. Once these stores are depleted, as they will be when the inflammation subsides, the hyperthyroidism disappears. The hyperthyroidism of subacute thyroiditis should be differentiated from the hyperthyroidism of Graves' disease. The short history, mild nature, tender thyromegaly, and lack of gravesian stigmata are the clinical features of subacute thyroiditis that permit differentiation from Graves' hyperthyroidism.

16.2.2.2. The Transition Phase

This phase can be recognized only if the patient is carefully followed after the initial phase. The key feature of this phase is improvement. Improvement in the pain, disappearance of constitutional symptoms, and improvement of the hyperthyroidism, even without therapy, are features recognizable during this phase. The thyromegaly may still be evident, but pain and tenderness are gone. The thyroid indices may still be elevated; hence, if the patient presents for the first time during this phase, it is easy to see how the diagnosis of subacute thyroiditis can be missed, since pain and tenderness are no longer evident.

16.2.2.3. The Hypothyroid Phase

This stage is the compensatory one. Following the "acute" phase, the gland has released all its stored hormone. The serum level of thyroid hor-

TABLE 44
Laboratory Studies in Subacute Thyroiditis

Phase	T_4, T_3	TSH	^{131}I uptake	Other studies
Hyperthyroid phase	↑ ↑	↓ ↓	Low (0–2%)	Low intrathyroid iodine content as shown by the fluorescent scan
Transition phase	↑	↓	Still low (2–5%)	
Hypothyroidal phase	↓	↑	Rebound ↑	Rising intrathyroidal iodine content as shown by the fluorescent scan
Recovery phase	N	N	May remain slightly ↑	Intrathyroidal iodine content will plateau eventually

mones gradually declines. The gland, depleted of all its hormonal and iodine stores, must start synthesizing new hormone to replete these stores. The stimulus to do so comes from TSH, which has been provoked by the declining thyroid hormone level. The clinical picture of mild hypothyroidism coupled with the elevated TSH in this phase resembles that of primary hypothyroidism.

16.2.2.4. The Recovery Phase

Under the stimulation of TSH, the thyroid gland is gradually restored to its normal status, since no permanent damage has been done. Once the glandular stores of hormone are repleted, functional euthyroidism is achieved, and the TSH is turned off.

16.2.3. Diagnostic Studies

The diagnostic tests will depend on the phase. Table 44 outlines these changes. Three important points are made by this table:

1. During the hyperthyroid phase, the hallmark of subacute thyroiditis is the low to undetectable radioactive iodine uptake. This finding clearly excludes Graves' hyperthyroidism.
2. The intrathyroid iodine content, measured by a fluorescent scan, can be used as a parameter to follow recovery.
3. During the hypothyroid phase, the radioactive iodine uptake increases. This can easily be differentiated from the high radioactive iodine uptake of Graves' disease because of the low T_4 and high TSH that accompany the high RAIU in this phase of subacute thyroiditis.

16.2.4. Treatment

Since subacute thyroiditis is a self-limiting disorder, the only treatments required are pain relief and symptomatic therapy for the hyperthyroidism.

Pain relief usually can be accomplished by analgesics, and symptomatic relief of hyperthyroidism can be attained by the use of propranolol. In severe cases, steroids have been tried with variable results. During the hypothyroid phase, the patient should be reassured, and no treatment is needed if the hypothyroidism is mild. If it is severe, *levo*-thyroxine therapy should be instituted but discontinued within 6 months to a year. Lifelong therapy with *levo*-thyroxine is not necessary.

16.3. Silent Thyroiditis

Silent thyroiditis (also referred to as "painless thyroiditis" and "lymphocytic thyroiditis with spontaneously resolving hyperthyroidism") has emerged as an important cause of self-limited hyperthyroidism, especially in pregnant and postpartum women.

16.3.1. Etiology

Although considered autoimmune in nature, silent thyroiditis is different from Hashimoto's thyroiditis, another autoimmune thyroid disorder, which rarely can present with self-limited hyperthyroidism (Hashitoxicosis). The significant difference between the two is the outcome following the hyperthyroid phase: Hashitoxicosis rapidly and inexorably progresses to eventual hypothyroidism, whereas silent thyroiditis does not.

16.3.2. Clinical and Diagnostic Features

The clinical presentation of silent thyroiditis is characterized by the triad of painless diffuse thyromegaly, transient, mild hyperthyroidism, and a temporal relationship to pregnancy or puerperium. The laboratory triad of silent thyroiditis is characterized by transiently elevated thyroid hormones, markedly decreased radioiodine uptake, and depleted intrathyroid iodine stores as determined by the fluorescent scan. Antithyroid antibodies are usually positive in modest titers. The histological appearance on needle biopsy consists of focal or diffuse lymphocytic infiltration reminiscent of Hashimoto's thyroiditis minus the fibrosis.

16.3.3. Differential Diagnosis

The differential diagnosis of this entity extends over a wide range of disorders including Graves' hyperthyroidism, subacute thyroiditis, Hashitoxicosis, and compensated Hashimoto's disease. The transient nature of the hyperthyroidism and the characteristically low radioactive iodine uptake help to differentiate silent thyroiditis from Graves' hyperthyroidism, in which the radioactive iodine uptake is high. The distinction between subacute thyroiditis and silent thyroiditis can be difficult, since both present with self-limited hyperthyroidism, low radioiodine uptake, depleted intrathyroid iodine content, and identical evolution in terms of the natural history. When pain and

TABLE 45
Transient Hyperthyroidism

	Subacute thyroiditis	Silent thyroiditis	Hashitoxicosis
1. Relationship to pregnancy	−	+	−
2. Degree of hyperthyroidism	Mild	Mild	Mild
3. Ophthalmopathy	Absent	Absent	Occasionally may be +
4. Thryomegaly	Mild	Mild	Mild
5. Pain and tenderness over the thyroid	Often present in the classic case; 10–15% "silent"	−	−
6. T_4, T_3	Elevated	Elevated	Elevated
7. RAI uptake	Low (0–3%)	Low (0–3%)	Normal to minimally elevated
8. Antithyroid antibodies	Negative	Elevated in modest titers	Elevated in high titers
9. Leucocytosis, sed. rate, fever	+	−	−
10. Outcome	Transient hypo- followed by euthyroidism	Transient hypo- followed by euthyroidism	Transient euthyroidism followed by permanent hypothyroidism
11. Etiology	Acute viral	Autoimmune	Autoimmune
12. Recurrence	−	10–20% recurrence	−

tenderness over the thyroid gland are present, the diagnosis is obviously subacute thyroiditis. The distinction between the painless form of subacute thyroiditis and silent thyroiditis can be established with certainty only by needle biopsy of the thyroid, where the granulomatous appearance of subacute thyroiditis contrasts sharply with the intense lymphocytic infiltration seen in silent thyroiditis.

Silent thyroiditis can be differentiated from Hashitoxicosis by three features: the radioactive iodine uptake in Hashitoxicosis is normal or minimally elevated, the antimicrosomal antibody titers are markedly elevated (greater than 1 : 28,000), and, most importantly, Hashitoxicosis progresses rapidly to permanent hypothyroidism. Since patients with silent thyroiditis may also go through a transient phase of hypothyroidism prior to restoration of euthyroidism, follow-up studies are crucial to establish the distinction. Finally, silent thyroiditis may, during its recovery phase, mimic Hashimoto's thyroiditis; both conditions may be associated with decreased thyroid hormone levels and an elevated TSH. The transient nature of such phenomena in silent thyroiditis helps to distinguish it from Hashimoto's thyroiditis, in which the disease progresses relentlessly to permanent hypothyroidism. Table 45 outlines the similarities and differences among silent thyroiditis, subacute thyroiditis, and Hashitoxicosis.

16.3.4. Course and Prognosis

The eventual outcome of silent thyroiditis is restoration of euthyroidism. As indicated above, a brief period of transient hypothyroidism is seen prior to such restoration. Recurrence of silent thyroiditis occurs in a small but significant proportion of patients.

16.3.5. Treatment

Treatment of silent thyroiditis is identical to that of subacute thyroiditis: temporary measures to treat the hyper- and hypothyroidism during their respective phases.

16.4. Hashitoxicosis

Hashitoxicosis is considered to be a phase in some patients with Hashimoto's thyroiditis. During this short-lived phase, the patient with Hashimoto's thyroiditis actually experiences hyperthyroidism. This phase is transient, soon giving way to the development of permanent hypothyroidism. It is presumed that Hashitoxicosis represents an unique instance in which Graves' disease and Hashimoto's cohabit the same gland, but the eventual dominance of the latter results in permanent hypothyroidism.

Hashitoxicosis is rare, most patients initially being diagnosed as Graves' hyperthyroidism. Its recognition often occurs when the radioiodine uptake by the thyroid is found to be unimpressively normal or when the patient rapidly becomes hypothyroid spontaneously or with minimal antithyroid therapy. Once the patient becomes hypothyroid, the clinical features and course are identical to Hashimoto's thyroiditis.

16.5. Hashimoto's Thyroiditis

Hashimoto's thyroiditis (struma lymphomatosa, autoimmune thyroiditis, chronic lymphocytic thyroiditis) is the most common etiology of spontaneous hypothyroidism in adults and children.

16.5.1. Etiology

Hashimoto's thyroiditis is a classic example of an autoimmune disease characterized by the development of autoantibodies against the thyroglobulin and microsomal components of the follicular cell of the thyroid. The destruction of the follicles occurs with lymphocytic infiltration and eventually fibrosis. The strong association between Hashimoto's thyroiditis and other autoimmune disease is legendary, including pernicious anemia, rheumatoid arthritis, systemic lupus, Addison's disease, diabetes, etc.

16.5.2. Clinical Features

Hashimoto's thyroiditis occurs more frequently in females. The two major presentations are goiter and varying degrees of hypothyroidism.

16.5.2.1. Goiter

Thyromegaly is evident in more than two-thirds of patients with Hashimoto's thyroiditis. The enlargement is mild to modest, rarely reaching sizes in excess of 80 g. The enlargement is usually symmetrical and diffuse, with the pyramidal lobe especially enlarging. The consistency of the enlarged gland is soft (rubbery). In one variant of Hashimoto's thyroiditis, called the fibrous variant, the gland assumes a firm or even hard consistency because of the inordinate increase in the fibrotic component. When these changes are focal, the distinction from malignant disease is extremely difficult. Thyromegaly may be absent in the atrophic variety of autoimmune thyroiditis. The thyroid lobes, in these instances, are represented by fibrous slices of atrophied thyroid tissue. Thus, the enlargement of the thyroid gland in this disorder is highly variable, with goitrous, fibrous, and atrophic variants all representing different facets in the evolution of the autoimmune process.

It is essential to understand the reasons for goiter formation in Hashimoto's thyroiditis. The major reason for thyromegaly is compensatory growth of the gland driven by TSH stimulation. When thyroid hormone production declines, the resultant decline in hormone levels signals the pituitary thyrotroph to secrete TSH; the thyroid gland responds to this by increasing function and growth. In fact, this "compensated euthyroid" state can maintain the patient in a reasonably good functional state for extended periods of time. Euthyroidism, in these instances, is maintained at the expense of a high TSH and a goitrous gland. The increase in cellular infiltrate and proliferation of fibrous tissue also contribute to the thyromegaly. Eventually, when the thyroid tissue can no longer maintain adequate function despite TSH stimulation, subclinical or overt hypothyroidism develops.

16.5.2.2. Hypothyroidism

The hypothyroidism of Hashimoto's thyroiditis can be subclinical, subtle, or overt (Table 46).

1. Subclinical hypothyroidism. The subclinical phase of hypothyroidism is a common disorder according to population survey studies, which indicate an overall prevalence of 2–7% for this disorder in the general population. Subclinical hypothyroidism represents the phase of compensated euthyroidism and is characterized by an absence of symptoms and normal levels of serum thyroxine, free thyroxine, and triiodothyronine. The only biochemical abnormality is an elevated TSH.

TABLE 46
Biochemical and Clinical Spectrum of Hashimoto's Thyroiditis

Type of hypothyroidism	T_4	T_3	TSH	TSH response to TRH	Symptoms	Signs
Subclinical (compensated)	N	N	↑	Exaggerated	None	None
Subtle	N	N	↑ (occasionally upper normal)	Exaggerated	Mild	None
Overt	↓	↓	↑	Exaggerated	+	+

2. Subtle hypothyroidism. Patients with this entity complain of mild symptoms of hypothyroidism, no signs of thyroid deficiency, "normal" thyroid hormone levels (but probably lower in comparison to their customary basal level), and an elevated TSH.

3. Overt hypothyroidism. This is characterized by obvious features of hypothyroidism: low hormone levels and elevated TSH levels.

Rarely, Hashimoto's thyroiditis may be associated with unusual manifestations, which include:

1. A transient phase of hyperthyroidism (Hashitoxicosis), which rapidly evolves into permanent hypothyroidism.

2. Infiltrative ophthalmopathy identical to that seen with Graves' disease.

3. Focal thyroiditis resulting in a palpable nodule that appears cold on scan.

4. The fibrous variant, which may present as a firm or hard thyroid lump.

16.5.3. Diagnostic Studies

16.5.3.1. Thyroid Hormones

The levels of serum thyroxine and serum triiodothyronine in Hashimoto's thyroiditis vary, depending on the stage in the evolution of the disease (Table 46). Thus, the serum hormone levels can be clearly low (as in the overtly hypothyroid patient), low normal (as in patients with subtle hypothyroidism), or clearly normal (as in the subclinical hypothyroid patient).

16.5.3.2. The Serum TSH

The serum level of TSH is clearly elevated in nearly all patients with Hashimoto's disease. Indeed, this is the only abnormality seen in patients with subclinical (compensated) hypothyroidism. In a small number of patients with subclinical or subtle hypothyroidism, the serum TSH may be in the upper limits of the normal range.

16.5.3.3. Antithyroid Antibodies

Antithyroglobulin or antimicrosomal antibodies are present in the circulation of more than 90% of patients with Hashimoto's thyroiditis. Antithyroglobulin antibodies are measured by the tanned red-cell agglutination method and are relatively nonspecific; antimicrosomal antibodies measured by complement fixation or a solid-phase immunoassay are more specific. Rarely, patients with biopsy-proven Hashimoto's thyroiditis may not demonstrate significant antibody titers. This is often seen in children, geriatric patients, very early disease, or end-stage disease characterized by extreme fibrosis or atrophy. A mild to modest increase in titers may be seen in patients with other thyroid disorders, particularly Graves' hyperthyroidism.

16.5.3.4. The TRH Study

The response of TSH to an intravenous bolus of TRH is always abnormal in Hashimoto's disease and is characterized by an exaggerated response. This is so even when the basal TSH is in the upper normal range. The TRH study is not indicated when the basal TSH is clearly elevated. It need be performed only when mild hypothyroidism is suspected and the basal TSH is in the upper normal range.

16.5.3.5. ^{131}I Uptake

Patients with Hashimoto's thyroiditis may have a normal, low, or even a high 24-hr radioactive iodine uptake. The apparent paradox of a high uptake in a hypothyroid patient (or in a gland bound for eventual myxedema) is explained on the basis that many of these patients demonstrate a defect in organification. The combination of a TSH-activated thyroid trap and an organification block results in an accumulation of unorganified iodine within the gland following administration of radioactive iodine.

16.5.4. Course and Prognosis

Hashimoto's disease is a benign disease characterized by relentless progression to hypothyroidism. Contrary to earlier opinions, Hashimoto's thyroiditis does not predispose to thyroid cancer. There is, however, an association between Hashimoto's thyroiditis and lymphoma of the thyroid, a condition being diagnosed with increasing frequency with the widespread application of diagnostic needle biopsy of the thyroid.

16.5.5. Treatment

The treatment for the hypothyroidism caused by Hashimoto's thyroiditis is lifelong replacement therapy with *levo*-thyroxine. Replacement therapy is indicated even in the "compensated," euthyroid patient with goiter to reduce the size and prevent further enlargement. Since the Hashimoto's goiter is caused by TSH, *levo*-thyroxine therapy is usually associated with impressive reduction in the goiter size. Very rarely, the goiter may fail to decrease in size or may even continue to enlarge when replacement thyroxine (100 to 150 μg) is given. In these rare instances, suppressive doses of thyroxine (up to 300 μg) may be necessary.

17

Thyroid Nodules

17.1. Introduction

Thyroid nodules represent an extremely common clinical problem, occurring in approximately 4% of the population. Thyroid nodules occur within the substance of the thyroid tissue, solid nodules representing localized areas of increased cell growth. Solitary thyroid nodules are more common than multinodular goiters.

17.2. Etiology

The three most common causes for solitary thyroid nodules are adenoma (benign neoplastic growth), thyroid cyst, and thyroid carcinoma. The relative preponderance of each of these entities varies with age. Overall, cysts account for nearly 20% of all solitary nodules, and adenomas represent nearly half. The incidence of carcinoma occurring in a thyroid nodule is variable, ranging from 5% to 35% depending on the patient's age—the younger the age the higher the incidence. Less common causes for thyroid nodules include focal thyroiditis, lymphoma of the thyroid, and metastatic disease from any distant primary, in particular breast or lung. Rare causes include granulomatous diseases such as tuberculosis, sarcoidosis, or parasitic diseases.

The etiology of nodular disease of the thyroid is unclear. Although TSH has been implicated in the development and maintenance of thyroid nodules, this is far from proven. Although it is an accepted fact that in many instances suppression of TSH by *levo*-thyroxine therapy results in an impressive shrinking in the size of a single nodule or even some multinodular goiters, the etiologic role of TSH as the primary culprit is unsettled. A similarly unsettled issue is the role of iodine deficiency. Since iodine is plentiful in our diet, one must assume that such deficiency probably operates at an intrathyroidal level. Proof for such a phenomenon is conspicuously lacking. The role of dietary or pharmacological goitrogens is even less certain. The only etiologic factor that has been definitively linked to thyroid nodules is the prior exposure to head and neck radiation (for acne or tonsils) during childhood. The growing thyroid of children and adolescents is extremely sensitive to the effects of low-dose radiation. The incidence of developing thyroid nodules following head and neck radiation in childhood is 20–26%, and of these 4–10% may harbor a well-differentiated malignancy.

17.3. Clinical Features

Most thyroid nodules are asymptomatic, often discovered during a routine physical examination. Frequently, in males, the nodules are detected while shaving. Pain is generally not a feature of thyroid nodules unless complicated by hemorrhage or infection. The presence of pressure symptoms such as dysphagia, hoarseness (resulting from recurrent laryngeal nerve infiltration), or dyspnea (from tracheal compression) is a sign of malignancy. Table 47

TABLE 47
The Thyroid Nodule: Clinical Evaluation

Finding	Comment
Age	The incidence of carcinoma in a nodule is inversely related to the age of the patient: the incidence in patients below 30 years of age ranges between 20% and 40%
Recent onset and rapid growth	Suspicious of malignancy
Rapid growth of a lump in a preexisting, longstanding multinodular goiter	Suggestive of the behavior pattern observed in anaplastic carcinoma
Presence of pain	Less likely to be malignancy
Past history of head and neck radiation in childhood for acne, tonsils, or thymic enlargement	25–28% incidence of nodule formation; 10–20% of these nodules will be malignant, usually papillary or follicular
Pressure effects (hoarseness, dysphagia)	Highly suggestive of malignancy
Past history of renal stones or a history of paroxysmal hypertension	Suggestive of MEA-II (Sipple syndrome)
Single nodule vs. multinodular gland	Multinodular gland is less likely to be malignant
Firm to hard consistency, especially in a nodule >3 cm	Suggestive of malignancy
Presence of lymphadenopathy	Virtually diagnostic (postcervical, submandibular, midline submental, and rarely supraclavicular)
Presence of thyrotoxicosis	Makes the diagnosis of thyroid cancer extremely unlikely (exception is metastatic functional thyroid carcinoma)

illustrates the importance of the history and physical examination in the evaluation of a thyroid nodule.

17.4. Diagnostic Studies

The diagnostic studies for the evaluation of thyroid nodules can be classified into isotopic, ultrasonographic, hormonal, cytological, and miscellaneous studies.

17.4.1. Isotopic Studies: Thyroid Scintigraphy

The thyroid scan is one of the most important and basic studies in the evaluation of the thyroid nodule, especially when it is solitary. It should be remembered that the purpose of the scintigraphic study is not to detect the nodule but rather to evaluate clinically palpated nodules in terms of their ability to concentrate radionuclide. Depending on this ability, the clinically palpated nodule can be classified as "hot," "cold," or "indeterminate." When the nodule concentrates the radionuclide to a greater extent than the surrounding paranodular tissue, it is referred to as a "hot" or hyperfunctional nodule (Figure 10); such nodules tend to evolve into autonomously functioning thyroid nodules (AFTN) when the function of the paranodular tissue is completely suppressed. The AFTN, while demonstrating a negligibly low potential for harboring malignancy, also demonstrates a heightened proclivity to cause hyperthyroidism (Plummer's disease). Thus, demonstration of a "hot"

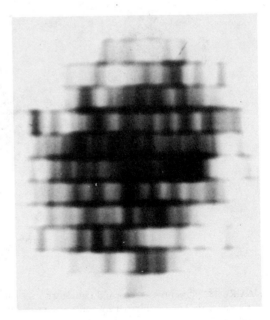

FIGURE 10. Patient with 3-cm nodule palpable on the left lobe of the thyroid gland. Thyroid scan demonstrates isotopic concentration limited to the palpable nodule with no visualization of paranodular tissue.

nodule obviates the need for ultrasonography (since it is unlikely to be a cyst) or aspiration biopsy (since it is unlikely to harbor cancer).

When the nodule concentrates radionuclide to a lesser extent than the surrounding tissue, it is referred to as "cold" or hypofunctional nodule (Figure 13). A cold nodule can be cystic or solid. Although most malignant lesions tend to be "cold," the reverse does not hold true. The likelihood of a solitary, solid, cold nodule being malignant is greater in younger patients. When the nodule concentrates the radionuclide to the same extent as the adjoining tissue, it is termed "indeterminate" or functional (Figure 14). The malignant potential in such a nodule is quite variable, the most common type being the follicular carcinoma.

The single most important reason to obtain a thyroid scan is to exclude the "hot nodule," because the demonstration of a hyperfunctional nodule greatly minimizes the need to pursue a "malignancy work-up." The additional reasons for performing a thyroid scan in a patient with a thyroid nodule are:

1. To identify the patients who would require further tests such as ultrasonography. The demonstration of a "cold" nodule is a clear indication for ultrasonography, which can effectively exclude a cyst.
2. To identify diffuse disease coexisting with the thyroid nodule. The demonstration of diffuse thyromegaly in addition to the nodule should raise the possibility of coexistent Graves' or Hashimoto's diseases.

Thyroid scans are performed with the use of radioactive iodine or tech-

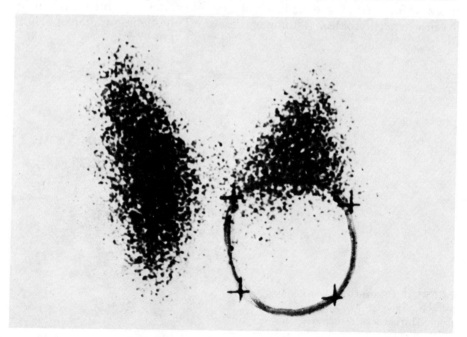

FIGURE 13. Twenty-two-year-old female with a 4-cm nodule in the lower pole of the left lobe of the thyroid. The nodule hardly concentrates radionuclide and is hence termed "hypofunctional" or "cold."

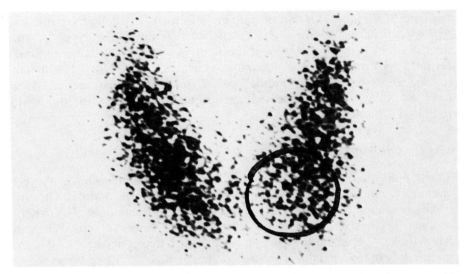

FIGURE 14. Forty-year-old female with 2.5-cm nodule in the left lower pole. Radionuclide scan demonstrates that the palpable nodule concentrates the isotope to the same extent as the adjacent tissue and hence is termed "functional" or "warm."

netium pertechnetate. Although the scans obtained with both isotopes are generally concordant, occasionally a nodule may appear functional with technetium but "cold" with radioactive iodine. The differentiation of benign from malignant disease cannot be made on the basis of the thyroid scan.

17.4.2. Ultrasonography

Although the scintiscan provides information regarding the functional ability of the nodule, gray-scale ultrasonography provides accurate information regarding the internal anatomy of the thyroid gland. All "cold" nodules should be scanned with ultrasound for diagnostic, prognostic, and therapeutic purposes. The demonstration of a completely cystic lesion corresponding to the palpated nodule almost eliminates the possibility of malignancy. Approximately 20% of cold nodules turn out to be cystic, and the incidence of malignancy in a completely cystic lesion under 4 cm is below 1%. The same cannot be said for a "mixed" (solid and cystic) lesion by ultrasonography. These lesions should be approached in the same manner as "solid" lesions. When a simple cyst is demonstrated, the therapeutic option, if chosen, is limited to aspiration of cyst with a large-bore needle. Such aspiration can be facilitated under ultrasonographic control.

17.4.3. Hormonal Studies

Screening for hyperthyroidism is particularly essential when an autonomously functioning nodule is demonstrated by scan. It should be pointed out that the screening should include measurement of triiodothyronine level in the serum because of the high incidence of T_3 toxicosis in the setting. When diffuse enlargement coexists with the nodule, antithyroid antibodies and a serum TSH level should be obtained to exclude compensated Hashimoto's thyroiditis presenting as a "nodule" with thyromegaly. When medullary carcinoma of the thyroid is suspected, measurement of serum calcitonin level is indicated (Chapter 52).

17.4.4. Cytological Studies

Fine-needle aspiration biopsy has added a new dimension in the preoperative evaluation of the solitary solid "cold" thyroid nodule. The fine-needle aspiration is a method to obtain cells shed by the nodule. The material obtained is smeared, stained, and evaluated for abnormal cells. When the cytopathology expertise is excellent, the ability to detect malignancy in a thyroid nodule by fine-needle aspiration is approximately 85% to 90%.

17.4.5. Miscellaneous Tests

Radiographs of the neck (for calcification), thoracic inlet films (for tracheal narrowing), and indirect laryngoscopy (for vocal cord movement) may be periodically indicated in the evaluation of a thyroid nodule. Figure 15 outlines the algorithmic approach for investigating the thyroid nodule.

17.5. Course and Prognosis

The "hot" (AFTN) nodule, as indicated above, is seldom malignant. The only risk in patients harboring an autonomous nodule is the development of hyperthyroidism (toxic adenoma); patients who are older and harboring nodules larger than 3 cm are at highest risk.

Among "cold nodules," 20% will prove to be benign cysts, 9–35% will turn out to be carcinoma or lymphoma, and the remainder are benign lesions such as adenomas or focal thyroiditis. The prognosis for malignant thyroid nodules is discussed elsewhere (Section 18.5). Thyroid cysts may remain stationary, may continue to grow, or may become infected. The course of benign adenomas presenting as cold nodules is variable. Bleeding into the adenoma with degenerative changes is a rare event and is characterized by sudden pain, swelling in the region of the nodule, and fever.

17.6. Treatment

The treatment of the thyroid nodule depends on the etiology. Thyroid cysts may require no treatment unless progressive enlargement occurs. Simple aspiration with a large-bone needle is curative in many instances; when re-

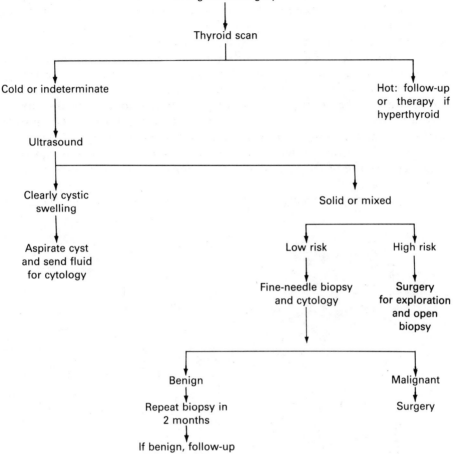

Careful history and physical examination to determine whether patient falls under low-risk or high-risk category

Thyroid scan

Cold or indeterminate

Hot: follow-up or therapy if hyperthyroid

Ultrasound

Clearly cystic swelling

Solid or mixed

Aspirate cyst and send fluid for cytology

Low risk

High risk

Fine-needle biopsy and cytology

Surgery for exploration and open biopsy

Benign

Malignant

Repeat biopsy in 2 months

Surgery

If benign, follow-up

FIGURE 15. Algorithm for diagnosis of a solitary thyroid nodule. Additional miscellaneous tests may include plain X ray of neck, thyroid function tests, serum calcitonin, serum calcium and phosphorus, and lymph node biopsy.

currence or repeated infection is a problem, surgical excision of the cyst, or sclerotherapy with tetracycline can be contemplated.

The treatment of euthyroid hot nodules is controversial. Observation is recommended by most, but prophylactic surgical ablation is recommended by some for patients who are at high risk of developing hyperthyroidism. (Suppression therapy with levothyroxine does not have any place in the treatment of the autonomously functioning nodule with euthyroidism.) The treatment of hot nodule complicated by hyperthyroidism (Plummer's disease) is discussed in Section 14.4.

The treatment of benign but cold thyroid nodules ranges among observation with no intervention, long-term suppression therapy with *levo*-thyroxine, and surgical removal. When the benignity of the nodule has been proven by repeated needle biopsy, the next step is to observe whether the nodule progresses or remains stationary. A nongrowing benign thyroid nodule does not require any therapeutic intervention. Benign nodules that continue to grow deserve to be treated with a trial of suppressive therapy with 0.3 mg of *levo*-thyroxine. The response usually ranges from good to excellent. In patients with benign nodules who cannot tolerate *levo*-thyroxine, or when a contraindication such as coronary heart disease precludes the use of suppressive doses of levothyroxine, the choice between no therapy and surgery will depend on the rate of growth of the nodule. It should be noted that stable iodine does not have any role in the treatment of nodular thyroid disease. In fact, its use is contraindicated, since the use of iodine in this setting may result in the occurrence of the Jod–Basedow phenomenon, i.e., iodine-induced hyperthyroidism.

The treatment of malignant thyroid nodules is discussed in Chapter 18.

18

Thyroid Cancer

18.1. Introduction

Cancer of the thyroid is a relatively uncommon malignancy; the incidence of clinically presenting thyroid carcinoma is approximately 36 per million population per year. A definite etiologic link exists between the development of thyroid cancer and a history of prior exposure to head and neck radiation. The incidence of differentiated thyroid carcinoma following head and neck radiation is 3–7%.

18.2. Classification

The four major types of thyroid carcinoma are papillary, follicular, anaplastic, and medullary. Papillary and follicular carcinomas are differentiated thyroid cancers arising from the follicular epithelium, whereas anaplastic cancer is undifferentiated. Medullary carcinoma of the thyroid arises from the C cells (parafollicular cells) and is discussed separately in Chapter 52.

18.3. Clinical Features

Some general characteristics of papillary, follicular, and medullary thyroid carcinoma are outlined in Table 48. The clinical presentation of thyroid carcinoma can include any of the following:

1. Nodule in the thyroid gland. The most common presentation of thyroid cancer is that of a solitary nodule in the thyroid gland. In terms of the anatomic and functional characteristics that are helpful in predicting benignity of a thyroid nodule, two facts are noteworthy. First, the incidence of malignancy is extremely low (below 1%) in completely

TABLE 48
Thyroid Carcinoma

Feature	Papillary (60%)	Follicular (20%)	Anaplastic (10%)
Peak incidence (age)	Second, third, and fourth decade	Fourth decade	Fifth
Sex preponderance	Female	Female	Either sex
Usual presentation	Single nodule	Single nodule	Irregular, hard lump
Scan	Hypofunctional nodule	Hypofunctional or functional	Hypofunctional
Metastases	Lymph nodes Local invasion Systemic (bone lungs)	Systemic Lymph nodes Local	Locally invasive, distant spread
Multicentric origin	+	+	?
TSH dependence	Yes	Yes	No
Sensitivity to ^{131}I	Yes	Yes	No
Prognosis	Good if properly treated	Fair if properly treated	Poor

cystic thyroid nodules. Second, the incidence of malignancy is negligible in a solitary "hot" nodule (autonomously functioning thyroid nodule). Although it is generally agreed that the incidence of malignancy is low in multinodular glands, this statement should be tempered by observations that anaplastic cancer may develop in patients with longstanding multinodular goiters and medullary carcinoma can manifest as bilateral thyroid nodules. The incidence of malignancy in thyroid nodules is inversely related to the patient's age. The clinical variables that influence this incidence have been outlined in Table 48 and mainly consist of age, size and growth rate of the nodule, presence of lymphadenopathy, and pressure effects.

2. Lymphadenopathy. Occasionally, thyroid cancer may present with lymph node enlargement involving the posterior cervical or submental group of nodes. Careful palpation of the thyroid gland often reveals the presence of an abnormality such as a palpable nodule. Very rarely, the palpatory findings may be normal.

3. Horseness. This symptom, resulting from involvement of the recurrent laryngeal nerve, can be encountered in any type of thyroid carcinoma.

4. Functional abnormalities. Although primary malignancy of the thyroid is characteristically associated with euthyroidism, rarely, the patient with thyroid cancer may manifest clinical or biochemical hyperthyroidism through one of three mechanisms. Disseminated disease (particularly to bones) with hyperfunctional metastases can result in hy-

perthyroidism. Rarely, malignant nodules can be functional and secrete hormone, particularly T_3, resulting in T_3 hyperthyroidism. Occasionally, an entity called "malignant pseudothyroiditis" can result in transient hyperthyroidism. In this setting, tissue necrosis with accentuated hormonal release may result in transient hyperthyroidism analogous to subacute thyroiditis.

18.4. Diagnostic Studies

18.4.1. Thyroid Imaging

Most thyroid carcinomas appear relatively "cold" on thyroid scan. However, carcinoma can and does occur in patients with functional nodules, most notably in the case of follicular carcinoma.

18.4.2. Fine-Needle Aspiration Biopsy

In this procedure, the nodule is aspirated by a fine needle to examine for cells that may have been "shed" by the neoplasm. The value of the procedure, to a large degree, is influenced by the experience of the aspirator and the expertise of the cytopathologist. In the hands of experts, the procedure can predict the presence of malignancy in a nodule with 85% to even 90% accuracy.

18.4.3. Thyroid Function Tests

These are usually normal except in the rare cases of thyroid carcinoma associated with hyperthyroidism.

18.4.4. Metastatic Study

An abnormal chest X ray, abnormal bone scan, abnormal lymph node biopsy, and an immobile vocal cord on indirect laryngoscopy are all indicators of distant or local spread. Two important observations pertain as they relate to the metastatic workup of differentiated thyroid carcinoma. First, searching for "functional" metastases with the use of ^{131}I is futile as long as functional thyroid tissue is present in the neck. Even a small amount of functioning thyroid tissue in the neck can compete for the tracer dose of isotope, minimizing the chances of the metastatic lesions picking up the tracer dose. This is one of the main reasons for removing as much thyroid tissue as possible during surgery (by near-total thyroidectomy) to facilitate detection of functional metastases. Second, plasma thyroglobulin does not help in the distinction between benign and malignant lesions. This measurement assumes importance only after the thyroid gland is completely ablated. Serial measurements of thyroglobulin in the plasma following complete ablation are an extremely useful adjunctive aid in detecting metastases of differentiated thyroid cancer (Section 18.6).

The diagnostic tests used in the evaluation of medullary thyroid cancer are discussed in Chapter 52.

18.5. Prognosis

The prognosis of papillary, follicular, and anaplastic cancer of the thyroid should be viewed separately, since they vary considerably. Papillary thyroid carcinoma is the least aggressive of all thyroid cancers. When the size of the initial lesion (nodule) is below 1.5 cm, the prognostic outcome following treatment is excellent. Even though nearly a third of patients with papillary carcinoma show local lymph node involvement at the time of initial surgery, this does not adversely affect the outcome. In the absence of distant metastases (bone, lung), papillary carcinomas, treated properly, do not adversely affect life expectancy. The prognosis is less satisfactory when there is capsular invasion or distant spread and in older patients, particularly males.

Follicular carcinoma, has a greater propensity for vascular spread than papillary cancer. The survival rate 10 to 15 years following initial surgery is 50–60% in the absence of distant metastases. The prognosis is adversely affected by nodule size (>3.5 cm), histological evidence of vascular invasion, the presence of distant spread, and older age.

Anaplastic carcinoma, an undifferentiated variety of malignancy, is extremely aggressive, spreading by contiguity and causing obstruction to the trachea, esophagus, or mediastinum. Most patients with anaplastic carcinoma are dead within a year following diagnosis.

Since differentiated carcinomas of thyroid (papillary, follicular) show a favorable outcome when detected early and when contained within the neck, attempts at early detection and aggressive treatment are crucial. Experience in the past decade has dispelled the myth that differentiated thyroid carcinoma is really a "benign cancer." Unless treated effectively, papillary thyroid cancer can and does kill.

18.6. Treatment

The treatment of differentiated carcinomas of the thyroid (papillary and follicular) can be viewed together. The proper application of the three modalities of therapy—surgery, radioactive iodine, and *levo*-thyroxine suppression—forms the basis of treatment.

The primary treatment modality for differentiated thyroid carcinoma, whether it is limited to a small palpable nodule or associated with metastases, is surgery. The recommended procedure is near-total thyroidectomy, i.e., removal of all but a rim of tissue to preserve parathyroids. The reasons for recommending near-total thyroidectomy are threefold. First and foremost, unless the "normal" functioning tissue is removed, early detection of distant metastases with use of the ^{131}I will be precluded because of competition by the thyroid tissue for ^{131}I. Second, even if distant metastases are evident by other means (bone films, conventional bone scans, etc.), treatment of these metastases cannot satisfactorily be achieved unless the thyroid gland is out of the way. Third, differentiated thyroid cancers are multicentric and often tend to recur in the contralateral lobe. Thus, the preferred surgical recommendation for treatment of differentiated thyroid cancer is near-total thyroidectomy with one possible exception: when the papillary cancer is below 1.5 cm, the outcome following lobectomy is as good as that following more extensive surgery.

After surgery the most crucial step is the detection of distant, early metastases, since this is a major determinant of the prognosis. The best means of achieving this is to deliberately allow the patient to become hypothyroid. The primary hypothyroid state with its elevated TSH level, affords the best setting to detect functioning TSH-dependent metastases by the use of ^{131}I. Thus, 6 weeks after surgery, the serum levels of T_4 and TSH are obtained; if primary hypothyroidism is established, additional blood is drawn for baseline thyroglobulin level, and the patient is evaluated with whole body scan. The demonstration of residual tissue in the thyroid bed or documentation of isotopic pick up in bones or lungs is an indication for radioactive iodine therapy.

Following surgical (and, if needed, radioactive iodine) ablation, the patient with differentiated thyroid carcinoma should be placed on suppressive doses of *levo*-thyroxine, 300 μg daily.

A progressive increase in serum thyroglobulin (performed after withdrawal of *levo*-thyroxine) is indicative of local recurrence or distal metastases; combined with whole-body scan, serum thyroglobulin determination serves as a good adjunctive tool in the follow-up evaluation of these patients.

The treatment for anaplastic carcinoma is disappointing. Palliative resection of the thyroid may be necessary to alleviate respiratory distress. Chemotherapy with adriamycin has been tried with limited success.

Selected Readings

Ashcraft, M. W., and Van Herle, A. J.: Management of thyroid nodules II, *Head Neck Surg.* **3:**297, 1981.

Beierwaltes, W. H.: The treatment of hyperthyroidism with iodine 131, *Semin. Nucl. Med.* **8:**95, 1978.

Beierwaltes, W. H.: The treatment of thyroid carcinoma with radioactive iodine, *Semin. Nucl. Med.* **1:**79, 1978.

Borst, G. C., Eil, C., and Butman, K. D.: Euthyroid hyperthyroxinemia, *Ann. Intern. Med.* **98:**366, 1983.

Brennan, M. D.: Thyroid hormones, *Mayo Clin. Proc.* **55:**33, 1980.

Brooks, M. H., and Waldstein, S. S.: Free thyroxine concentrations in thyroid storm, *Ann. Intern. Med.* **93:**694, 1980.

Burrow, G. N.: Hyperthyroidism during pregnancy, *N. Engl. J. Med.* **298:**150, 1978.

Cheron, R. G., Kaplan, M. M., Larsen, P. R., *et al.*: Neonatal thyroid function after propylthiouracil therapy for maternal Graves' disease, *N. Engl. J. Med.* **304:**525, 1981.

Chopra, I. J., and Solomon, D. H.: Thyroid function tests and their alteration by drugs, *Pharmacol. Ther.* **1:**367, 1976.

Chopra, I. J., Hershman, J. M., Paardridge, W. M., *et al.*: Thyroid function in nonthyroidal illness (U.C.I.A. conference), *Ann. Intern. Med.* **98:**946, 1983.

Cooper, D. S.: Antithyroid drugs, *N. Engl. J. Med.* **311:**1353, 1984.

Crowley, W. F., Ridgway, E. C., Bough, E. W., *et al.*: Noninvasive evaluation of cardiac function in hypothyroidism, *N. Engl. J. Med.* **296:**1, 1977.

Davis, P. J., and Davis, F. B.: Hyperthyroidism in patients over the age of 60 years, *Medicine (Baltimore)* **53:**161, 1974.

Evered, D., and Hall, R.: Hypothyroidism, *Br. Med. J.* **2:**290, 1972.

Glennon, J. A., Gordon, E. S., and Sawin, C. T.: Hypothyroidism after low dose ^{131}I treatment of hyperthyroidism, *Ann. Intern. Med.* **76:**721, 1972.

Gluck, F. B., Nusynowitz, M. L., Plymate, S., *et al.*: Chronic lymphocytic thyroiditis thyrotoxicosis, and low radioactive iodine uptake, *N. Engl. J. Med.* **293:**624, 1975.

Gobien, R. P.: Aspiration biopsy of the solitary thyroid nodule, *Radiol. Clin. North Am.* **17:**543, 1979.

Hall, R., and Scanlon, M. F.: Hypothyroidism: Clinical features and complications, *Clin. Endocrinol. Metab.* **8:**29, 1979.

Hamburger, J. I.: Evaluation of toxicity in solitary nontoxic autonomously functioning thyroid nodules, *J. Clin. Endocrinol. Metab.* **50:**1089, 1980.

Hershman, J. M., and Pittman, J. A., Jr.: Utility of the radioimmunoassay of serum thyrotrophin in man, *Ann. Intern. Med.* **74:**481, 1971.

Hothem, A. L., Thomas, C. G., and Van Wyk, J. J.: Selection of treatment in the management of thyrotoxicosis in childhood and adolescence, *Ann. Surg.* **187:**593, 1978.

Katz, S. M., and Vickery, A. L.: The fibrous variant of Hashimoto's thyroiditis, *Hum. Pathol.* **5:**161, 1974.

Klein, I., and Levey, G. S.: New perspectives on thyroid hormone, catecholamines, and the heart, *Am. J. Med.* **76:**167, 1984.

Klein, I., and Levey, G. S.: Unusual manifestations of hypothyroidism, *Arch. Intern. Med.* **144:**123, 1984.

Klein, I., Parker, M., Shebert, R., *et al.*: Hypothyroidism presenting as muscle stiffness and pseudohypertrophy: Hoffman's syndrome, *Am. J. Med.* **70:**891, 1981.

Larsen, P. R.: Tests of thyroid function, *Med. Clin. North Am.* **59:**1063, 1973.

Levine, H. D.: Compromise therapy in the patient with angina pectoris and hypothyroidism—a clinical assessment, *Am. J. Med.* **69:**411, 1980.

Levine, S. N.: Current concepts of thyroiditis,, *Arch. Intern. Med.* **143:**1952, 1983.

Locke, W.: Unusual manifestations of Graves' disease, *Med. Clin. North Am.* **51:**915, 1967.

Mazzaferri, E. L., and Skillman, T. G.: Thyroid storm, *Arch. Intern. Med.* **124:**684, 1969.

Mazzaferri, E. L., and Young, R. L.: Papillary thyroid carcinoma—a ten year follow-up report of impact of therapy in 576 patients, *Am. J. Med.* **70:**511, 1981.

Mazzaferri, E. L., Young, R. L., Oertel, J. E., *et al.*: Papillary thyroid carcinoma the impact of therapy in 576 patients, *Medicine* **56:**171, 1977.

Nofal, M. M., Beierwaltes, W. H., and Patno, M. E.: Treatment of hyperthyroidism with sodium iodide I^{131}, *J.A.M.A.* **197:**87, 1966.

Rosenbaum, R. L., and Barzel, U. S.: Levothyroxine replacement for primary hypothyroidism decreases with age, *Ann. Intern. Med.* **96:**53, 1982.

Scheible, W., Leopold, G. R., Woo, V. L., *et al.*: High resolution real-time ultrasonography of thyroid nodules, *Radiology* **133:**413, 1979.

Schimmel, M., and Utiger, R.: Thyroidal and peripheral production of thyroid hormones, *Ann. Intern. Med.* **87:**760, 1977.

Schneider, A. B., Favus, M. J., Stachura, M. E., *et al.*: Incidence, prevalence, and characteristics of radiation induced thyroid tumors, *Am. J. Med.* **64:**243, 1978.

Senior, R. M., Birge, S. J., Wessler, S., et al.: The recognition and management of myxedema coma, J.A.M.A. **217:**61, 1971.

Solomon, D. H., Chopra, I. J., Chopra, U., et al.: Identification of subgroups of euthyroid Graves' ophthalmopathy, N. Engl. J. Med. **296:**181, 1977.

Sridama, V., McCormick, M., Kaplan, E. L., et al.: Long term follow-up study of compensated low dose ^{131}I therapy for Graves' disease, N. Engl. J. Med. **311:**426, 1984.

Sterling, K., Refetoff, S., and Selenkow, H. A.: T_3 toxicosis–thyrotoxicosis due to elevated triiodothyronine levels, J.A.M.A. **213:**571, 1970.

Stock, J. M., Surks, M. I., and Oppenheimer, J. H.: Replacement doseage of l-thyroxine in hypothyroidism: A re-evaluation, N. Engl. J. Med. **290:**529, 1974.

Swanson, J. W., Kelly, J. J., Jr., and McConahey, W. M.: Neurologic aspects of thyroid dysfunction, Mayo Clin. Proc. **56:**504, 1981.

Thomas, F. B., Mazzaferri, E. L., and Skillman, T. G.: Apathetic thyrotoxicosis: A distinctive clinical and laboratory entity, Ann. Intern. Med. **72:**679, 1970.

Thompson, N. W., Dunn, E. L., Freitas, J. E., et al.: Surgical treatment of thyrotoxicosis in children and adolescents, J. Pediatr. Surg. **12:**1009, 1977.

Totten, M. A., and Wool, M. S.: Medical treatment of hyperthyroidism. Med. Clin. North Am. **63:**321, 1979.

Tunbridge, W. M. G., Evered, D. C., Hall, R., et al.: The spectrum of thyroid disease in a community. The Whickam survey, Clin. Endocrinol. **7:**481, 1977.

Van Herle, A. J., Rich, P., Ljung, B. E., et al.: The thyroid nodule, Ann. Intern. Med. **96:**221, 1982.

Waldstein, S. S., Slodki, S. J., Kaginiec, G. I., et al.: A clinical study of thyroid storm, Ann. Intern. Med. **52:**626, 1960.

Woolf, P. D.: Transient painless thyroiditis with hyperthyroidism. A variant of lymphocytic thyroiditis, Endocrinol. Rev. **1:**411, 1980.

III

The Parathyroids

The Parathyroids

III

19

Anatomy of the Parathyroids

The parathyroid glands are usually four in number, two superior and two inferior. Embryologically, the parathyroid glands are derived from the fourth and the third branchial pouches. The two superior parathyroids, which are derived from the fourth branchial pouch, are located at the posterior aspect of the lateral lobes of the thyroid, corresponding to the cricothyroid junction. Positional variations are less frequent with the superior parathyroid glands, and hence they are easily identifiable during neck exploration. The inferior parathyroids, which are derived from the third branchial pouch, follow the origin and descent of the thymus very closely until they reach their eventual destination at the lower poles of the thyroid gland. Considerable anatomic variations can occur in the position of the inferior parathyroids, and they are found in their expected location (lower poles of the thyroid) in only half of all cases. The lower glands are very often found in the thymic tongue; rarely, they may be located in the mediastinum within the thymus or high in the neck adjacent to the carotid sheath because of an arrest in descent. In 2% to 4% of subjects, a fifth (or sixth) parathyroid gland may be present.

The anatomic relationships of the parathyroid glands are extremely crucial. The major landmarks of the superior parathyroid glands are the recurrent laryngeal nerve and the middle thyroid artery, since the gland is located at the junction of these two extremely important structures. The posterior thyroid capsule lies anterior to the upper parathyroid, which is often firmly attached to this capsule. When the upper parathyroid is embedded in the superior pole of the lobe, a rim of thyroid tissue surrounds the gland. The inferior parathyroid is located slightly below the lower pole of the thyroid lobes and just lateral to the trachea.

The parathyroid glands, both upper and lower, are supplied by branches of the inferior thyroid artery. The venous drainage, however, is different for the upper and lower parathyroids. The superior parathyroids are drained by the superior thyroid veins, whereas the inferior parathyroids are drained by the inferior thyroid veins. Occasionally, however, some crossover can be seen, resulting in the superior parathyroid being drained by both superior and inferior thyroid veins.

Macroscopically, the parathyroids are elliptical, flat structures measuring 6 mm in their longest diameter. *In vivo,* because of its fat content, the gland can be mistaken for fat tissue by the inexperienced eye.

Microscopically, the parathyroid glands consist of two types of cells— chief cells and oxyphill cells—dispersed within a variable amount of fatty tissue. The chief cells contain secretory granules and are responsible for the synthesis and secretion of PTH. They can easily be recognized by the presence of a prominent cell membrane and a dark, centrally located nucleus. The secretory apparatus of the chief cells—the endoplasmic reticulum and Golgi apparatus—can be readily identified by election microscopy. The oxyphilic cells do not synthesize or secrete hormone.

20

Physiology
The Control, Regulation, and Actions of Parathyroid Hormone

20.1. Introduction

Parathyroid hormone (PTH) is the predominant regulator of calcium and phosphorus metabolism. It maintains calcium (and phosphorus) homeostasis by performing a delicate balancing act mediated by its direct actions on the renal tubules and bone cells and by its indirect action on the intestines.

20.2. Secretion

Parathyroid hormone is synthesized in the parathyroid glands from a precursor prepro-PTH (115 amino acids). Intraglandular conversion of pre-pro-PTH into pro-PTH (90 amino acids) and PTH (84 amino acids) probably takes place in the rough endoplasmic reticulum. The native hormone is released as such into the circulation, undergoing immediate cleavage into a carboxy (C) terminal and an amino (N) terminal. Under normal circumstances very little pro-PTH or prepro-PTH is released into the circulation. The secretion of PTH by the secretory granules within the parathyroid cells is mediated through cyclic AMP. *In vitro* evidence suggests that the magnitude of PTH secretion parallels the quantity of cyclic AMP generated within the secretory cells.

20.3. Control of Secretion

The single most important regulator of PTH secretion by the parathyroids is the ambient calcium level in the serum. Thus, hypocalcemia stimulates

PTH secretion and release, whereas hypercalcemia suppresses these phenomena. However, it is important to recognize that this inverse relationship between PTH and serum calcium operates over a narrow range of serum calcium (7.5 to 10.5 mg/dl). When the serum calcium concentration exceeds or decreases below this range, the changes in PTH secretory rate are only minimally affected. It is now evident that the parathyroid glands do continue to secrete a basal amount of hormone despite hypercalcemia and that this basal, "nonsuppressible" secretory process continues independent of hypercalcemia. Maximal secretory responses occur during early hypocalcemia, and, notably, there is a lack of progressive increase in the secretory rate in response to profound hypocalcemia. Thus, although it is true that a low calcium stimulates and a high calcium suppresses PTH secretion, the magnitude of the secretory response does not correlate with the magnitude of the changes in serum calcium.

Magnesium, another divalent cation, controls PTH secretion in a variable fashion. Acute hypomagnesemia stimulates PTH release, whereas chronic hypomagnesemia impairs PTH secretion and blunts the ability of the parathyroids to respond to the hypocalcemic stimulus.

Inorganic phosphate does not directly influence PTH secretion or release. The changes in PTH secretion following phosphate infusion are a reflection of the changes in serum calcium levels consequent to hyperphosphatemia.

Catecholamines also play a role in the secretion and release of PTH. *In vitro* studies indicate that PTH release in augmented by catecholamines. In humans, evidence to imply a role for catecholamines in the mediation of PTH release is supported by three lines of evidence: first, asthmatics using isoproterenol, a β-adrenergic agent, demonstrate a heightened tendency for hyperparathyroidism; second, the use of β blockers such as propranolol evokes a lowering in PTH levels; third, transient hyperparathyroidism can be observed in patients with pheochromocytoma, reversible on removing the adrenal tumor.

20.4. Immunoheterogeneity

Parathyroid hormone released into the blood circulates as different fragments. Immediately after release, PTH is cleaved into a carboxy terminal (C terminal) and an amino terminal (N terminal). The C terminal has a long half-life, is excreted by the kidneys, and is biologically inactive. The N terminal has an extremely short half-life, is internalized by target cells, and is the biologically active fragment. In addition to these two fragments, there are small fragments that contribute to C-terminal reactivity.

The immunoreactive PTH measures the fragments "seen" by the antisera employed. Figure 16 illustrates the amino acid sequence of the intact molecule (1–84), the N terminal (1–34), and the C terminal (35–84) (35–65) of the parathyroid hormone. Also shown are the characteristics of these fragments (Table 49).

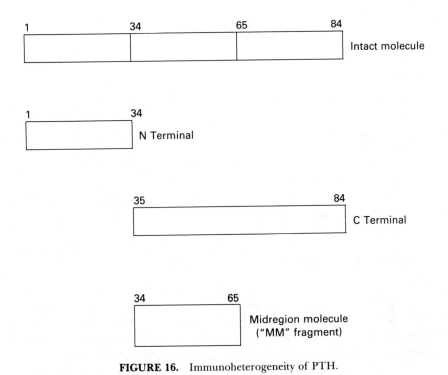

FIGURE 16.   Immunoheterogeneity of PTH.

TABLE 49
Comparison of PTH Fragments

N Terminal	C Terminal	MM Fraction
Metabolically active	Inactive	Inactive
Very short half-life	Longer half-life	Longer half-life
Metabolized in target tissues	Degraded by the kidney and liver	Degraded by the kidney and liver
Not sensitive for Dx of 1° HPT	80% sensitive for Dx of 1° HPT	Combined C-terminal and MM assays 90% sensitive for Dx of 1° HPT
Minimally elevated in CRF	Markedly elevated in CRF	Markedly elevated in CRF
Does not separate normals from 1° HPT	Clear separation of normals and 1° HPT	Extremely clear separation of normals and 1° HPT when combined C-terminal and MM assays are performed
No cross reactivity with "tumor PTH"	Some cross reactivity with tumor PTH (as low as 2% to as high as 18%)	Unknown

20.5. Actions

The actions of PTH on the renal tubules, the bone tissue, and the gut are as follows:

1. PTH decreases tubular reabsorption of phosphorus by the renal tubules and thus causes phosphaturia.
2. PTH increases tubular reabsorption of calcium and thus promotes calcium retention.
3. PTH stimulates osteoclastic bone resorption and thus facilitates mobilization of calcium from bone (osteolysis).
4. PTH promotes intestinal absorption of calcium (and phosphorus) indirectly through stimulation of renal hydroxylation of 25-hydroxycholecalciferol to 1,25-dihydroxycholecalciferol.
5. PTH also has an anabolic effect on bone mass, an action seen only during near-normal secretory rates of the hormone.

The action of PTH on the target cell is mediatd by activation of adenylate cyclase with the subsequent generation of cyclic AMP. At least three components are needed for the activation of adenylate cyclase responsible for catalyzing cyclic AMP production: the hormone receptor, a guanine nucleotide-binding regulatory protein called the N protein/G unit, and the catalytic unit of the adenylate cyclase enzyme. The action of PTH on the target cell is exerted by a series of steps (Figure 17):

1. The first step is binding of the hormone (PTH) to its specific receptor located in the cell membrane.
2. The hormone–receptor complex associates with the N protein, which is part of the N protein/G unit, also located in the cell membrane.
3. As a result, the N protein binds GTP (guanosine triphosphate).
4. The N protein–GTP activates the GTPase activity, resulting in the association of the N–GTP complex with the catalytic moiety of adenylate cyclase, an enzyme that converts intracellular ATP into cyclic AMP.
5. The subsequent action of cyclic AMP is on protein kinases. These are phosphorylating enzymes composed of catalytic (C) and regulatory (R) subunits. Binding of cyclic AMP to the regulatory subunit frees the catalytic subunit.
6. The freed catalytic subunit allows phosphorylation of various proteins (S) within the cell. The activated proteins express hormone action.
7. The GTPase activity of N protein then converts GTP to GDP, which terminates activation.

With the above framework of the actions of PTH in perspective, each of the five major effects of the hormone on calcium (and phosphorus) homeostasis can be reviewed.

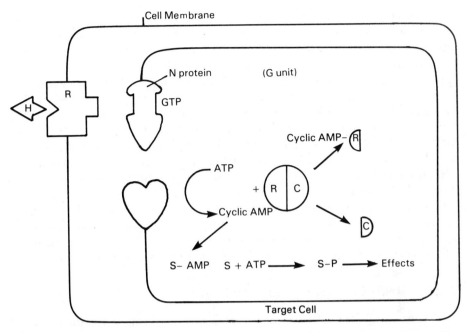

FIGURE 17. Mechanism of the action of PTH. H, hormone; R, receptor or cyclic-AMP-binding subunit of protein kinase; C, catalytic subunit.

20.5.1. Phosphaturic Effect of PTH

Parathyroid hormone is the predominant hormonal factor that controls the ambient serum phosphorus level by modulating the renal phosphorus threshold. Increased PTH secretion lowers this threshold and causes phosphaturia, whereas suppressed or absent PTH function is attended with marked increase in the threshold and consequently reduced phosphate excretion. This action of PTH was the earliest discovered action of that hormone, yet its biological significance is relatively unclear. It is felt that PTH-induced phosphaturia may reflect an adaptive mechanism to its calcium-mobilizing effect on bone. The PTH-induced phosphaturic action is associated with other ionic fluxes, the most significant of which is bicarbonate. The phosphate and bicarbonate rejected by the proximal tubule are not reabsorbed by the distal tubule, resulting in phosphate and bicarbonate losses. Since bicarbonate and phosphate are also liberated as counterions during PTH-induced calcium mobilization from the bone reservoir, it is tenable that the effect of the hormone on the tubules is a counteradaptive phenomenon to help excrete phosphate and bicarbonate.

Regardless of the physiological basis for the PTH-induced phosphaturia, this phenomenon serves as the index for PTH responsiveness. Administration of exogenous parathyroid extract and observation of the phosphate excretion in urine constituted the Ellsworth–Howard test to determine renal responsiveness to PTH. The test, today, has been modified by the additional measurement of cyclic AMP in urine after PTH administration. Cyclic AMP generation constitutes the first portion of PTH effect on the tubule, whereas phosphaturia is the second. Patients with pseudohypoparathyroidism represent a classic example of target organ resistance to the action of PTH. The mechanism may involve failure to generate cyclic AMP (and therefore phosphaturia as well) or failure to respond to the generated cyclic AMP because of a breakdown in intracellular signals distal to cyclic AMP formation.

Renal resistance to the action of PTH can be encountered under several circumstances: pseudohypoparathyroidism types I and II, which are congenital conditions characterized by inherent target organ resistance; renal failure resulting in loss of population of responsive tubules; or chronic hypomagnesemia, which may also impair tubular responsiveness to PTH, but to a lesser extent than it impairs bone responsiveness to PTH. The phosphaturic effect of PTH can be mimicked by severe hypercalcemia *per se* and by "tumor PTH."

20.5.2. Renal Calcium Retention by PTH

Although PTH causes decreased reabsorption of calcium by the proximal tubule (analogous to phosphate and bicarbonate), the hormone markedly enhances the distal tubular reabsorption of calcium (unlike phosphorus and bicarbonate). Therefore, the net effect of PTH on calcium handling by the renal tubules is one of calcium retention. The magnitude of the effect of PTH even overrides the calciuric response of mild to moderate hypercalcemia. Normally, since calcium is a threshold substance, hypercalcemia results in an increased filtered load of calcium. However, in the presence of concomitant PTH excess, increased tubular reabsorption of calcium predominates, resulting in calcium retention rather than calciuria. When the rise in the serum calcium level is profound and chronic, the PTH effect on the tubules can be overcome, resulting in calcium excretion in urine.

20.5.3. Bone Resorption Induced by PTH

The third major effect of PTH is its catabolic effect on bone. This osteolytic effect of PTH consists of a fast and a slow component, the latter involving enzymes synthesis. The rapid component mobilizes calcium from the bone without bone destruction, whereas the slow component is characterized by destruction of bone matrix. Administration of PTH to experimental animals results in enhanced uridine incorporation into the osteoclasts with increased synthesis of cytoplasmic and nuclear RNA. With continued PTH administration, there is an increase in the proliferation of the osteoclasts and their precursors. The initial calcium-mobilizing effect of PTH does not involve phosphorus mobilization, but with a chronic, slow effect, both calcium and phosphorus are released from the bone into the circulation.

The resorptive effect of PTH on the bone can be modified by several factors:

1. Resistance to the action of PTH can be congenital, as in pseudohypoparathyroidism.
2. Hyperphosphatemia *per se* can blunt the calcium-mobilizing effect of PTH on bone. Such is the case in the skeletal resistance seen with chronic renal failure.
3. Chronic hypomagnesemia also impairs bone responsiveness to PTH. Such is the case in the hypocalcemia secondary to chronic hypomagnesemia seen in several clinical states (alcoholism, diarrhea, etc.).
4. The presence of "osteoid tissue" also impairs the calcium-mobilizing effect of PTH. Such is the case is osteomalacia or rickets, where the calcium is low despite high PTH concentrations. When the condition is treated with vitamin D and the osteoid tissue decreases, there may be a sudden flooding of calcium into the circulation because of the already high PTH, resulting in hypercalcemia. Osteoid tissue probably poses an anatomic or functional barrier to the release of calcium from bone.

The calcium-mobilizing as well as bone resorptive actions of parathyroid hormone are shared and mimicked by several "humoral mediators." These include "tumor PTH," osteoclast-activating factor, prostaglandins, and vitamin-D-like sterols, particularly 1,25-dihydroxycholecalciferol. The mechanism of hypercalcemia in the "humoral hypercalcemic syndromes of cancer" is thus identical to the mechanism of hypercalcemia in primary hyperparathyroidism.

20.5.4. Action of PTH on Intestinal Calcium Absorption

Parathyroid hormone enhances the fractional absorption of calcium and phosphorus by the intestines. This action is slow and indirectly mediated by the metabolite 1,25-dihydroxycholecalciferol, which is PTH dependent. The synthetic steps involved in the formation of the potent vitamin D metabolite are shown in Figure 18.

Hydroxylation of the hepatic metabolite 25-hydroxycholecalciferol to the renal metabolite 1,25-dihydroxylcholecalciferol is a crucial step, since the latter is at least 10 times more potent than the parent compound. The formation of 1,25-dihydroxylcholecalciferol is dependent on several factors:

1. Availability of adequate renal tissue and renal function, since the renal mitochondrial enzymes, 1-α-hydroxylase is essential for the conversion; the source of the enzyme is probably the proximal convoluted tubule.
2. Parathyroid hormone, which stimulates the 1-α-hydroxylase to convert 25-hydroxycholecalciferol to 1,25-dihydroxycholecalciferol.

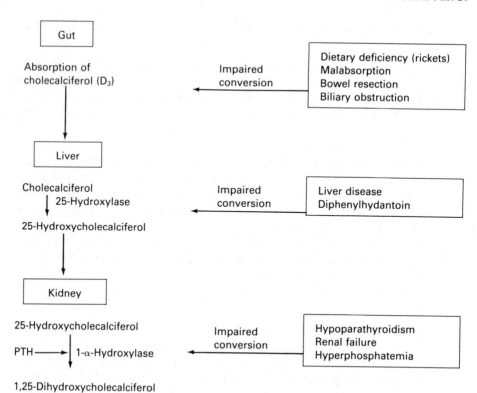

FIGURE 18. Vitamin D metabolism and disorders affecting the various steps in synthesis.

3. Optimum phosphorus concentrations within the renal cells. Hyperphosphatemia suppresses the enzyme activity of 1-α-hydroxylase.
4. Optimum calcium concentrations within the renal cells. Hypocalcemia stimulates, and hypercalcemia suppresses, the enzyme activity of 1-α-hydroxylase.

Thus, renal failure, hypoparathyroidism, and hyperphosphatemia from any cause suppress the formation of 1,25-dihydroxycholecalciferol, resulting in vitamin D insufficiency resistant to vitamin D administration. In the absence of parathyroid hormone (or in the presence of hypercalcemia), 24,25-dihydroxy-D_3 is produced, which has variable biological activity depending on the species tested. The actions of 1,25-dihydroxycholecalciferol are threefold:

1. This most potent vitamin D analogue stimulates intestinal absorption of calcium.
2. 1,25-Dihydroxycholecalciferol also stimulates intestinal absorption of phosphorus.
3. This metabolite is a powerful mobilizer of calcium from bone.

The mechanism of action of 1,25-dihydroxycholecalciferol on its target cells, particularly the intestine, resembles that of other steroid hormones. Hence, the term "hormone D_3" is often used to denote 1,25-dihydroxycholecalciferol. This steroid combines with a receptor protein in the cytosol of the intestinal cell with subsequent interaction with the nuclear protein, resulting in the transcription of messenger RNA. The effect is the formation of calcium transport proteins within the cell. These calcium transport proteins move to the brush border surface and facilitate calcium absorption.

The similarities and differences between PTH and 1,25-dihydroxycholecalciferol are intriguing. Both possess similar effects on the bone in terms of mobilizing calcium. However, the predominant role of 1,25-dihydroxycholecalciferol is to mineralize the osteoid and form bone. In regard to intestinal transport of calcium and phosphorus, PTH does not have a direct action but plays a crucial role in stimulating the formation of the most potent vitamin D_3 to effectively carry out this function. Finally, as far as the effects on the renal tubule are concerned, 1,25-dihydroxycholecalciferol does not share the phosphaturic effects of PTH. In physiological doses the vitamin analogue facilitates calcium retention similarly to PTH.

20.5.5. The Anabolic Effect of PTH

This effect of PTH, a hormone traditionally associated with bone destruction, has recently come to light. It probably represents the action of PTH when present in normal concentrations as opposed to the catabolic bone effects that are manifestly predominant when the hormone is present in high concentrations. The anabolic effects of PTH consist of promoting bone formation and proper mineralization. In animal experimental models using bone biopsy studies, high concentration of PTH inhibit bone formation, but as the levels decline, uridine incorporation by the osteoblasts begin to increase.

Collectively, the actions of PTH on the skeleton are geared in different directions when the hormone is secreted at a physiologically normal rate as opposed to a hypersecretory state. When the hormone is secreted at a near-normal rate, the predominant role of the hormone is anabolic in terms of the skeleton. Parathyroid hormone stimulates bone formation and gears up its action to promote calcification of the newly formed matrix. This is done by calling on vitamin D to provide the necessary calcium flux via an increase in intestinal calcium absorption, a PTH-dependent phenomenon. Parathyroid hormone also maintains a positive calcium balance by renal conservation of calcium. The net effect, it appears, in the physiological state is to promote bone formation and facilitate all the mechanisms required to mineralize the bone. When a period of calcium stress is superimposed (pregnancy, lactation, etc.), PTH adapts the role of calcium mobilizer, by moving the calcium out of the skeleton and supplying the other tissues with the mobilized calcium. When an autonomous hypersecretory state develops (primary hyperparathyroidism), the gears shift in the direction of bone catabolism, resulting in inappropriate and unnecessary calcium mobilization and, consequently, hypercalcemia. The negative balance in the skeleton and the bone turnover can become exceedingly catabolic in extreme situations, resulting in "excretion of the skeleton through the kidneys."

The differential actions of PTH during physiological and pathological states are typical of many hormonal situations wherein too much of a good thing becomes deleterious.

21

Hypercalcemia

21.1. Introduction

In Chapter 20, the regulatory mechanisms that control calcium homeostasis are outlined. This chapter focuses on hypercalcemia to provide a general overview in terms of etiology, mechanisms involved in causation, and clinical presentation. Also, the general principles in the diagnostic and therapeutic approach to hypercalcemia are discussed.

Hypercalcemia is defined as a persistent increase in the serum calcium levels above the upper limits of normal established for the particular laboratory. For most laboratories, this is 10.8 mg/dl. The calcium measured in the serum is the fraction bound to serum proteins, particularly albumin. In most circumstances, there is an excellent correlation between the bound fraction of the calcium in serum and the "free" ionic calcium. The only circumstances characterized by significant discordance between the bound and free calciums are alterations in the pH of blood, which affect the binding of calcium to proteins.

The interpretation of the serum calcium should take into consideration the serum albumin level and the status of hydration. A drop in serum albumin by 1 g is associated with a decline in the measured "total" calcium by 0.8 mg/dl; alterations in serum globulins can occasionally affect the serum calcium level, the most striking example being represented by multiple myeloma, a condition that is associated with an extremely high incidence of "true" hypercalcemia as well. Also, the status of hydration affects the serum calcium to a small but significant extent; severe volume contraction can increase the serum calcium by as much as 1 mg/dl, underscoring the need to repeat the calcium after restoring volume expansion.

The demonstration of "persistent" hypercalcemia on at least three consecutive occasions clearly denotes an underlying perturbation in calcium homeostasis.

21.2. Etiology

Instead of a review of the etiology of hypercalcemia in terms of a list of conditions that elevate the calcium, a classification based on the mechanism of hypercalcemia provides a better perspective. There are four major mechanisms that can lead to hypercalcemia: increased mobilization from bone by resorption, increased absorption from the gut, decreased excretion by the kidneys, and increased dietary calcium. Table 50 illustrates the conditions that cause hypercalcemia based on mechanism. As can be seen, some etiologies for hypercalcemia operate by more than one mechanism.

Since more than 90% of calcium reserve in the body is in the bone pool, it is not surprising that the most frequent mechanism for hypercalcemia is increased mobilization of calcium from the bones by resorption. The two most frequent disorders that cause hypercalcemia by bone resorption as the major mechanism are primary hyperparathyroidism and malignant disease. The mechanisms and the nature of hypercalcemia caused by specific etiologies are discussed below.

Primary hyperparathyroidism, the single most frequent etiology for hypercalcemia in individuals under the age of 50, causes hypercalcemia by two crucial mechanisms: by osteoclastic stimulation and by increasing the absorption of calcium through the gut by stimulating the renal mitochondrial conversion of 25-hydroxy-D_3 to 1,25-dihydroxy-D_3. The hypercalcemia of primary hyperparathyroidism is usually mild, asymptomatic, and sustained.

TABLE 50
The Mechanisms and Etiology of Hypercalcemia

Mechanism of hypercalcemia	Etiologic disorder
Increased bone resorption	Primary hyperparathyroidism
	Metastatic bone disease
	Multiple myeloma
	Humoral hypercalcemia of cancer
	Vitamin D (or A) intoxication
	Hyperthyroidism
	Paget's with immobilization
	Secondary hyperparathyroidism
	Sarcoidosis
	Thiazides, estrogens(?)
Increased gut absorption	Sarcoidosis
	Hypervitaminosis D
	Granulomatous lung disease (TB, fungi, berylliosis)
	Primary hyperparathyroidism
Decreased renal excretion	Acute renal failure
	Thiazides, lithium, etc.
	Milk alkali syndrome
Increased dietary calcium	Milk alkali syndrome
	Overmedication with replacement

Occasionally the serum calcium in primary hyperthyroidism can exceed 15 mg/dl with serious sequelae and significant symptoms. Intermittency of hypercalcemia may rarely be seen with primary hyperparathyroidism. Adenoma of the parathyroid accounts for the primary hyperparathyroidism in more than 85% of cases.

Malignancy-related hypercalcemia is the single most frequent etiology of hypercalcemia in individuals over the age 50, especially in hospitalized patients. There are two mechanisms whereby malignant diseases cause hypercalcemia: by bone destruction secondary to metastases and by secretion of a variety of humoral mediators that stimulate bone resorption. In many instances both of these mechanisms prevail. Metastatic bone disease can occur from any primary malignancy, the three most common ones being malignancies of the breast, lung, and kidneys, followed by prostate, thyroid, and gastrointestinal neoplasms. Humoral mediation of hypercalcemia can be secondary to secretion of PTH, osteoclast-activating factor (OAF), the prostaglandins, or vitamin-D-like sterols. Parathyroid hormone secretion by neoplastic disease (pseudohyperparathyroidism) can occur with any malignancy but is most frequently associated with renal cell carcinoma, bronchogenic carcinoma (squamous), and uterine cancer. The prototype of OAF secretion is multiple myeloma, followed by Hodgkins's and non-Hodgkin's lymphomas. Prostaglandin secretion by cancer is best exemplified by bronchogenic cancer, particularly the oat cell type. Secretion of 1,25-dihydroxycholecalciferol is being recognized with increasing frequency, particularly with lymphomas. In addition to these two major mechanisms (metastases to bone and secretion of "humors by tumors"), another mechanism is the secretion of a "parathyrotropic substance" by neoplastic tissue, accounting for the remarkable frequency with which primary hyperparathyroidism occurs in association with cancer. The hypercalcemia of malignancy is usually of moderate to severe degree, evolves rapidly, and causes severe clinical effects.

Multiple myeloma deserves separate emphasis for several reasons. The hypercalcemia in myeloma is caused by direct effects of osteolytic lesions on the bone (often demonstrable as "punched-out" lesions by X ray) as well as by secretion of the humoral mediator osteoclast-activating factor. The hypercalcemia in myeloma assumes importance in staging the disease and is often responsible for deterioration in the already compromised renal function seen in this disease. Finally, although the hypercalcemia in myeloma can attain dangerous levels, it often responds remarkably well to aggressive therapeutic modalities.

Hypercalcemia in sarcoidosis is a consequence of increased absorption of calcium across the gut, an effect secondary to increased formation of 1,25-dihydroxycholecalciferol by sarcoid tissue. The hypercalcemia of sarcoidosis is associated with marked hypercalciuria, a phenomenon shared by hypervitaminosis D. Hypercalcemia in sarcoidosis usually indicates active disease and is seen in conjunction with abnormal chest radiography or abnormal liver function and with an elevated level of angiotensin-converting enzyme (ACE) in the serum.

The hypercalcemia seen in hyperthyroidism is characteristically mild, asymptomatic, and responds excellently to β blockers such as propranolol. Very rarely, the association of parathyroid adenoma and Graves' hyperthyroidism has been described. The mechanism underlying the hypercalcemia of hyperthyroidism is unclear and is presumed to be an effect of excess thyroid hormone on bone resorption.

Drug-induced hypercalcemia is self-limited. The hypercalcemia of thiazide diuretics results from a combination of factors: a primary effect on the renal tubules resulting in decreased excretion of calcium coupled with an adjunctive effect on the bone characterized by increased osteoclast responsiveness to PTH. The hallmarks of thiazide-diuretic-induced hypercalcemia are its mild degree and nonsustained nature. The demonstration of sustained hypercalcemia with thiazides is indicative of an underlying abnormality in calcium homeostasis. The other drug that causes hypercalcemia when abused is vitamin D. Hypervitaminosis D is encountered in food faddists on megavitamin therapy and during overzealous replacement therapy for hypoparathyroidism with vitamin D. The rapid evolution of hypercalcemia results at least in part from the concomitant renal compromise caused by hypervitaminosis D. Rare causes of drug-induced hypercalcemia include vitamin A overdose and lithium carbonate. The abandonment of the use of calcium carbonate and milk in treatment of peptic ulcer disease has resulted in the milk alkali syndrome being relegated to the status of a historical footnote.

The hypercalcemia of acute renal failure is also transient, occurring as a consequence of failure to excrete calcium by the renal tubules. An exception, it should be noted, is the acute renal failure of rhabdomyolysis (crush injury), which is associated with hypocalcemia during the phase of renal failure.

21.3. Clinical Features

The clinical consequences of hypercalcemia depend on the magnitude of elevation in the serum calcium and the rapidity with which the elevation occurred. The four major organ systems involved are the gastrointestinal, cardiovascular, renal, and neuropsychiatric systems.

The gastrointestinal manifestations of hypercalcemia are the most frequently encountered symptoms and include nausea, vomiting, anorexia, and constipation. The constipation, which can become quite severe, is often the reason for consulting the physician.

The cadiovascular features of hypercalcemia are variable, ranging on one extreme from mild hypertension to, on the other extreme, cardiac arrhythmias and sudden cardiac arrest during systole. The most common electrocardiographic abnormality is a shortened Q–T interval. Hypercalcemia renders patients with cardiac failure more susceptible to digitalis intoxication. Finally, chronic hypercalcemia has been etiologically linked to the development of coronary heart disease.

The effects of chronic hypercalcemia on the kidneys and tubules are threefold: nephrocalcinosis, polyuria, and the development of nephrogenic diabetes insipidus. Nephrocalcinosis, the fine crystallization of calcium deposits in the renal interstitium, is a sign of chronicity and is usually seen in primary hyperparathyroidism. When calcium levels in the serum are persistently elevated, the tubules tend to excrete calcium along with water, resulting in osmotic diuresis. Protracted hypercalcemia renders the collecting tubules insensitive to vasopressin, resulting in severe polyuria (nephrogenic DI) with dehydration and further worsening of the serum calcium.

The effects of hypercalcemia on the central nervous system are also variable. In its most severe form, hypercalcemia causes drowsiness, lethargy, and even coma, representing an important etiology of metabolic encephelopathy. Other effects of hypercalcemia include changes in behavior such as depression or irritability, easy fatigability, and muscle weakness with decreased tendon reflexes.

21.4. Diagnostic Studies

The diagnostic workup employed in arriving at the cause of hypercalcemia is highly variable; in some patients the etiology of hypercalcemia can be readily established by a single blood test (PTH assay), whereas in others an exhaustive array of diagnostic studies may be required to arrive at the precise etiology. There are three categories of tests that may be required in the evaluation of patients with hypercalcemia.

1. Tests that establish a parathyroid origin for hypercalcemia.
2. Tests that indicate a nonparathyroid origin for hypercalcemia.
3. Tests that are nonspecific.

The tests that establish a parathyroid origin include measurement of PTH level in the serum and other parameters that suggest increased bioactivity of PTH in the serum. These include measurement of nephrogenous cyclic AMP and phosphorus excretion indices (%TRP). Also included in this category are tests that unequivocally establish the effects of chronic primary hyperparathyroidism on target organs (subperiosteal bone resorption, renal calculus disease, or peptic ulcer disease). These and other tests of parathyroid hyperfunction are discussed in Chapter 22.

The tests that indicate a nonparathyroid etiology are studies that disclose evidence of metastatic disease of the bone (bone scan), multiple myeloma (serum and urine protein immunoelectrophoresis), malignant disease elsewhere, sarcoidosis, or hyperthyroidism.

The nonspecific tests that are of "nonhelp" are serum phosphorus, serum chloride, serum alkaline phosphatase, etc. The serum phosphorus is expected to be low in primary hyperparathyroidism but is so only in 30–35% of patients with this disease. Further, patients with malignancy-associated hypercalcemia may have hypophosphatemia, although generally it is normal or even high in this entity. The serum chloride is usually elevated in parathyroid-mediated hypercalcemia and is normal or low in non-PTH-mediated hypercalcemia. The calculation of chloride/phosphorus ratio may suggest PTH-mediated hypercalcemia, a ratio greater than 34 often favoring that entity. As for elevated alkaline phosphatase, this may be encountered in hypercalcemic states secondary to primary hyperparathyroidism, metastatic bone disease, or sarcoidosis.

21.5. Treatment

Aside from the primary therapy directed against the etiology that caused hypercalcemia, the measures aimed at reduction of the serum calcium include volume repletion using normal saline combined with furosemide, the use of calcitonin, and the administration of mithramycin.

The use of saline diuresis employing the combination of normal saline and furosemide is based on the principle of the shared pathway of sodium and calcium excretion by the renal tubules. When saline is used for volume expansion, the proximal tubular reabsorbtion of sodium is decreased, resulting in natriuresis. The use of the loop diuretic furosemide magnifies this natriuretic response. When sodium is lost, calcium is also lost in the urine because of the common transport system shared by sodium and calcium. The only hazard with this therapy is that the doses (80 to 120 mg four times a day) of furosemide used can result in dehydration unless normal saline is infused in adequate amounts, approximately 4 liters a day. Saline diuresis is effective in lowering calcium by as much as 2.5 mg/dl compared to the base line.

Calcitonin administration acutely lowers calcium by inhibiting osteoclast activity. The effect can be seen within hours after the intramuscular administration of 100 to 200 U of salmon calcitonin. The effectiveness of calcitonin diminishes after a few days through blunting of receptor sensitivity to calcitonin. This can, to some extent, be restored by the use of corticosteroids. Corticosteroids are also useful in the treatment of hypercalcemia secondary to sarcoidosis, hypervitaminosis D, and multiple myeloma.

When the serum calcium level is dangerously high (>15–16 mg/dl), attempts can be made to lower the calcium with the use of intravenous mithramycin. Given in the dose of 25 μg/kg body weight, this inhibitor of osteoclast function lowers the calcium effectively. The effects of mithramycin take 16 to 48 hr to manifest and may last as long as 5–7 days. When the calcium level is critical, the use of "triple therapy"—saline diuresis, calcitonin, and mithramycin—ensures immediate as well as sustained modalities at work. The toxic effects of mithramycin include thrombocytopenia and nephrotoxicity.

The intravenous use of diphosphonates has provided a safe modality for lowering calcium. The use of hemodialysis to lower calcium is limited to cases of extreme elevation and/or refractoriness to other forms of therapy.

22

Primary Hyperparathyroidism

22.1. Introduction

Primary hyperparathyroidism is an extremely frequent disorder, representing the most common cause for hypercalcemia in individuals under 50 years of age.

22.2. Etiology

In 85% of instances, primary hyperparathyroidism is caused by a single adenoma of the parathyroid secreting excessive quantities of PTH. In the rest, hyperparathyroidism is caused by diffuse hyperplasia of all four glands, multiple adenomas, and, rarely, by clear-cell hyperplasia or carcinoma of the parathyroid glands. In approximately one out of 15 patients with primary hyperparathyroidism, a familial tendency may be observed. The familial hyperparathyroidism may be isolated or may be part of the MEA-I or MEA-II syndromes (Chapter 52). A higher incidence of parathyroid adenomas has been noted following head and neck radiation for acne or tonsils during childhood.

22.3. Clinical Features

There are three major presentations of primary hyperparathyroidism: the asymptomatic variety, the hypercalcemic syndrome, and the syndrome caused by target organ effects of chronic hyperparathyroidism.

22.3.1. Asymptomatic Hyperparathyroidism

The most common presentation today is the asymptomatic variety detected serendipitously during routine multichannel screening. The changing picture of this disorder is a reflection of the early diagnosis made by routine screening.

22.3.2. Hypercalcemic Syndrome

Primary hyperparathyroidism may present with the symptoms of hypercalcemia (Section 21.3) and represents the most frequent etiology for hypercalcemia in younger individuals.

22.3.3. The Syndrome of Target Organ Disease

The five target organs that bear the brunt of chronic hyperparathyroidism are the renal system, the bones, the gastrointestinal tract, the joints, and muscular systems.

22.3.3.1. The Renal Effects

The incidence of renal disease in primary hyperparathyroidism is approximately 30–33% and may take one of three forms: calculous disease (or nephrocalcinosis) of the urinary tract, decreasing GFR, and renal tubular disease. The incidence of renal stones in primary hyperparathyroidism has considerably decreased in the past decade, occurring in perhaps no more than 18–20% of patients with hyperparathyroidism today. The real threat, in terms of renal disease, is the progressive decrease in creatinine clearance that occurs in untreated patients with primary hyperparathyroidism. Declining renal function, which may occur in one-fourth to one-third of untreated patients with primary hyperparathyroidism, even in those with mild, asymptomatic disease, constitutes the major argument for therapeutic intervention. Renal tubular defects and an increased susceptibility to urinary tract infections may be related to interstitial disease seen with chronic primary hyperparathyroidism.

22.3.3.2. The Skeletal Manifestations

The skeletal manifestations of primary hyperparathyroidism have considerably decreased, representing a classic example of a disease changing with time. The classic bone changes of primary hyperparathyroidism (osteitis fibrosa cystica, deformities, "Brown tumors," etc.) have become rare and are only of historical interest. The most important manifestation of hyperparathyroidism today is osteopenia (and back pain), especially in older patients with the disease. Subperiosteal bone resorption of the metacarpal bones or phalanges may be seen in fewer than 10% of patients, a sign that is pathognomonic of hyperparathyroidism when present.

22.3.3.3. The Gastrointestinal Manifestations

The two gastrointestinal manifestations of primary hyperparathyroidism are peptic ulcer disease and pancreatitis. The association between peptic ulcer disease and primary hyperparathyroidism is intriguing. When primary hyperparathyroidism is part of the MEA-I syndrome, peptic ulcer is often an integral part of that syndrome (ulcerogenic tumor of pancreas, primary hyperparathyroidism, and pituitary tumor). The association between peptic ulcer and the nonfamilial, isolated variety of hyperparathyroidism is controversial, since both disorders occur with a high frequency in the general population. The bulk of evidence favors a causal relationship between primary hyperparathyroidism and peptic ulcer disease; chronic hypercalcemia serves as a physiological stimulus for release of gastrin by the G cells of the antrum, resulting in secondary hyperacidity and ulcer diathesis.

The relationship between pancreatitis and primary hyperparathyroidism is a well-established one and may take several forms; acute, recurrent, chronic with pain, chronic painless, and postoperative varieties of pancreatitis have been described in association with primary hyperparathyroidism. It is noteworthy that the serum calcium levels in primary hyperparathyroidism with acute pancreatitis may be normalized during the acute episode. This is because of the tendency for calcium to be locally sequestered by saponification in the pancreatic bed.

22.3.3.4. The Articular Manifestations

Pseudogout (chondrocalcinosis) and uric acid arthropathy are the two articular manifestations of primary hyperparathyroidism. Pseudogout, presenting with painful swelling of major joints, may manifest for the first time in the postoperative period after parathyroid surgery for hyperparathyroidism; the reason for this peculiar phenomenon is unclear.

Mild hyperuricemia is fairly common, but gout occurs only in the genetically predisposed individual.

22.3.3.5. Myopathic Manifestations

Rarely, primary hyperparathyroidism may manifest with a severe form of proximal myopathy characterized by severe muscle weakness, usually involving the proximal group of muscles but occasionally being generalized. This unusual presentation is associated with severe weakness, profound weight loss bordering on cachexia, and mild anemia. The presentation mimics neurological syndromes, malignancy, and apathetic hyperthyroidism. The entire syndrome is reversible after surgical cure of the hyperparathyroidism. Thus, primary hyperparathyroidism should be included in the differential diagnosis of myopathic syndromes, weakness, and weight loss.

22.4. Diagnostic Studies

The diagnostic studies involved in primary hyperparathyroidism fall under three categories: studies that directly or indirectly establish excess parathormone; studies that demonstrate classic target-organ involvement by chronic

TABLE 51
Diagnostic Studies in Primary Hyperparathyroidism

Studies that directly or indirectly establish excess PTH
    Direct
        Radioimmunoassay for PTH
    Indirect
        Nephrogenous cyclic AMP
        TRP studies
        1,25-dihydroxy-D_3 in plasma
Studies that demonstrate target organ effects of chronic hyperparathyroidism
    Kidney
        Creatinine clearance
        IVP
    Bone
        Hand films (for subperiosteal resorption)
        Spine films (for osteoporosis)
        Alkaline phosphatase in serum
        Bone densitometry (for osteopenia)
    GI tract
        Upper gastrointestinal series (for peptic ulcer)
Studies to exclude common causes for hypercalcemia
    Serum and urine immunoelectrophoresis
    Chest X ray
    Bone scan
    Thyroid profile

hyperparathyroidism; and studies that exclude some common causes of hypercalcemia (Table 51).

22.4.1. Studies That Directly or Indirectly Establish Excess PTH

Measurement of the immunoreactive PTH with a simultaneous calcium level is the most direct method of establishing the diagnosis of primary hyperparathyroidism. The diagnosis of primary hyperparathyroidism can be established by radioimmunoassay of PTH in 80% of instances. The immunoassay of PTH and its interpretation require a basic understanding of the immunoheterogeneity of PTH. Parathyroid hormone is synthesized in the parathyroid glands as a prohormone (pro-PTH, molecular weight 12,000). Within the gland, pro-PTH is converted into PTH, an 84-amino-acid peptide with a molecular weight of 9500. This is the form in which the hormone is secreted into the circulation. In the circulation, PTH is immediately cleaved into a carboxy or C terminal (COOH) and an amino terminal (NH_2 or N terminal). The N terminal has an extremely short half-life, is biologically active, and is internalized by target cells. The C terminal, in contrast, circulates longer, is biologically inactive, and is excreted by the kidneys. In addition to these two fragments, there are other "small fragments" with long half-lives that contribute to the immunoreactivity of the C-terminal fragments. The immunoreactive PTH measured in the plasma, depends on the ability of the antisera to "see" the different fragments of PTH in the circulation (Figure 16).

In the hypercalcemic patient with an elevated immunoreactive PTH in the absence of renal failure, the diagnosis of primary hyperparathyroidism is very strong. In the hypercalcemic patient with a suppressed PTH, the diagnosis of primary hyperparathyroidism is almost excluded. In the hypercalcemic patient with normal PTH, primary hyperparathyroidism or ectopic secretion of PTH by neoplasms are both equally possible.

Table 52 outlines several dictums that need to be kept in mind in interpreting the immunoreactive PTH.

Despite the abovementioned instances in which the assay falls short of diagnostic expectations, the PTH assay can accurately predict the diagnosis of hyperparathyroidism in 80–85% of instances and hence constitutes the initial diagnostic procedure.

Indirect methods that evaluate the bioeffects of excess PTH secretion are measurement of nephrogenous cyclic AMP, the tubular reabsorption of phosphorus, and the measurement of 1,25-dihydroxy-D_3. The two sources of urinary cyclic AMP are the fraction filtered from plasma and the nephrogenous cyclic AMP derived from renal synthesis of the nucleotide. In general, the plasma level of cyclic AMP and the glomerular filtration of cyclic AMP are relatively constant. The nephrogenous cyclic AMP is greatly influenced by endogenous PTH levels, and the latter accounts for 90–100% of the nephro-

TABLE 52
Clinical Dictums to Remember When Interpreting the PTH Immunoassay

1. The PTH assay should always be interpreted in light of the serum calcium level.
2. A 100% reliance cannot be placed on the immunoassay because of the inherent immunoheterogeneity of PTH.
3. In 80% of patients with primary hyperparathyroidism, the C-terminal assay would disclose clearly elevated PTH values.
4. A suppressed PTH value in a hypercalcemic patient points against primary hyperparathyroidism as the etiology.
5. A "normal" PTH in a hypercalcemic patient is consistent with primary hyperparathyroidism as well as "ectopic hyperparathyroidism."
6. A minimally elevated PTH level in a hypercalcemic patient poses diagnositc problems, since tumor PTH may cross react with the C-terminal–MM assay. The frequency of such a phenomenon varies with different laboratories.
7. Very few labs are capable of measuring "tumor PTH."
8. When the serum calcium is in excess of 16 mg/dl, even the "autonomous" parathyroid adenoma may "turn off," giving spurious results in the assays.
9. Occasionally, a parathyroid adenoma may preferentially secrete midregion molecule or N-terminal, resulting in low levels by C-terminal assay.
10. Occasionally, suppressed parathyroid glands may continue to secrete inactive C terminals into the circulation, giving values suggestive of primary hyperparathyroidism.

genous component in the urine. Elevated nephrogenous cyclic AMP is encountered in 90–95% of patients with primary hyperparathyroidism. Unfortunately, the nephrogenous cyclic AMP is also elevated in 40–50% of patients with humoral hypercalcemic syndromes associated with cancer. The test is done by determining plasma cyclic AMP, urinary cyclic AMP, and the creatinine clearance. The nephrogenous cyclic AMP is expressed in terms of the GFR and the clearance of cyclic AMP.

The percentage tubular reabsorption of phosphorus (TRP) is an index of the phosphaturic effect of PTH. The TRP, measured by calculating the clearances of creatinine and phosphorus, is expressed in terms of the amount of phosphate reabsorbed for a given creatinine clearance. The percentage TRP is lowered in primary hyperparathyroidism. A recent modification of the percentage TRP is the determination of the renal phosphate threshold (RPT). This is the ratio of tubular maximal reabsorption of phosphorus to the glomerular filtration rate, TMP : GFR. This ratio may be regarded as the "set point" for phosphorus absorption by the tubules and is the principal determinant of plasma levels of phosphorus. Parathyroid hormone lowers this set point, inducing phosphaturia. The test is done by measuring plasma phosphorus and creatinine in timed urine samples. After the tubular resorption of phosphorus and TRP are calculated, the TMP is derived from a nomogram. The normal range is between 2.5 and 4.2 mg/dl. In patients with primary hyperparathyroidism, the values are generally under 2.5 mg/dl.

The third indirect parameter of PTH action is the plasma level of 1,25-dihydroxy-D_3, the metabolite of 25-hydroxy-D_3 derived by 1-α-hydroxylation by the kidneys. This metabolite is elevated in all patients with primary hyperparathyroidism.

22.4.2. Studies That Demonstrate Target Organ Effects

Even if the immunoreactive PTH assay has established the diagnosis of primary hyperparathyroidism, it is essential to perform studies to evaluate the damage from hyperparathyroidism. Subperiosteal resorption, renal calculi, decreased creatinine clearance, osteopenia, and peptic ulceration are effects of chronic disease and indicative of target organ damage.

22.4.3. Tests to Exclude Common Causes of Hypercalcemia

Since hypercalcemia is a very common marker of cancer in patients over 50, a quick search for a few frequently occurring neoplasms is indicated. At the very least, a chest X ray, immunoelectrophoresis, bone scan, and thyroid profile are indicated, even when the immunoreactive PTH is diagnostic. Often, dual reasons for hypercalcemia complicate the picture. When the PTH is nondiagnostic, the diagnostic search for malignancy becomes more extensive.

22.5. Differential Diagnosis

The most important differential diagnosis of primary hyperparathyroidism is hypercalcemia of malignancy. The age of the patient, the clinical picture, the associated physical findings, the degree of hypercalcemia, the presence of underlying malignancy, the presence of target organ damage from chronic hyperparathyroidism, and the PTH assay can all assist in making that diagnosis.

22.6. Prognosis

Primary hyperparathyroidism is entirely curable with surgery. Untreated, the target organ damage occurring in the bones and kidneys can lead to considerable disability.

22.7. Treatment

The only therapy for primary hyperparathyroidism is surgery. The indications for surgical intervention are:

1. Persistent elevation of serum calcium in excess of 1 mg/dl over the upper limits of normal for the particular laboratory (>12 mg/dl).
2. Clinical or laboratory evidence of target organ involvement regardless of the degree of hypercalcemia (metabolically active renal calculi, bone disease, declining creatinine clearance, etc.).
3. When the serum calcium is below 12 mg/dl, the indications for surgical intervention are the demonstration of a gradual upward trend in calcium, the development of sudden bouts of hypercalcemia over 13 mg/dl punctuating milder hypercalcemia on a chronic basis, and a declining creatinine clearance.

Preoperative localization is not necessary; the diagnostic accuracy of the study cannot match the expertise of digital exploration by the experienced surgeon. The ease in identification of the parathyroid glands and recognition of an adenoma are a reflection of surgical expertise. If a single adenoma is identified, biopsy of one other gland is necessary to exclude hyperplasia. If the biopsy of the uninvolved gland is "normal," the surgical recommendation is excision of the adenomatous gland.

For hyperplasia of four glands, the surgical recommendation is three-and-a-half parathyrodectomy. If on exploration no adenoma can be found, and the biopsy of the glands shows no evidence of hyperplasia, the search for the adenoma should be high and low: high in the superior cervical region and low in the mediastinum. If still no adenoma is found, intraoperative localization procedures should be recommended.

Transient hypoparathyroidism following removal of adenoma is frequently seen and is self-limiting. Permanent hypoparathyroidism should not occur after adenomectomy, since the surgery involves removal of only a single gland. Permanent hypoparathyroidism may be seen following surgery for hyperplasia, which involves surgery on all the glands.

Medical treatment for primary hyperparathyroidism employing cimetidine, propranolol, phosphates, and calcitonin does not provide an alternative to surgery.

23

Hypocalcemia

23.1 Introduction

Hypocalcemia, a lowering of the serum calcium level, signifies considerable depletion of total body calcium. Unlike hypercalcemia, which is a very frequent perturbation, hypocalcemia is relatively less frequent because of the interplay of excellent adaptive mechanisms in calcium homeostasis. The major counterregulatory mechanism that comes into play is parathyroid hormone. This hormone counteracts hypocalcemia by mobilizing calcium from bone and by promoting calcium absorption from the gut via 1,25-dihydroxycholecalciferol.

The normal range of calcium in the serum is 9 to 10.8 mg/dl. The interpretation of serum calcium should take into consideration the level of albumin in the serum, since the major portion of calcium in the serum circulates bound to albumin. The measured serum calcium drops by 0.8 mg/dl per gram of decline in serum albumin. Since the homeostatic mechanisms to maintain serum calcium are exquisitely sensitive, hypocalcemia below 7 mg/dl indicates a serious underlying problem.

23.2. Etiology

The several etiologies that cause hypocalcemia can be viewed in perspective of the causative mechanisms. The two major mechanisms that usually underlie hypocalcemia are calcium malabsorption and hyperphosphatemia; less commonly, hypocalcemia can result from increased accretion of calcium in the bone, losses of calcium in the urine, or as a consequence of humoral mediators. Each of these mechanisms is briefly outlined below.

23.2.1. Malabsorption of Calcium

One of the major mechanisms for hypocalcemia is faulty absorption of calcium by the intestines. Since vitamin D is mandatory for transport of calcium across the small intestinal mucosa, it is not surprising that calcium malabsorption is intimately linked to vitamin D deficiency. There are several disorders characterized by an absolute or relative failure in vitamin D metabolism.

1. Dietary deficiency of vitamin D results in rickets, an uncommon disorder in the western world.
2. Since vitamin D is a fat-soluble vitamin and requires bile for absorption, any condition that causes obstruction to the biliary outflow tract can result in malabsorption of vitamin D; this is the mechanism of hypocalcemia in obstructive jaundice.
3. Vitamin D absorption can be greatly impaired by inherent intestinal malabsorption, which interferes with the mucosal function of the small bowel; this is the mechanism of hypocalcemia associated with celiac sprue, bowel resection, extensive Crohn's disease, generalized lymphoma of the bowel, etc., resulting in osteomalacia.
4. Vitamin D metabolism can be affected at the hepatic level, a site at which hydroxylation of cholecalciferol to 25-hydroxycholecalciferol takes place. This is the mechanism of hypocalcemia in extensive liver disease or with the use of diphenylhydantoin ("anticonvulsant osteomalacia").
5. Vitamin D metabolism may also be affected by faulty generation of 1,25-dihydroxycholecalciferol from the hepatic precursor, 25-hydroxycholecalciferol. This is the mechanism of hypocalcemia in chronic renal disease and hypoparathyroidism.
6. Finally, vitamin D resistance, especially the hereditary hypophosphatemic vitamin-D-resistant rickets, causes calcium malabsorption because of target organ resistance at the gut level to the action of vitamin D.

Calcium malabsorption can also result from non-vitamin-D-dependent mechanisms; the hypocalcemias of extreme malnutrition, alcoholism, and hypomagnesemia fall in this category. Generally, when hypocalcemia is secondary to intestinal malabsorption, there is hypophosphatemia as well because of impaired absorption of phosphorus in addition to calcium.

23.2.2. Phosphate Retention

The second major mechanism for hypocalcemia is phosphate retention. Hyperphosphatemia lowers the calcium in an effort to maintain a normal $Ca \times P$ product. This "see-saw" relationship with hyperphosphatemia can be seen with acute and chronic elevations of serum phosphate. Acute hyperphosphatemia is the underlying mechanism of hypocalcemia following phosphate infusions, phosphate burns, and sudden "flooding" with phosphate following chemotherapy for acute blast cell leukemia. The hypocalcemia of chronic renal failure results in part from phosphate retention.

23.2.3. Rarer Mechanisms of Hypocalcemia

Rarely, hypocalcemia may result from increased bone accretion. Three situations exemplify hypocalcemia from such a mechanism: the development of "hungry bone syndrome" following surgery for hyperparathyroidism may lead to an avid "siphoning" of calcium from the blood into the "hungry" osteopenic bone that has been released from the influence of PTH excess; increased bone accretion associated with osteoblastic metastases, particularly of the prostate; and increased calcitonin in the absence of parathyroid glands, as in recurrent medullary carcinoma of thyroid after thyroid and parathyroid surgery.

Hypocalcemia from renal losses is extremely unusual and may be the mechanism of hypocalcemia during the polyuric phase of acute renal failure.

Finally, hypocalcemia can occur as a consequence of humoral mediators secreted by tumors. This rare entity, referred to as "oncogenic hypocalcemia," has been described in association with tumors of mesenchymal origin and may be related to secretion of "osteoblast-activating factor," which promotes calcium movement into the bone.

Table 53 outlines the various mechanisms of hypocalcemia discussed above.

23.3. Clinical Features

Since calcium is a divalent cation that is ubiquitously distributed throughout the body, it is not surprising that the effects of hypocalcemia are far-reaching and diverse. The symptomology of hypocalcemia is highly variable and dependent on the severity as well as the rapidity of evolution. When hypocalcemia evolves rapidly (as in postoperative hypoparathyroidism), the symptoms are profound even with mild hypocalcemia, whereas patients with chronic hypocalcemia adjust to their low level of calcium and may show a surprising paucity of impressive symptoms despite very low levels of calcium in the circulation.

The hallmark of hypocalcemia is increased neuromuscular excitability. This effect may result in widespread effects involving the CNS as well as the smooth muscle in the bronchi, intestine, gallbladder, and even the larynx. In addition, chronic hypocalcemia can affect practically every organ system, causing an array of effects involving the skin, teeth, gastrointestinal tract, heart, and eyes.

The term "tetany" is used to describe a constellation of features occurring as a consequence of increased neuromuscular excitability. Overt, classic tetany (carpopedal spasm) is characterized by three components: sensory, motor, and involuntary. The attacks begin with sensory symptoms, usually tingling and numbness of the mouth and extremities. The paresthesias are often associated with pain. The motor component, characterized by weakness often described as "leadlike heaviness," may not be evident in all patients. The sensorimotor components are followed by carpopedal spasm that slowly evolves

TABLE 53
Mechanisms of Hypocalcemia

Malabsorption of calcium
    Vitamin D related
        Dietary deficiency (rickets)
        Lack of availability of bile
            (intra- or extrahepatic biliary obstruction)
        Intestinal malabsorption syndrome
            (sprue, resection, Crohn's, lymphoma, etc.)
        Hepatic
            (anticonvulsants, cirrhosis, etc.)
        Renal
            Chronic renal failure
            Hypoparathyroidism
    Vitamin D unrelated
        Alcoholism
        Malnutrition
        Hypomagnesemia
Hyperphosphatemia
    Acute
        Phosphate infusions
        Phosphate burns
        Chemotherapy for blast cell tumors
        Rhabdomyolysis
    Chronic
        Chronic renal failure
        Hypoparathyroidism
Increased bone accretion
    "Hungry bone syndrome"
    Osteoblastic metastases
        (prostate)
    Calcitonin excess in absence of parathyroids
Increased renal loss
    Polyuric phase of acute renal failure
Oncogenic hypocalcemia
    Mesenchymal tumors

as the patient watches in horror and disbelief, without any control in stopping these movements. The classic response is adduction of thumb, extension at the interphalangeal joints, flexion at the metacarpophalangeal joints, followed by flexion at the wrist and even at the elbow. The fully developed abnormality is graphically and aptly described by the French as "main de accoucheur" or the "obstetrician's hand." Tetany can also involve the feet. When the neuromuscular irritability is severe, convulsions (cerebral tetany), wheezing (bronchial), biliary colic, abdominal pain (intestinal tetany), and laryngeal spasm with dysphonia, stridor, and cyanosis can cause an alarming picture.

Although hypocalcemia represents the most frequent etiology of tetany, hypokalemia, hypomagnesemia, alkalosis, and, rarely, hyperkalemia may cause an identical clinical picture. The effects of hypocalcemia and alkalosis are additive. Such is the case when the patient with early hypocalcemic tetany panics and hyperventilates and develops alkalosis, which aggravates the tetany. The mechanism of alkalosis-induced tetany in normocalcemic individuals is that alkalosis increases the binding of calcium to proteins, thereby decreasing ionic calcium. Alkalosis also increases organic acids that bind calcium. These effects are detrimental to the patient with borderline hypocalcemia, resulting in precipitation of overt tetany.

Although overt tetany occurs spontaneously, latent tetany can be unmasked by the Chvostek's (tapping on the facial nerve in front of the zygoma) and Trousseau's signs (inflating the pressure in the cuff of the sphygmomanometer and observing for carpal spasm).

In addition to the increased neuromuscular irritability, chronic hypocalcemia has protean systemic expressions. Decreased intelligence and depression are features of chronic hypocalcemia regardless of etiology, reversible on restoration of eucalcemia. Somatic and intellectual retardation may be seen.

The skin changes of hypocalcemia include dryness and a tendency to contract mucocutaneous candidiasis. The nails are brittle with a tendency to break. The teeth are affected only during the deciduous phase.

The ocular manifestations of hypocalcemia are usually seen in chronic undertreated hypocalcemia and consist of the development of premature cataracts and papilledema. The cataracts are small, dotlike, and mulitlayered, occurring in the posterior aspect. The papilledema is a result of benign intracranial hypertension and causes headaches.

The effects of hypocalcemia on the gastrointestinal tract are striking and may result in diarrhea and even steatorrhea, mimicking nontropical sprue, a condition notorious for causing malabsorption of calcium. The radiologic features of hypocalcemic enteropathy can be identical to those of sprue and consist of flocculation ("puddling") of the barium. Further, the small bowel biopsy may demonstrate villous atrophy, making the similarity between the two disorders striking. The distinction can be made by observing the effect of gluten-free diet on the diarrhea–steatorrhea complex; patients with hypocalcemic enteropathy obviously show no response to this diet and respond only to restoration of eucalcemia.

The effects of chronic hypocalcemia on the central nervous system are extremely important. Grand mal, focal, and even petit mal seizures can occur as a consequence of hypocalcemia. If the mistaken diagnosis of epilepsy is made, and the error is compounded by the use of diphenylhydantoin, which can further lower the calcium, the consequences are obvious. Hypocalcemia lowers the seizure threshold in patients with subclinical idiopathic epilepsy.

The cardiovascular effects of hypocalcemia primarily include ECG abnormalities: prolongation of the Q–T interval, ST and T depression, and the development of Q waves. The association between chronic hypocalcemia and a cardiomyopathy (hypocalcemic cardiomyopathy) is debatable.

Thus, the clinical spectrum of hypocalcemia encompasses several disciplines of medicine, and the patient may seek consultation from the neurologist, dermatologist, dentist, psychiatrist, or gastroenterologist before the endocrine nature of the problem is discovered by the simple test of measuring serum calcium in blood.

23.4. Diagnostic Tests

The three sets of tests that help in evaluating the etiology of hypocalcemia are measurement of serum phosphorus, assay of PTH, and radiologic studies.

23.4.1. Serum Phosphorus

The measurement of the serum phosphorus in the hypocalcemic patient provides an excellent clue to the underlying disorder in most instances.

TABLE 54
Radiologic Studies in Hypocalcemia

X ray	Significance
1. Teeth	Delay in eruption
2. Bone survey	Renal osteodystrophy
	Osteosclerosis (hypoparathyroidism)
	Cysts (pseudohypo-/hyperpara)
	Osteoblastic lesions (prostatic cancer)
	Osteomalacia (vitamin D deficiency)
	Osteopenia (vitamin D deficiency)
3. GI series	Primary malabsorption
	Hypocalcemic enteropathy
4. Flat plate abdomen	Calculi in common bile duct (obstructive biliary disease)
	Pancreatic calcification (chronic pancreatitis)
5. Shoulders	Soft tissue calcification (pseudohypoparathyroidism)
6. Skull	Basal ganglion calcification (pseudo- or idiopathic hypoparathyroidism)
	Choroid plexus calcification (pseudo- or idiopathic hypoparathyroidism)
7. Hand	Brachydactyly (pseudohypoparathyroidism)

Hypocalcemia with hyperphosphatemia is indicative of chronic renal failure or parathyroid failure. Rare causes for such a combination are hypomagnesemia, phosphorus burns, cytotoxic therapy, rhabdomyolysis, and hyperphosphatemic osteomalacia.

Hypocalcemia with hypophosphatemia is indicative of vitamin D deficiency from any mechanism, intestinal malabsorption, or acute pancreatitis.

23.4.2. Assay of PTH

Since hypocalcemia is a powerful stimulus for PTH release, the demonstration of a low PTH in the presence of a low calcium clearly signals hypoparathyroidism. The different variants of hypoparathyroidism and the various tests available to delineate these variants are described in Chapter 24.

23.4.3. Radiologic Studies

These are summarized in Table 54.

23.5. Treatment

The treatment for acute hypocalcemia is intravenous administration of 10% calcium gluconate. The treatment for chronic hypocalcemia, the prototype of which is hypoparathyroidism, is discussed in Chapter 24.

24

Hypoparathyroidism

24.1. Introduction

Hypoparathyroidism includes a spectrum of disorders characterized by hypocalcemia and hyperphosphatemia in the absence of chronic renal failure, osteomalacia, or rickets. This disease can occur either as a result of impaired secretion of PTH by the parathyroid glands (hormonopenic) or as a consequence of target organ resistance to the action of PTH (hormonoplethoric).

24.2. Etiology

The classification of various hypoparathyroid states is outlined in Table 55.

Hypoparathyroidism resulting from congenital maldevelopment of the parathyroid glands usually manifests with severe hypocalcemia at birth or during the neonatal period. This condition is often associated with thymic aplasia, since the thymus and the parathyroid glands originate from common embryologic pouches. The infant succumbs to a variety devastating opportunistic infections because of congenital immune deficiency.

Postsurgical hypoparathyroidism represents the most common variety of hypoparathyroidism and results from inadvertent removal of the parathyroids during thyroid or parathyroid surgery. The incidence of hypoparathyroidism after subtotal thyroidectomy for Graves' hyperthyroidism ranges from 1% to 3%. A higher proportion of patients tend to demonstrate limited PTH reserve despite a low-normal basal calcium level. Permanent hypoparathyroidism following removal of single parathyroid adenoma is extremely unusual.

Idiopathic hypoparathyroidism is one of the most common varieties of hypoparathyroidism seen in adulthood. An autoimmune etiology is strongly supported by the following observations: familial aggregation, the demonstration of autoantibodies against parathyroid tissue in at least some cases,

223

TABLE 55
Diagnostic Tests in Various Hypoparathyroid States

Condition	Calcium	Phos–phorus	PTH levels	Phospha–turia in response to PTH	Cyclic AMP excretion in response to PTH	Bone survey
Idiopathic hypoparathyroidism	↓	↑	↓	+	+	Osteosclerosis
Pseudohypoparathyroidism I	↓	↑	↑	−	−	Osteosclerosis
Pseudohypoparathyroidism II	↓	↑	↑	−	+	Osteosclerosis
Pseudoidiopathic hypoparathyroidism	↓	↑	↑	+	+	
Pseudohypo-hyperparathyroidism	↓ or normal	↑	↑	−	−	Osteitis fibrosa cystica
Pseudohypoparathyroidism	N	N	N	N	N	Short metacarpals

and the association with other autoimmunopathies involving other endocrine glands. The most notable examples of pluriglandular failure associated with idiopatic hypoparathyroidism are autoimmune adrenal failure, ovarian failure, insulin-dependent diabetes mellitus, and autoimmune thyroiditis. Vitiligo and candidiasis also occur with a higher frequency in these individuals.

Hypoparathyroidism following ^{131}I therapy for thyroid carcinoma is an extremely rare phenomenon and may be a result of radiation fibrosis or vascular insufficiency secondary to endarteritis.

Hypoparathyroidism secondary to infiltrative disorders such as hemochromatosis, sarcoidosis, or metastases is extremely rare, constituting only sporadic reports in the literature.

Pseudohypoparathyroidism and its variants represent examples of target organ resistance to the effects of PTH. Often inherited as a sex-linked recessive condition, this disorder, in its fully expressed form, is highlighted by the triad of hypocalcemia, somatic stigmata, and soft tissue calcification. The resistance can be partial or complete, can involve the kidneys, bone, or both, and, surprisingly, can wax and wane in severity. All varieties of pseudohypoparathyroidism are characterized by renal resistance to the action of PTH. The resistance to PTH may result from failure of the hormone to stimulate cyclic AMP, as a consequence of which there is failure to elicit a phosphaturic response (pseudohypoparathyroidism I); or the failure can be in the events distal to generation of cyclic AMP response, which is preserved, but the phosphaturic response is lost (pseudohypoparathyroidism II).

Pseudohypoparathyroidism I can be further categorized into pseudohypoparathyroidism I-A or I-B, depending on the N-protein level. This "coupling protein" is responsible for coupling the signal generated by PTH with the intracellular ability to generate cyclic AMP. Patients with pseudohypoparathyroidism 1-A have low N protein, whereas those with pseudohypoparathyrodidism 1-B have normal N protein.

Rarely, the patient may show only renal resistance with preservation of the skeletal responsiveness. As a consequence of the elevated PTH, a feature common to all forms of pseudohypoparathyroidism, the bones suffer the ill effects of hyperparathyroidism. This entity is aptly called pseudohypo-hyperparathyroidism. Very rarely, the patient may show resistance to endogenous PTH (probably an abnormal molecule without receptor affinity) but may respond to exogenous PTH, a condition termed pseudoidiopathic hypoparathyroidism. The term pseudopseudohypoparathyroidism refers to the presence of somatic stigmata of pseudohypoparathyroidism in the absence of any biochemical or hormonal abnormalities.

24.3. Clinical Features

The clinical features of hypoparathyroidism can be divided into three categories: those caused by the metabolic abnormality, i.e., hypocalcemia, those related to somatic stigmata, and those secondary to associated disorders.

The clinical effects of acute and chronic hypocalcemia are outlined in Chapter 23. Hypoparathyroidism should be suspected in any patient with overt or latent tetany or with systemic effects of chronic hypocalcemia such as cataracts, papilledema, convulsive disorder, diarrhea–steatorrhea, or recurrent mucocutaneous candidiasis.

Somatic stigmata, when present, identify pseudohypoparathyroidism (PsHP). Approximately 85% of patients with PsHP demonstrate these stigmata, which consist of short stature, brachydactyly, rounding of face, short neck, and intellectual retardation. Of these, brachydactyly (short fourth and fifth metacarpal bones) is the most frequent abnormality, often evident when the patient makes a fist (Albright's sign or "knuckle-knuckle-dimple-dimple sign"). It should be underscored that not all patients with PsHP show the somatic stigmata, in the absence of which the clinical presentation resembles idiopathic or pseudoidiopathic forms of hypoparathyroidism. The somatic abnormalities are usually present in PsHP type I-A, i.e., patients with low N–protein level.

The associated features that may help identify the etiology of hypoparathyroidism include a scar of previous neck surgery, vitiligo, or associated endocrine pluriglandular failure.

24.4. Diagnostic Studies

The four categories of diagnostic studies employed in patients with hypoparathyroidism are biochemical, hormonal, renal response studies, and radiologic studies. These tests not only help establish the diagnosis of hypoparathyroidism but also identify the etiology.

24.4.1. Biochemical Tests

Hypocalcemia and hyperphosphatemia are common to all forms of hypoparathyroidism and indicate the classic consequences of absence of hormone or absence of its effect. An identical picture is seen with chronic renal failure.

24.4.2. Hormonal Tests

Measurement of the immunoreactive PTH constitutes the first step in the diagnostic evaluation of hypocalcemia. Parathyroid hormone levels are undetectable or low when hypocalcemia is caused by idiopathic hypoparathyroidism, whereas the levels are high in the pseudo- and the pseudoidiopathic varieties. Again, a low calcium and a high phosphorus with an elevated PTH value may also be encountered in chronic renal failure.

24.4.3. Renal Response Studies

These are studies that evaluate the renal response to exogenous administration of PTH.

The binding of the hormone to specific membrane receptors causes activation of adenylate cyclase, which converts ATP to cyclic AMP. Cyclic AMP binds to specific intracellular receptor proteins and generates protein kinases that mediate the effect of the PTH, in this instance, phosphaturia. Thus, the two parameters that are evaluated following exogenous administration of PTH are cyclic AMP excretion and phosphaturia. In PsHP I, in which the block in hormone action is proximal, there is no increase in the excretion of cyclic AMP or phosphate. In PsHP II, a condition characterized by adequate cyclic AMP generation but a failure in the reception of the cyclic AMP message, phosphaturia is absent although cyclic AMP excretion is preserved. Patients with pseudoidiopathic hypoparathyroidism classically demonstrate a normal response to exogenous PTH in terms of both cyclic AMP and phosphate.

24.4.4. Radiological Studies

These are aimed at demonstrating brachydactyly (hands), osteosclerosis (femur), and soft tissue calcification (skull).

Table 55 summarizes the biochemical, hormonal, radiologic and renal responsiveness studies in the various types of hypoparathyroidism.

24.5. Treatment

The treatment of hypoparathyroidism is replacement of calcium by supplementations, lowering the phosphorus level by antacids containing aluminum hydroxide, and vitamin D therapy to promote calcium absorption by the gut.

Calcium replacement should be aimed at providing 1.5 to 2g of elemental calcium per day. One gram of elemental calcium is provided by 5.5 g of calcium chloride, 8 g calcium lactate, or 11 g of calcium gluconate. Thus, 16 to 24 tablets of calcium need to be taken on a daily basis, life long—a Herculean task for even the most compliant of patients. Besides, calcium lactate dissolves poorly, and calcium gluconate predisposes to alkalosis, a situation that may lower free calcium.

Vitamin D is required to treat patients with hypoparathyroidism, since these patients are unable to produce 1,25-dihydroxycholecalciferol. The renal hydroxylation of 25-hydroxycholecalciferol to its 1,25 metabolite requires PTH. Further, hyperphosphatemia poses an added burden, suppressing the enzyme 1-α-hydroxylase, required for such conversion. Therefore, the most physiological vitamin D therapy for patients with any form of hypoparathyroidism is with 1,25-dihydroxycholecalciferol (calcitriol) in doses of 0.5 to 1 μg daily. Alternately, 1α-calcidiol or dihydrotachysterol can be used, since these analogues do not require renal hydroxylation.

The adverse effect of chronic replacement therapy with calcium and vitamin D is the development of vitamin D intoxication. The symptoms of hypervitaminosis D are polyuria, thirst, and other symptoms of hypercalcemia, with the eventual development of renal failure. The symptoms are quickly reversible when analogues with a short half-life are used (calcitriol). Discontinuation of the therapy on a temporary basis, vigorous hydration, and glucocorticoids are usually effective in reversing the vitamin D intoxication.

Selected Readings

Arnaud, C. D., Goldsmith, R. S., Border, P. J., *et al.:* Influence of immunoheterogeneity of circulating parathyroid hormone on results of radioimmunoassays of serum in man, *Am. J. Med.* **56:**785, 1974.

Avioli, L. V.: The therapeutic approach to hypoparathyroidism, *Am. J. Med.* **57:**34, 1974.

Barreras, R. F.: Calcium and gastric secretion, *Gastroenterology* **64:**1168, 1973.

Barzel, U. S.: Systemic alkalosis in hypoparathroidism, *J. Clin. Endocrinol. Metab.* **29:**917, 1969.

Baxter J. D., and Bondy, P. K.: Hypercalcemia of thyrotoxicosis, *Ann. Intern. Med.* **65:**429, 1966.

Benson, R. C., Jr., Riggs, B. L., Pickard, B. M., *et al.:* Immunoreactive forms of circulating parathyroid hormone in primary and ectopic hyperparathyroidism, *J. Clin. Invest.* **54:**175, 1974.

Berson, S. A., and Yalow, R. S.: Heterogeneity of parathyroid hormone in plasma, *J. Clin. Endocrinol. Metab.* **28:**1037, 1968.

Binstock, M. L., and Mundy, G. R.: Effect of calcitonin and glucocorticoids in combination on the hypercalcemia of malignancy, *Ann. Intern. Med.* **93:**269, 1980.

Boyd, J. C., Lewis, J. C., Slatopolsky, E., *et al.:* Parathyrin measured concurrently with free or total calcium in the differential diagnosis of hypercalcemia, *Clin. Chem.* **27:**574, 1981.

Broadus, A. E., and Rasmussen, H.: Evaluation of parathyroid function, *Am. J. Med.* **70:**475, 1981.

Chase, L. R., and Aurbach, G. D.: Parathyroid function and renal excretion of 3'5'-adenylic acid, *Proc. Natl. Acad. Sci. U.S.A.* **58:**518, 1967.

Chase, L. R., Melson, G. L., and Aurbach, G. D.: Pseudohypoparathyroidism: Defective excretion of 3'5' cAMP in response to parathyroid hormone, *J. Clin. Invest.* **48:**1832, 1969.

Dauphine, R. T., Riggs, B. L., Scholz, D. A., *et al.:* Back pain and vertebral crush fractures: An unemphasized mode of presentation for primary hyperparathyrodism, *Ann. Intern. Med.* **83:**365, 1975.

DeLuca, H.: Vitamin D endocrinology, *Ann. Intern. Med.* **85:**367, 1976.

Drezner, M., Neelon, F. A., Lebovitz, H. E., *et al.:* Pseudohypoparathyroidism type II: A possible defect in the reception of the cyclic AMP signal, *N. Engl. J. Med.* **289:**1056, 1973.

Duarte, C. G., Winnaker, J. L., Becker, K. L., *et al.:* Thiazide induced hypercalcemia, *N. Engl. J. Med* **284:**828, 1971.

Eisenberg, H., Pallotta, J., Sherwood, L. M., *et al.:* Selective arteriography, venography and venous hormone assay in diagnosis and localization of parathyroid lesions, *Am. J. Med.* **56:**810, 1974.

Farfel, Z., Brickman, A. S., Kaslow, H. R., *et al.:* Defect of receptor–cyclase coupling protein in pseudohypoparathyroidism, *N. Engl. J. Med.* **303:**237, 1980.

Farr, H. W., Fahey, T. J., Nash, A. G., *et al.:* Primary hyperparathyroidism and cancer, *Am. J. Surg.* **126:**539, 1973.

Gittler, R. D., and Maier, H.: Carcinoma of the parathyroid, *Arch. Intern. Med.* **130:**413, 1972.

Heath, H., Hodgson, S. F., and Kennedy, M. A.: Primary hyperparathyroidism. incidence, morbidity, and potential economic impact in a community, *N. Engl. J. Med.* **302:**189, 1980.

Jacobs, T. P., Siris, E. S., Bilezikian, J. P., *et al.:* Hypercalcemia of malignancy: Treatment with intravenous dichloromethylene diphosphonate, *Ann. Intern. Med.* **94:**312, 1981.

Kiang, D. T., Loken, M. K., Kennedy, B. J., *et al.:* Mechanism of the hypocalcemic effect of mithramycin, *J. Clin. Endocrinol. Metab.* **48:**341, 1979.

Kodiciek, E.: The story of vitamin D from vitamin to hormone, *Lancet* **1:**325, 1974.

Mixter, G., Keynes, W. M., Coper, O., *et al.:* Further experience with pancreatitis as a diagnostic clue to hyperparathyroidism, *N. Engl. J. Med.* **266:**265, 1962.

Mundy, G. R., Eilon, G., Orr, W., *et al.:* Osteoclast activating factor: Its role in myeloma and other types of hypercalcemia of malignancy, *Metab. Bone. Dis. Rel. Res.* **2:**173, 1980.

Mundy, G. R., Ibbotson, K. J., D'Souzar, S. M., *et al.:* The hypercalcemia of cancer—clinical implications and pathogenic mechanisms, *N. Engl. J. Med.* **310:**1718, 1984.

Nusynowitz, M. L., and Klein, M. H.: Pseudoidiopathic hypoparathyrodism, *Am. J. Med.* **55:**677, 1973.

Palmer, F. J., Nelson, J. C., Bacchus, H., *et al.:* The chloride–phosphate ratio in hypercalcemia, *Ann. Intern. Med.* **80:**200, 1974.

Paloyan, E., Paloyan, D., Pickleman, J. R., *et al.:* Hyperparathyroidism today, *Surg. Clin. North Am.* **53:**211, 1973.

Parsons, J. A., and Potts, J. T., Jr.: Physiology and chemistry of parathyroid hormone, *Clin. Endocrinol. Metab.* **1:**33, 1972.

Patten, B. M., Bilezikian, J. P., Mallette, L. E., *et al.:* Neuromuscular disease in primary hyperparathyroidism, *Ann. Intern. Med.* **80:**182, 1974.

Powell, D., Singer, F. R., Murray, T. M., *et al.:* Nonparathyroid humoral hypercalcemia in patients with neoplastic diseases, *N. Engl. J. Med.* **289:**176, 1973.

Purnell, D. C., Smith, L. H., Scholz, D. A., *et al.:* Primary hyperparathyroidism—a prospective clinical study, *Am. J. Med.* **50:**670, 1971.

Raisz, L. G., Yajnik, C. H., Bockman, R. S., *et al.:* Comparison of commercially available parathyroid hormone immunoassays in the differential diagnosis of hypercalcemia due to primary hyperparathyroidism or malignancy, *Ann. Intern. Med.* **91:**739, 1979.

Roof, B. S., Carpenter, B., Finle, D. J., *et al.:* Some thoughts on the nature of ectopic parathyroid hormones, *Am. J. Med.* **50:**686, 1971.

Scholz, D. A., and Purnell, D. C.: Asymptomatic primary hyperparathyroidism. A 10 year prospective study, *Mayo Clin. Proc.* **56:**473, 1981.

Seyberth, H. W., Segre, G. V., Morgan, J. L., *et al.:* Prostaglandins as mediators of hypercalcemia associated with certain types of cancer, *N. Engl. J. Med.* **293:**1278, 1975.

Stewart, A. F., Horst, R. A., Deftos, L. J., *et al.:* Biochemical evaluation of patients with cancer associated hypercalcemia; evidence for humoral and nonhumoral groups, *N. Engl. J. Med.* **303:**1377, 1980.

Suki, W. M., Yium, J. J., Von Minden, M., *et al.:* Acute treatment of hypercalcemia with furosemide, *N. Engl. J. Med.* **283:**836, 1970.

Van Dop, C., and Bourne, H. R.: Pseudohypoparathyroidism, *Annu. Rev. Med.* **34:**259, 1983.

Wang, C. A.: The anatomic basis of parathyroid surgery, *Ann. Surg.* **183:**271, 1975.

Wang, C. A.: Parathyroid re-exploration: A clinical and pathological study of 112 patients, *Ann. Surg.* **186:**140, 1977

IV

The Adrenal Glands

25

Anatomy of the Adrenal Glands

The adrenal (or suprarenal) glands, two in number, are located retroperitoneally atop the superiomedial pole of each kidney. Each gland weighs approximately 3 to 5 g and measures 2.5 × 0.6 cm. The left adrenal is larger and assumes a crescentlike shape in contrast to the right, which is triangular. Each adrenal gland consists of two portions—an outer cortex and an inner medulla. These two parts differ in their embryology, histology, and secretory functions. The adrenal cortex is derived from the celomic epithelium (mesoderm), whereas adrenal medulla is derived from the neural crest (neurectoderm). The adrenal cortex is composed of three clearly defined zones with separate secretory activity, whereas the adrenal medulla is composed of chromaffin tissue with histological characteristics of sympathetic ganglia. The adrenal cortex synthesizes steroids (mineralocorticoids, glucocorticoids, and sex steroids), whereas the medulla synthesizes catecholamines.

The adrenal cortex constitutes 80–85% of the adrenal gland and consists of three layers, the zona glomerulosa, the zona fasciculata, and the zona reticularis. Histologically, the zona glomerulosa, which is the outermost layer of the adrenal cortex, is composed of small epithelioid cells. The electron microscopic hallmark of the cells in this zone is the presence of elongated mitochondria with cristae arranged in a lamellar fashion. The zona glomerulosa secretes mineralocorticoids, the prototype of which is aldosterone. The zona fasciculata, the middle zone, is composed of polygonal columnar cells arranged as long cords. The electron microscopic features of these cells include a vacuolated cytoplasm and an agranular endoplasmic reticulum. The cells of the zona fasciculata synthesize and secrete glucocorticoids, the prototype of which is cortisol. The zona reticularis is the innermost layer of the cortex and is in close proximity to the adrenal medulla. The cells of this zone demonstrate extreme variability in size and shape. The secretory products of this zone are the adrenal androgens, the prototype of which is dehydro-epiandrosterone (DHEA).

The adrenal gland is related inferiorly to the kidneys, and superiorly to the undersurface of the diaphragm. The left adrenal is in close proximity to the spleen, whereas the right adrenal is very close to the inferior vena cava. Both adrenals lie retroperitoneally at the level of the 12th thoracic vertebra.

Both adrenal glands are supplied by branches of the splenic, renal, intercostal, and diaphragmatic arteries arising from the aorta. The left adrenal, in addition, receives arterial blood supply from branches of the ovarian or internal spermatic arteries. The adrenals are drained by the adrenal veins, the right one draining into the inferior vena cava and the left adrenal vein draining into the left renal vein.

Physiology
The Secretion, Regulatory Control, and Actions of the Adrenal Steroids

The adrenal cortex secretes three distinct types of steroids. The zona glomerulosa secretes mineralocorticoids, the zona fasciculata secretes glucocorticoids, and the zona reticularis secretes androgens. Each of these compounds possesses distinctly different actions, with different regulatory mechanisms controlling their secretion and release.

The substrate for steroidogenesis by the adrenal cortex is cholesterol. Conceptually, adrenal steroidogenesis is visualized as a three-tier synthetic system, the top panel consisting of mineralocorticoids, the middle panel representing glucocorticoids, and the lower, third panel consisting of androgens (Figure 19). The mineralocorticoid synthesis at the zona glomerulosa originates by the conversion of cholesterol into pregnenolone and progesterone, precursors that do not possess any mineralocorticoid activity. The next step is the formation of desoxycorticosterone (DOC), a weak mineralocorticoid. This step is mediated by an important enzyme, 21-hyroxylase. The DOC serves as the substrate for the formation of corticosterone through the action of a very important enzyme 11-β-hydroxylase. Corticosterone, a fairly effective mineralocorticoid, is further hydroxylated and dehydrogenated at the 18th position into aldosterone, the most potent mineralocorticoid.

Glucocorticoid synthesis originates by hydroxylation of pregnenolone and progesterone at the 17th position into 17-α-hydroxypregnenolone and 17-α-hydroxyprogesterone. These two important but inactive precursors will serve as substrates for glucocorticoid synthesis on one end and for androgen synthesis on the other. 17-α-Hydroxy progesterone is acted on by the enzyme 21-hydroxylase and converted to 11-deoxycortisol, an important but biologically inert precursor (compound S). By the action of the enzyme 11-hydrox-

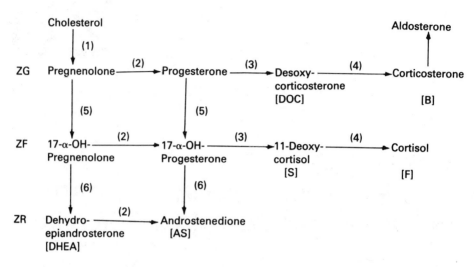

FIGURE 19. Adrenal steroidogenesis. Enzymes: (1) desmolase, (2) 11-β-ol-dehydrogenase, (3) 21-hydroxylase, (4) 11-hydroxylase, (5) 17-α-hydroxylase, (6) 17,20-desmolase. ZG, zona glomerulosa; ZF, zona fasciculata; ZR, zona reticularis.

ylase, this compound is converted into cortisol (compound F), a most potent glucocorticoid.

The synthesis of androgens by the zona reticularis begins by using the substrate 17-α-hydroxyprogesterone that originated at the zona fasciculata. These compounds, by the action of an enzyme called 17,20-desmolase, are converted to dehydroepiandrosterone (DHEA) and androstenedione, the two most important adrenal androgens.

Three important facts should be stressed regarding the substrates, enzymes, and zones involved in adrenal steroidogenesis. First, although the same enzymes are present throughout all layers of the adrenal cortex, these enzymes produce different steroids at different zones depending on the substrate; for example, the enzyme 11-hydroxylase in the zona glomerulosa converts DOC to corticosterone, whereas in the zona fasciculata the same enzyme converts 11-deoxycortisol to cortisol. Second, although the three zones function as independent units, the substances formed in one zone serve as substrates for synthesis of the products in an adjacent zone; for example, pregnenolone and progesterone synthesized by the zona glomerulosa are not only essential for the synthesis of mineralocorticoids by that zone but are also utilized by the zona fasciculata as substrates for the synthesis of glucocorticoid precursors. Third, adequate steroidogenesis requires ACTH stimulation, particularly for synthesis of glucocorticoids and adrenal androgens.

Following synthesis, these steroids are released into the bloodstream. Aldosterone undergoes reduction to tetrahydroaldosterone, which is conjugated in the liver to form a water-soluble glucuronide and is excreted as such in the urine. Cortisol circulates in the plasma bound to a globulin called transcortin. This carrier protein, to a lesser extent, also transports other steroids such as 11-deoxycortisol, 11-deoxycorticosterone, and corticosterone. The glucocorticoids are mainly inactivated in the liver by a series of reduction reactions, resulting in the formation of dihydro- and tetrahydrocortisol, which are further conjugated to become tetrahydrocortisol glucuronide. Approximately 30% of the cortisol secreted is converted to tetrahydrocortisol glucuronide. Compound S (11-deoxycortisol) is similarly converted into tetrahydro-11-deoxycortisol glucuronide. These two compounds are excreted in the urine as 17-hydroxycorticosteroids (17-OHCS).

Dehydroepiandrosterone, the prototype adrenal androgen, circulates in the plasma as such and by a series of reactions is excreted in the urine as 17-ketosteroids. It should be remembered that testosterone, the most potent androgen, is not a 17-ketosteroid.

The control of the secretion and release of the adrenal steroids is complex and should be viewed separately for each set of hormones. The mineralocorticoid synthesis and release is primarily mediated by the renin–angiotensin–aldosterone system (RAAS). Renin is an enzyme secreted by the juxtaglomerular (JG) cells of the kidney. These cells are exquisitely sensitive to changes in blood volume and changes in plasma sodium concentrations. When hypovolemia or hyponatremia develops, the JG cells are stimulated to secrete renin, which acts on the renin substrate (angiotensinogen) to form angiotensin I, an inactive decapeptide. Angiotensin I is converted to angiotensin II, an octapeptide, by the enzyme angiotensin-converting enzyme (ACE). Angiotensin II, besides being a powerful pressor agent, also is a potent stimulator of the zona glomerulosa to synthesize and release aldosterone.

In addition to the RAAS, the zona glomerulosa is controlled, but to a lesser extent, by two other factors: serum potassium and ACTH. Potassium exerts its control on aldosterone secretion independent of the RAAS. Hy-

TABLE 56
Actions of Adrenal Steroids

Steroid	Action	Clinical correlation
Mineralocorticoids	Conserve Na and excrete potassium at the distal tubule	Lack of aldosterone (Addison's) results in ↓ Na and ↑ K; Excess (tumor) results in ↓ K
Glucocorticoids	Combat stress Anabolic Pressor effect Promotes gluconeogenesis and glycogenolysis	Cortisol deficiency results in an inability to combat stress, wasting, hypotension, and fasting hypoglycemia
	Counterinsulin effect	Cortisol excess results in glucose intolerance
Androgens	Initiation of "adrenarche" (development of axillary and pubic hair)	Excess can cause premature puberty or virilization

perkalemia releases, and hypokalemia inhibits, the secretion of aldosterone. The role of ACTH in the control of aldosterone secretion is complex. The zona glomerulosa cells clearly demonstrate specific receptors for both angiotensin II and ACTH. However, in the day-to-day physiological control, the dominant role is played by angiotensin II and not ACTH. Pharmacological doses of ACTH, when given intravenously, cause a brisk and prompt release of aldosterone from the zona glomerulosa.

The glucocorticoid synthesis and release are entirely governed by ACTH. The reciprocal relationship between circulating cortisol level and ACTH, the negative feedback effect of cortisol on both the hypothalamus and the pituitary, the role of stress in overcoming this negative reciprocal relationship, and the general principles that underlie ACTH control are discussed in Chapter 2. ACTH stimulates glucocorticoid synthesis by binding to membrane receptors, followed by stimulation of adenylate cyclase and the generation of intracellular cyclic AMP. The utilization of this principle in the evaluation of adrenal reserve is discussed in Chapter 27, dealing with testing of the adrenal function. Cortisol is secreted in a pulsatile pattern, a fact that should be remembered when one interprets a single sample of blood drawn at an isolated period in time.

The adrenal androgens are also under the stimulatory influence of ACTH. However, these androgens do not play a role in control of ACTH secretion.

The actions of adrenal steroids are outlined in Table 56.

27

Testing Adrenocortical Function

27.1. Introduction

The availability of highly specific radioimmunoassays for measurement of practically every steroid synthesized by the adrenal cortex has greatly enhanced and simplified evaluation of adrenal function. The next section of this chapter focuses on the basal tests available to evaluate adequacy of adrenocortical function. These tests employ collection of a single sample of blood or urine. The assays in the plasma or urine available to the clinician and the limitations of these tests are pointed out. The following section of this chapter deals with dynamic tests that are employed in the evaluation of adrenal dysfunction.

27.2. Basal Tests to Evaluate Adrenocortical Function

As indicated above, the emergence of sophisticated radioimmunoassays has facilitated accurate measurement of practically every steroid secreted by the adrenal cortex. The convenience factor involved in measuring a single sample of blood or urine to establish the suspected clinical diagnosis is the singular advantage of basal tests. However, despite this advantage, basal tests have not eliminated the need for more elaborate testing. The two reasons for this are the pulsatile nature of secretion of these steroids and the great overlap in the ranges of basal hormones between normal and abnormal subjects, resulting in an unacceptable rate of false positives and negatives.

Table 57 illustrates the adrenal steroids in plasma and their products measured in the 24-hr urine. The three commonly used basal tests that involve plasma assays are cortisol, DHEA, and 17-hydroxylprogesterone. The three commonly used basal tests that involve urinary asays are 17-hydroxycortico-

TABLE 57
Adrenal Steroids in Blood and Urine

Steroids	Blood	Urine
Mineralocorticoids	Aldosterone	Tetrahydroaldosterone
Glucocorticoids	Cortisol (compound F)	17-Hydroxycorticosteroids (S and F)
		Urinary free cortisol
Androgens	Dehydroepiandrosterone (DHEA)	17-Ketosteroids
Precursors	17-Hydroxyprogesterone Compound S	Pregnanetriol

steroids, urine free cortisol, and 17-ketosteroids. A brief overview of each of these tests is necessary to help one understand the indications, use, and limitations involved.

27.2.1. Serum Cortisol (Compound F)

The availability of a radioimmunoassay for cortisol has eliminated the calorimetric and fluorometric methods for measurement of cortisol. The disadvantages of these older methods were several, including interference from other drugs as well as from other steroids, particularly 11-deoxycortisol. The currently available radioimmunoassay for cortisol is exquisitely sensitive and specific for compound F, the only biologically effective glucocorticoid.

The primary indication to obtain serum cortisol is when hypo- or hyperfunction of the adrenal cortex is suspected. Indeed, when the serum cortisol is extremely high or extremely low, the assay may adequately establish disordered function. Unfortunately, such instances in clinical practice are few. There are two basic difficulties in interpreting a single sample of serum cortisol. First, although cortisol secretion does follow a circadian pattern, it is secreted in episodic bursts with variable peaks and nadirs. Therefore, depending on sampling time, a high or low value may be encountered, obliterating the clear difference between normal and abnormal ranges. Second, since the radioimmunoassay measures the cortisol in the circulation that is bound to the globulin transcortin, any factor that increases this globulin (such as obesity, pregnancy, alcohol, or estrogens) would spuriously elevate the cortisol level in the serum as measured by radioimmunoassay.

The normal range for cortisol in the serum is 5–22 μg/dl.

27.2.2. Dehydroepiandrosterone

This steroid is the prototype of adrenal androgens and is an excellent indicator for the adequacy of androgen synthesis by the zona reticularis. The plasma level of DHEA is reasonably stable throughout the day but slightly higher in the morning. In females, the major source of DHEA is the adrenal cortex; in males, a small contribution (20%) is derived from testosterone secreted by the testes.

The assay of DHEA level in plasma has supplanted the cumbersome need for urine collections to estimate the 17-ketosteroids, the conventional indicator of adrenal androgen activity.

The primary indications to obtain DHEA level in plasma are in the evaluation of hirsutism or virilization in adult females, precocious puberty in boys, and premature adrenarche or virilization in girls. Since the adrenal androgens are "weak" androgens, the level of DHEA in plasma would be markedly elevated when virilization is secondary to adrenal androgen excess. The two important causes for increased synthesis of adrenal androgens by the zona reticularis are adrenogenital syndrome and tumors of the adrenal cortex, particularly carcinoma.

27.2.3. 17-α-Hydroxyprogesterone

This substance is an important precursor in glucocorticoid synthesis. Adequate channeling of 17-α-hydroxyprogesterone into compound S (11-deoxycortisol and compound F (cortisol) involves the integrity of two enzymes— 21-hydroxylase and 11-hydroxylase, respectively. Hence, when a partial or complete block in either one of these two enzymes occurs, there is accumulation of 17-hydroxyprogesterone, the precursor proximal to the block. The measurement of serum level of 17-α-hydroxyprogesterone has supplanted the cumbersome need for urine collections to estimate pregnanetriol in urine, the conventional indicator of enzymatic blocks involving 21- or 11-hydroxylase.

The primary indication to obtain 17-hydroxyprogesterone level in plasma is the evaluation of a patient suspected of having adrenogenital syndrome, i.e., ambiguous genitalia, hyponatremia, and hyperkalemia in the neonatal life, precocious puberty in the male child, virilization in the female child, hypertension and hypokalemia in young adults, and, most commonly, in the evaluation of hirsutism in adult females.

27.2.4. Urinary 17-Hydroxycorticosteroids

This measurement of the "Porter–Silber chromogens" in a 24-hr collection of urine estimates the metabolic products of glucocorticoid activity. Purportedly, this reflects the integrated secretory activity of cortisol in a 24-hr period as opposed to the serum cortisol, which merely reflects that activity at a given moment. Approximately one-third of the cortisol secreted during the day is excreted as 17-OHCS in the urine. Since this measurement depends on intact hepatic and renal mechanisms of inactivation and clearance, the presence of liver or kidney damage would alter these levels.

As a screening test for hypo- or hyperfunction of the adrenal cortex, the urinary 17-OHCS are of help only when the values are extremely low or extremely high. The recent availability of 24-hr urine free cortisol determination is a much superior screening test for hypercortisolism than the 17-OHCS. The most significant value of the 17-OHCS is related to the fact that all the major dynamic tests for adrenal dysfunction have been standardized on the basis of the 17-OHCS in urine. Thus, the standard dexamethasone suppression test, the standard ACTH stimulation test, and the standard metyrapone test are all interpreted using 17-OHCS in urine as the measured parameter.

27.2.5. Urinary 17-Ketosteroids

These compounds, measured in the urine by the Zimmerman reaction, reflect the metabolic products of adrenal androgens such as dehydroepiandrosterone, androstenedione, and etiocholanolone. The 17-KS level in the urine is not a measure of testosterone activity, since the contribution of this potent androgen to the urinary 17-KS is only minor. The advent of DHEA assays in plasma has decreased reliance on measuring urinary 17-KS to determine adrenal androgenicity.

27.2.6. Urinary Free Cortisol

In contrast to plasma cortisol, which is affected by changes in the level of transcortin, the urinary free cortisol parallels the true secretory rate of the glucocorticoids by the adrenal cortex. The measurement of "free" cortisol in the urine is a reflection of complete or near-complete saturation of transcortin by endogenously secreted cortisol. Thus, the only means of increasing free cortisol in the urine is by complete occupancy of transcortin by cortisol, resulting in a spillover "filterable" cortisol, which is measured in urine as free cortisol. The urinary free cortisol is considered a sensitive screening test for hypercortisolism since it is independent of perturbations in transcortin and since it is nearly always elevated in that disorder. However, it should be recognized that endogenous depression and stress can also elevate urinary free cortisol. As a screening test for hypofunction, urinary free cortisol is unreliable, since the levels in normals and hypoadrenal patients overlap considerably.

27.3. Dynamic Tests to Evaluate Adrenocortical Function

These are tests that employ various maneuvers to test the physiology of the hypothalamo–pituitary–adrenal (HPA) axis. As in other areas of endocrinology, stimulation tests are used when hypofunction is suspected, and suppression tests are used when hyperfunction is suspected. Table 58 summarizes the various dynamic tests employed in the evaluation of adrenocortical dysfunction. The stimulation test is first described, followed by an overview of the various suppression tests that have been devised. Finally, the metyrapone test and tests involving ACTH are mentioned.

TABLE 58
Dynamic Tests in the Evaluation of Adrenocortical
Dysfunction

Test	Comment
Rapid ACTH stimulation test	Screening test for hypoadrenalism
Standard ACTH stimulation test	Definitive test to document hypoadrenalism as well as its origin, i.e., pituitary versus adrenal
Metyrapone test	A test to document ACTH deficiency as the cause for hypoadrenalism; also useful in differentiating the etiologies of hypercortisolism
Overnight dexamethasone suppression tests	Screening test for hypercortisolism
Standard dexamethasone suppression test	Assists in delineating the etiology of hypercortisolism

27.3.1. The Stimulation Tests

27.3.1.1. Rapid ACTH Stimulation Test

This is a simple screening test to detect adrenal insufficiency. In its simplest form, the test involves measuring the basal plasma cortisol before and 30, 60, and 90 min following the administration of an intravenous bolus of 25 U (2.5 mg) of synthetic ACTH (cosyntropin). The normal response varies according to different workers, but one that is accepted by most is a cortisol level that doubles and increases by 10 μg over the base line following ACTH. The peak is usually evident in 60 min but occasionally takes longer. The test can also be performed in the ill patient who cannot tolerate a delay in therapy by administering methylprednisolone and fludrocortisone prior to the test. This provides gluco- and mineralocorticoid support to the ill patient while allowing the diagnostic study to be performed.

Three statements need to be emphasized regarding the rapid ACTH stimulation test. First, the test is, at best, a screening procedure and separates the normal responder from the abnormal one; i.e., the demonstration of a clearly normal response precludes the need for further workup in the direction of adrenal failure. Second, a blunted or flat response can be encountered in both primary (Addison's) and secondary (pituitary) hypoadrenal states; in the former, the lack of response results from a decreased reserve of the zona fasciculata, whereas in the latter condition, this layer of the cortex is dorment because of chronic ACTH deprivation. Third, and most importantly, the response patterns of patients with partial adrenal insufficiency (the limited adrenal reserve syndrome) and patients under stress can be quite variable and can defy interpretation. For instance, some patients with partial disease may show a near-normal response of the rapid test, whereas normal subjects under stress, whose adrenals already are working at full capacity, may not demonstrate the expected peak following ACTH. It is for these reasons that the rapid ACTH test should be considered only as a screening test. No patient should be placed on life-long steroid replacement solely on the basis of results of the rapid ACTH test performed in the simple manner described above. For definitive documentation of adrenal failure, one resorts to the standard ACTH stimulation test. We revisit the rapid test in its modified form following an overview of the standard ACTH stimulation test.

27.3.1.2. The Standard ACTH Stimulation Test

This test evaluates the ability of the adrenal cortex to secrete glucocorticoids in response to protracted stimulation with ACTH. The parameter evaluated is the 24-hr urinary 17-OHCS (and in some protocols the 17-KS as well). The test, which requires hospitalization and the meticulous collection of 24-hr urines for 7 days at a stretch, is performed as follows. Base-line 24-hr urinary 17-OHCS (and 17-KS) are collected for 2 days. Plasma cortisol and the plasma level of circulating ACTH are also assayed at the basal state. Then, 40 U of ACTH (crystalline, soluble ACTH) is infused in normal saline for an 8-hr period, usually from 8 a.m. to 4 p.m. The urinary 17-OHCS, 17-KS, and plasma cortisol are assayed daily and continuously during the 3 days of ACTH infusion as well as for 1 day thereafter. The total test period in this format is 7 days (Table 59).

In interpreting this cumbersome but "gold standard" of a test, three points are worth bearing in mind. First, the normal adrenal cortex puts out most of its glucocorticoids during the first day of ACTH administration, with the normal response defined as a two- to fourfold increase in the 17-OHCS following the infusion. Second, patients with Addison's disease demonstrate a characteristic flat response throughout the test, whereas patients with hypopituitarism (ACTH deficiency) demonstrate a "stepladder" pattern of increase, with responses after the second or third day of ACTH. Third, patients with "limited reserve" syndrome show their maximal response in the first day

TABLE 59
The Standard ACTH Stimulation Test

Day	ACTH	Cortisol	Urine 17-OHCS	17-KS
1 (Pretest)	Basal	Basal	Basal	Basal
2 (Pretest)	Basal	Basal	Basal	Basal
3 (40 U ACTH)	—	√	√	√
4 (40 U ACTH)	—	√	√	√
5 (40 U ACTH)	—	√	√	√
6 (Posttest)	—	√	√	√

of ACTH, after which the magnitude of response diminishes. This pattern may overlap with the response of some normal subjects.

In general, the standard ACTH stimulation test permits the differentiation to be made among normals, primary hypoadrenalism, secondary hypoadrenalism, and the limited adrenal reserve syndrome. The limitations of the test are the time and expense consumed as well as the cumbersome need for collecting seven 24-hr urines.

Since the sole purpose of the standard ACTH test is to evaluate the performance of adrenal cortex under repeated stimulation, the rapid test can be modified to suit such a purpose. The "rapid" ACTH test can be performed on three occasions, with sampling of plasma not only for cortisol but also for aldosterone and plasma DHEA.

The criteria that characterize Addison's disease are a low basal serum cortisol that repeatedly demonstrates a failure to respond to a bolus of intravenous ACTH, a low basal serum aldosterone that fails to respond to intravenous ACTH, and a low basal serum DHEA level that also fails to respond to ACTH.

In contrast to Addison's disease, hypopituitary patients demonstrate preservation of aldosterone response to ACTH even when the cortisol response is blunted because of dormancy.

27.3.2. The Suppression Tests

The suppression tests evaluate the ability of the hypothalamo–pituitary axis to suppress in response to orally administered dexamethasone, a potent glucocorticoid. Obviously, these tests assume importance only when hyperfunction is suspected. The overnight dexamethasone test evaluates the plasma cortisol level following 1 mg dexamethasone given at midnight (before sleep). The dexamethasone given before sleep abolishes the nycthemereal release of ACTH, and hence the cortisol level drawn at 8 a.m. will be below 5 μg/dl. Dexamethasone is potent at this dose but does not interfere with plasma measurements of cortisol. The value of the test lies in the fact that it is convenient, inexpensive, and if the patient suppresses below 5 μg, hypercortisolism is nearly completely excluded. Unfortunately, there is a wide variety of conditions characterized by "nonsuppression"—obesity (30–45%), drug intake (estrogens, diphenylhydantoin), alcoholism, and endogenous depression. Thus, the only valuable information provided by the test is when the results are suppressible, i.e., a decline below 5 μg following oral dexamethasone.

The low-dose dexamethasone test involves administering 0.5 mg of dexamethasone four times a day orally for 2 days and evaluating the 24-hr urinary 17-OHCS before and after; normal suppression is defined as a decrease in 17-OHCS below 3.5 mg after dexamethasone. The only group of patients who suppress to the low dose, in terms of those who showed nonsuppression to the overnight test, are the obese patients and some patients on medication; since the urinary free cortisol is a superior index for hypercortisolism because it is not affected by obesity or medications, the low-dose test has nothing more to offer in these circumstances than the urinary free cortisol does. Therefore, in many centers, the low-dose test is circumvented in favor of the 24-hr urinary free cortisol.

The high-dose dexamethasone test evaluates the 17-OHCS before and after the administration of 2 mg of oral dexamethasone four times a day for 2 days. Suppression here is defined as a drop in the 17-OHCS by at least 50% of the base line. This test has some discriminatory value in separating the various etiologies of hypercortisolism in the following manner:

1. The characteristic response of pituitary-dependent Cushing's is suppression to the high dose but nonsuppression to the low dose.
2. The characteristic response of adrenal tumors is nonsuppression to high dose, since endogenous ACTH is already maximally suppressed.
3. The characteristic response of ectopic ACTH-secreting tumor is also nonsuppression to the high dose.

Despite the above "classical" responses, it should be realized that there are several exceptions to the general rules outlined above:

1. Twenty to 25% of patients with pituitary dependent Cushing's may not suppress to a high dose, requiring a "high-high" dose, since they are functioning at a phenomenally higher threshold.
2. A small (5%) number of patients with adrenal tumors (micronodular disease) may demonstrate preservation of high-dose suppression, thus mimicking pituitary-dependent Cushing's.
3. The rare bronchial carcinoid ectopically secreting ACTH may also demonstrate preservation of suppression to the high-dose dexamethasone test.
4. Endogenous depression is often associated with abnormal steroid dynamics, the most frequent one being nonsuppression to the low dose but preservation of suppression to the high dose, mimicking pituitary disease. It is particularly important to keep this entity in mind, since the urinary free cortisol also can be elevated in depressed patients. The constellation of elevated urinary free cortisol and abnormal suppression data in such patients may result in an erroneous diagnosis of pituitary-dependent Cushing's.

Table 60 outlines the hormonal dynamic tests involving suppression tests in diverse conditions. The differential diagnosis of a "pituitary response," i.e., nonsuppression to low dose but preservation of suppression to a high dose of dexamethasone, includes the occasional adrenal adenoma, the rare bronchial carcinoid with ectopic ACTH secretion, the frequently encountered patient with endogenous depression, and the patient on anticonvulsants. The differential diagnosis of nonsuppression to high dose includes adenoma or carcinoma of adrenal, ectopic ACTH-secreting neoplasms, as well as the minority of patients with pituitary-dependent Cushing's functioning at a markedly high set point for negative feedback suppression.

TABLE 60
Dynamic Testing in States of Hypercortisolism: General Principles

Condition	Overnight DXM (1 mg DXM at midnight P.O.)	Low-dose DXM (0.5 mg q.i.d. for 2 days)	High-dose DXM (2 mg q.i.d. for 2 days)	Ancillary tests			
				ACTH Stim.	Metapyrone	Plasma ACTH	Other
Exogenous obesity	75% suppress, 25% may not	Suppression	Not indicated				
Endogenous depression and stress	Close to 40% may not show suppression	90% suppress	100% suppress				
Diphenylhydantoin, estrogens	No suppression	No suppression	Suppression				
Pituitary ACTH-dependent Cushing's	No suppression	No suppression	Suppression	Exaggerated response	Exaggerated response	"Normal" to modest ↑	
Adrenal adenoma	No suppression	No suppression	No suppression	50% show no response	May or may not respond	Suppressed	CT scan
Adrenal CA	No suppression	No suppression	No suppression	No response	No response	Suppressed	CT scan, 17-KS
Ectopic ACTH syndromes	No suppression	No suppression	No suppression	No response	No response	↑↑	
Definition of normal response	Post-DXM value under 5 µg is suppression	17-OHCS less than 3.5 mg in 24 hr is suppression	17-OHCS less than 50% of base line is suppression				

The algorithm for the workup of hypercortisolism is outlined in Figure 4 (Chapter 4).

From the foregoing, it becomes apparent that the various stimulation tests to evaluate hypoadrenalism and the diverse suppression tests to evaluate hypercortisolism are helpful in most instances. Two other adjuncts in evaluation of both hypo- and hypercortisolism are metyrapone test and the plasma ACTH assay. These are discussed in Chapter 3.

28

Hyperfunction of the Adrenal Cortex

28.1. Introduction

Hyperfunction of the adrenal cortex is associated with three distinct clinical syndromes. Hypersecretion of mineralocorticoids by the zona glomerulosa results in the syndrome of primary hyperaldosteronism; hyperfunction of the zona fasciculata is expressed as Cushing's syndrome; hyperfunction of zona reticularis results in virilizing syndromes.

28.2. Primary Hyperaldosteronism

The sustained hypersecretion of mineralocorticoids by the zona glomerulosa results in the development of the syndrome of primary hyperaldosteronism. Primary hyperaldosteronism probably represents 1% to 2% of all cases of hypertension. The most common mineralocorticoid that is hypersecreted is aldosterone, but, rarely, mineralocorticoid excess may involve selective hypersecretion of deoxycorticosterone (DOC). Currently hyperaldosteronism exists in the following three forms: (1) aldosterone-producing adenoma, (2) bilateral hyperplasia, and (3) glucocorticoid-suppressible hyperaldosteronism (GSH). As becomes apparent in Section 28.2.4, identification of each of the abovementioned entities is crucial because of the significant differences in therapy.

28.2.1. Clinical Features

The two classes of symptoms in patients with hyperaldosteronism are those related to hypertension and those related to hypokalemia. Both reflect the consequences of sustained production of aldosterone by the zona glomerulosa.

28.2.1.1. Hypertension

The most common symptom experienced by patients with hyperaldosteronism is headache. In general, the hypertension tends to be mild and nonprogressive in nature, with a paucity of significant target organ damage. Thus, it is unusual for these patients to develop grade III or grade IV retinopathy, cardiac failure, or renal insufficiency. However, exceptionally, there may be severe hypertension with sequelae.

28.2.1.2. Symptoms of Hypokalemia

The three symptoms of hypokalemia experienced by patients with primary hyperaldosteronism are weakness of extremities, polyuria, and parasthesias. The muscle weakness can be chronic and mild or may be manifested as sudden severe weakness. Polyuria is secondary to impaired conservation of water by the renal tubules, which are resistant to the effects of vasopressin (nephrogenic diabetes insipidus). The parasthesias result from increased neuromuscular excitability caused by chronic hypokalemia. In extreme cases, twitching and even tetany may develop.

The physical examination of patients with primary hyperaldosteronism is usually unremarkable.

28.2.2. Diagnostic Studies

The four diagnostic features of primary hyperaldosteronism are hypokalemia, kaliuresis, suppressed plasma renin activity (PRA), and an elevated, nonsuppressible aldosterone level in the serum.

28.2.2.1. Hypokalemia

The biochemical hallmark of primary hyperaldosteronism is hypokalemia. In instances of "normokalemic hyperaldosteronism," this abnormality is often unmasked by the administration of diuretics or by a salt load. The serum potassium usually ranges between 2 and 3.5 mEq/liter, occasionally declining to dangerously low levels.

28.2.2.2. Kaliuresis

The hypokalemia in primary aldosteronism results from loss of K^+ in the urine, an effect of excess aldosterone. Continuous potassium excretion in the urine in the presence of hypokalemia is inappropriate and is clearly indicative of renal losses of K^+ as the primary mechanism of hypokalemia. Such a combination is not unique to primary hyperaldosteronism and is encountered in diverse disease states (see Section 28.2.3).

28.2.2.3. Suppressed Plasma Renin Activity

The enzymatic hallmark of primary hyperaldosteronism is a low PRA, reflecting the suppression of this enzyme because of negative feedback from the sodium retention. Retention of sodium and volume expansion are features of hypersecretion of aldosterone. The suppressive effect on renin release is so profound that provocative stimuli fail to increase the PRA. Thus, assumption of upright posture and volume depletion induced by diuretics, powerful provocative stimuli that augment renin release, fail to increase renin level in patients with primary hyperaldosteronism. The test is performed by measuring plasma level of renin in the recumbent state and following ambulation for 2 to 4 hr. The failure to demonstrate an increase in PRA with upright posture and diuretics is the diagnostic hallmark of mineralocorticoid excess.

28.2.2.4. Nonsuppressible Aldosterone

The hormonal hallmark of primary hyperaldosteronism is increased secretion of aldosterone. Since the hypersecretion of aldosterone in these patients is autonomous, the level of the hormone, predictably, demonstrates inadequate suppression to salt administration, a maneuver that normally suppresses this hormone. The test is performed by evaluating the response of aldosterone in the plasma before and after the intravenous administration of 2 liters of normal saline in 4 hr. In normal subjects as well as in patients with essential hypertension, the serum level of aldosterone declines below 8.5 ng/dl following saline. Failure to do so is highly suspicious of mineralocorticoid excess. It should be pointed out that the aldosterone studies should be performed only after normalizing the serum potassium, since the aldosterone level can, even in "autonomous" states, be lowered by profound hypokalemia.

28.2.3. Differential Diagnosis

The four diagnostic features of primary hyperaldosteronism—hypokalemia, kaliuresis, suppressed PRA, and nonsuppressible aldosterone—are shared by several disorders (Table 61). The criteria for the diagnosis of primary aldosteronism are hypokalemia, kaliuresis, suppressed PRA, elevated, nonsuppressible aldosterone level, and exclusion of partial adrenogenital syndromes.

Once the diagnosis of primary aldosteronism has been established, the distinct etiology for mineralocorticoid excess needs to be delineated; this is crucial for therapy, since the three etiologic disorders that cause hyperaldosteronism, i.e., adenoma, hyperplasia, and GSH (glucocorticoid-suppressible hyperaldosteronism), respond to widely different therapeutic modalities. The

TABLE 61
Differential Diagnosis of Primary Aldosteronism

Feature	Common causes	Rare
Hypokalemia	Diuretic use Diarrhea Laxative abuse Vomiting Malignant hypertension	Primary aldosteronism Bartter's syndrome Cushing's syndrome Ectopic ACTH syndrome Renin-secreting tumors
Hypokalemia with kaliuresis	Diuretic use Malignant hypertension Ectopic ACTH- secreting tumors	Primary aldosteronism Low-renin essential hypertension Bartter's syndrome Cushing's syndrome Renin-secreting tumors Adrenogenital syndrome
Hypokalemia, kaliuresis, and suppressed PRA	Primary aldosteronism Low-renin essential hypertension	Partial adreno- genital syndrome
Hypokalemia, kaliuresis, suppressed PRA, and nonsuppressible aldosterone level	Primary hyperaldosteronism	Partial 17-hydroxylase deficiency

distinction can be made by hormonal maneuvers, noninvasive imaging techniques, therapeutic maneuvers, and invasive methods. This order is important to follow to save the patient needless invasive tests.

28.2.3.1. Hormonal Maneuvers

Patients with aldosterone-producing adenoma (Conn's syndrome) demonstrate an anomalous decline in the aldosterone level with posture, whereas patients with hyperplasia do not. Patients with GSH generally behave like those with hyperplasia, although they may occasionally demonstrate an anomalous decline, mimicking adenoma. The anomalous decline in patients with aldosterone-producing adenoma is believed to be a reflection of ACTH dependence of these tumors. Such a response is encountered in nearly 85% to 90% of patients with aldosteronomas.

28.2.3.2. Noninvasive Imaging Techniques

Computerized tomography of the adrenals detects a solitary adenoma in the zona glomerulosa in approximately 40–60% of instances. The small size of the tumor is the reason for the low yield. The success rate of localization using [131I]iodocholesterol to detect the adrenal adenoma is also variable, ranging from 30% to 70%.

28.2.3.3. Therapeutic Maneuvers

In patients with CT-negative hyperaldosteronism, a trial of dexamethasone for 4 weeks is indicated to exclude glucocorticoid-suppressible hyperaldosteronism. These patients demonstrate impressive improvement in blood pressure, hypokalemia, and abnormal aldosterone dynamics following dexamethasone.

28.2.3.4. Invasive Methods

Selective catheterization of adrenal veins with measurement of aldosterone in venous effluent is diagnostic; the level of aldosterone in the venous effluent from the side of the tumor is severalfold higher than that on the normal side. Since the adenoma responds in an exaggerated fashion to the administration of ACTH, the test can be performed with the use of ACTH, which magnifies the difference between the two sides.

Figure 20 explains the algorithm for investigating the patient with primary aldosteronism.

28.2.4. Treatment

The treatment for aldosterone-producing adenoma is surgical removal of the tumor. The results of such therapy in terms of normalizing the blood pressure are excellent and gratifying. The treatment for bilateral hyperplasia is medical, with the use of spironolactone, an aldosterone antagonist. The treatment for GSH is the chronic use of small doses of dexamethasone.

28.3. Cushing's Syndrome

The hypersecretion of glucocorticoids by the zona fasciculata is called "hypercortisolism" and can result either from increased ACTH drive from the pituitary or elsewhere (ectopic ACTH) or from autonomous hypersecretion of cortisol by a tumor in the adrenal cortex. The most common tumor of the adrenal cortex that causes Cushing's syndrome is an adenoma, but less frequently, carcinoma of the adrenal, a devastating disease, may underlie the hypersecretion.

28.3.1. Clinical Features

The clinical features that are associated with hypercortisolism were described in Chapter 4 in regard to pituitary-dependent Cushing's disease. The features of chronic sustained hypercortisolism are the same regardless of whether the reason for the hypersecretion is excess pituitary ACTH or autonomous secretion of glucocorticoids by a benign adrenal adenoma. Thus, the plethoric features of hypercortisolism (weight gain, truncal obesity, "mooning

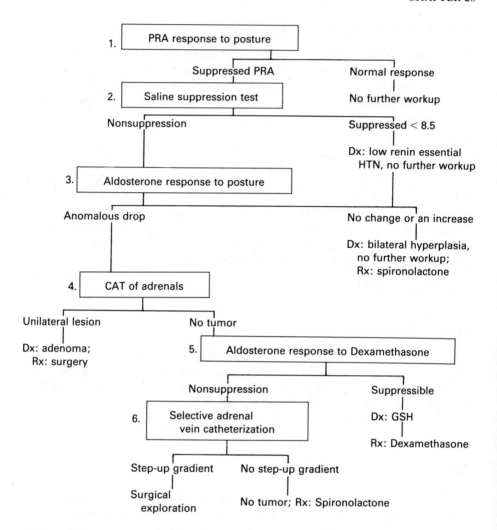

FIGURE 20. Algorithm for workup of mineralcorticoid excess. GSH, Glucocorticoid suppressible hyperaldosteronism.

of face," dorsocervical fat pads, striae, and flushed face) are identical in both diseases. The nonspecific features of central Cushing's disease, such as hypertension, glucose intolerance, mild hirsutism, etc., are also seen with the same frequency in Cushing's syndrome caused by adrenal adenomas. Further, the serious facets of hypercortisolism, such as myopathy, psychopathy, and osteoporosis, complicate the course of patients with both pituitary-dependent (central) and -nondependent (adrenal) Cushing's. Therefore, in most clinical settings it is difficult to differentiate the two entities on the basis of clinical findings alone. However, the presence of visual field cuts, severe headaches, galactorrhea, and pigmentation, when present, are suggestive of pituitary-dependent Cushing's disease.

When Cushing's syndrome is caused by adrenal carcinoma, the clinical presentation is highlighted by the presence of virilization. The combination of hypercortisolism and virilization in females is virtually diagnostic of this lethal disease. Virilization is characterized by amenorrhea, breast atrophy, temporal baldness, increased muscle mass, acne, clitoromegaly, and hirsutism. The rapid evolution is also striking.

When Cushing's syndrome is caused by ectopic ACTH secretion, three distinct syndromes evolve: cachectic, pigmentary, and plethoric. The most frequent ones are cachectic and pigmentary. The cachectic form of ectopic ACTH-secreting syndrome, the prototype of which is lung cancer, is characterized by severe weight loss, darkening of skin, and metabolic changes of profound cortisol excess (hypokalemic alkalosis and hyperglycemia). In the pigmentary form, the clinical picture is dominated by increased skin pigmentation with little or no clinical evidence of Cushing's syndrome. The reason for the paucity of plethoric findings in these circumstances is that the malignancy does not allow the patient enough time to develop cushingoid features. Occasionally, however, patients with ectopic ACTH secretion may indeed manifest the plethoric features of Cushing's; the four classical examples of such a phenomenon are represented by ectopic ACTH secretion by carcinoids of the bronchus, carcinoid tumors of the pancreatic islets, medullary carcinoma of the thyroid, and pheochromocytoma. The ectopic ACTH secreted by these tumors, which are benign or of a low-grade malignancy, results in chronic stimulation of both adrenal glands. In all cases of ectopic ACTH-secreting syndrome, the disease results in stimulation of both adrenal glands. To this extent, the disorder resembles pituitary-dependent Cushing's disease. The vast majority of tumors that secrete ACTH ectopically are indeed autonomous. A rare exception to this rule is bronchial carcinoid, which may demonstrate some degree of responsiveness to suppression tests. Whether these cases represent ectopic secretion of a corticotrophin-releasing factorlike peptide (CRF-like peptide) is a controversial issue.

When Cushing's syndrome is secondary to iatrogenic causes—the most common form of Cushing's—the clinical features are again identical to other forms of plethoric Cushing's. There is a higher incidence of certain physical findings when Cushing's syndrome is caused by exogenous steroid administration. These include a higher incidence of ocular findings such as cataracts and papilledema, painful myopathy, ischemic necrosis of the femoral head, and pancreatitis. The reasons for the above phenomena are not clear. It is also recognized that the incidence of fractures and opportunistic infections is greater in iatrogenic Cushing's syndrome. Table 62 outlines the clinical presentations of the four forms of hypercortisolism.

28.3.2. Diagnostic Studies

The principles of the dexamethasone suppression tests are outlined in Chapter 27. These general principles, as they apply to hypercortisolism, are further outlined in Chapter 4. The tests that are employed in the diagnostic

TABLE 62
Hypercortisolism: A Clinical Perspective

Pituitary-dependent Cushing's	Adrenal adenoma	Adrenal carcinoma	Ectopic ACTH syndrome	Iatrogenic
Slow evolution	Slow evolution	Rapid evolution	Cachexia	History of steroid therapy
Plethoric features	Plethoric features	Virilization	Pigmentation	Cataracts
Headaches	Unilateral disease	Absence of myopathy	Metabolic ($\downarrow$ K, $\uparrow$ glucose)	Papilledema
Field cuts		Dissemination to lung, bone	Rarely cushingoid	Fractures
Galactorrhea			(carcinoids of bronchus,	Femoral head
Pigmentation			islet cell tumors, MCT,	necrosis
Both adrenals enlarged			tumors, MCT, pheo)	

workup are classified into tests that reflect the presence of hypercortisolism, hormonal tests that indicate an adrenal etiology, and the tests for localization.

28.3.2.1. Tests to Demonstrate Hypercortisolism

The three parameters that indicate the presence of hypercortisolism are the urinary free cortisol, the 24-hr urinary 17-OHCS, and the serum cortisol. Usually, all three are elevated, the most sensitive and specific parameter being the urinary free cortisol.

28.3.2.2. Hormonal Tests to Determine the Adrenal Etiology

Here, again, the three tests to suggest an adrenal etiology are the high-dose dexamethasone suppression test, the metyrapone test, and the plasma level of circulating ACTH. Patients with Cushing's syndrome secondary to an adrenal tumor characteristically demonstrate nonsuppression to the high dose of oral dexamethasone because the endogenous ACTH level is already max-imally suppressed. The response of adrenal tumors to the administration of metyrapone is characterized by a lack of increase in compound S or 17-OHCS because the plasma ACTH in these patients cannot be stimulated. The cir-culating ACTH level, as measured by radioimmunoassay, is undetectable or extremely low (below 10 pg), a physiological negative feedback response to the autonomous production of cortisol by the adrenal tumor. Thus, all three tests—the high-dose dexamethasone test, the metyrapone test, and the plasma ACTH level—are based on a single phenomenon of suppressed corticotrophs of the pituitary gland. If all three tests turn out to be concordant, i.e., non-suppression to high-dose dexamethasone, nonresponse to metyrapone, and a plasma ACTH below 10 pg, the diagnosis of an autonomous adrenal tumor is unmistakable. The next step is to measure the adrenal androgen level, since an abnormally elevated DHEA (or 17-KS in the urine) is an ominous sign, raising the ugly specter of adrenal carcinoma.

28.3.2.3. The Tests for Localization

Computerized tomography is an excellent imaging technique to localize adrenal tumors, with yields as high as 100% for carcinoma and 85% to 90% for adenoma. High-resolution CT of adrenals has obviated the need for resorting to other imaging procedures such as iodocholesterol scans and invasive procedures such as selective venous catheterization, adrenal venography, or arteriography in the evaluation of adrenal tumors.

28.3.3. Prognosis

The complications of hypercortisolism—cosmetic, metabolic, and osseous—are related to the duration and severity of disease. The course is also complicated by opportunistic infections, particularly mycobacterial, fungal (*Cryptococcus, Candida*), and protozoal (*Pneumocystis*). The earlier the disease is detected, the better the outcome. Adrenal carcinoma carries and extremely gloomy prognosis despite the availability of aggressive measures to treat this devastating disease.

28.3.4. Treatment

The therapy for pituitary-dependent Cushing's disease is discussed in Section 4.3.4.

The therapy for adenoma of the adrenal cortex is surgical removal after localization. The cushingoid features ameliorate within a reasonable time (6 months).

The therapy for adrenal carcinoma is discussed in Section 30.2.4.

The treatment of ectopic ACTH-secreting tumors should be aimed at the primary tumor. Surgical debulking or radiation, when applicable, are at best palliative. The use of medical adrenalectomy with o',p'-DDD and the use of metyrapone in large doses to decrease the load of metabolically active compound F are additional medical measures that are available.

28.4. Virilizing Syndromes

Hypersecretion of adrenal androgens by the zona reticularis results in virilization of the female. "Adrenal virilism" can be secondary to bilateral disease, as in adrenogenital syndrome, or be caused by unilateral tumors such as carcinoma of the adrenal gland. The difference between the two conditions is that the adrenogenital syndrome, the hyperandrogenism is an ACTH-dependent phenomenon secondary to faulty cortisol production, whereas the androgen excess encountered in tumors is an example of autonomous hyperandrogenism. The virilizing syndrome caused by adrenal tumors is discussed in Chapter 30. This section deals with the hyperandrogenism of adrenogenital syndromes.

28.4.1. Pathophysiology

The pathophysiology of the adrenogenital syndromes is simple to understand if the disorder is viewed as a series of chain reactions consisting of the following links:

1. The point of origin is a partial or complete inability to secrete the glucocorticoid cortisol; this results from a partial or complete absence of certain enzymes required for steroidogenesis.
2. The lack of cortisol inevitably results in stimulation of pituitary ACTH, since the corticotrophs sense the lack of cortisol.
3. The ACTH release, a compensatory phenomenonon, stimulates both adrenal cortices to increase steroidogenesis in an attempt to overcome the block.
4. Under the vigorous stimulation by their trophic hormone, both adrenal cortices are driven to produce steroids, but production can proceed only up to the synthetic steps proximal to the block. Therefore, there is a marked increase in and accumulation of the products proximal to the block.
5. The final consequence involves the utilization of these precursors into synthesis of androgens, often the only pathway open. Since the zona reticularis is provided with the substrates (precursor products proximal to the block) and the stimulus (ACTH), excessive androgen synthesis occurs.

Two points should be obvious from the above phenomena. First, the entire chain reaction can be abolished by replacing glucocorticoid, the lack of which started the entire process; and second, the clinical effects of these adrenogenital syndromes depend on the severity of the block, because minor, partial blocks can be overcome by the powerful ACTH drive.

Figure 19 (Chapter 26) illustrates the pathway of adrenal steroidogenesis and the various enzymes involved. Some enzyme blocks are incompatible with life (for example, complete deficiency of desmolase); some enzyme deficiencies are rarely encountered (for example, 3-β-ol dehydrogenase deficiency). Some enzyme deficiencies share the dubious distinction of occurring in both the adrenals and the gonads (for example, 17-α-hydroxylase deficiency). But, by and large, the two most frequent enzyme blocks are 21-hydroxylase and 11-hydroxylase deficiencies. The pathophysiology as well as the clinical and hormonal consequences of these two important enzymatic blocks need to be considered individually.

28.4.1.1. 21-Hydroxylase Deficiency

The most frequent enzymatic deficiency is partial or complete lack of this important enzyme. The consequences depend on the severity of the deficiency as well as on the occurrence of deficiency in multiple zones. 21-Hydroxylase in the zona glomerulosa is responsible for converting progesterone into DOC, and in the zona fasciculata, it is responsible for converting 17-α-hydroxyprogesterone into 11-deoxycortisol (compound S). All patients with 21-hydroxylase deficiency lack the enzyme in the zona fasciculata, and when the lack is severe and complete, the enzyme is also absent in the zona glomerulosa. Table 63 summarizes the constellation of features that lead to the expression of the syndrome. The adrenogenital syndrome is a unique example of an adrenal disease in which one part of the gland is underproducing because of an enzyme block while an adjacent part of the same gland is hyperfunctioning. Thus, in 21-hydroxylase deficiency, the dual effects are, on one hand, lack of adequate synthesis of glucocorticoids (and mineralocorticoids), resulting in hypoadrenalism, while, on the other hand, the hyperfunctioning zona reticularis secretes increased androgens, resulting in virilization.

28.4.1.2 11-Hydroxylase Deficiency

This enzyme deficiency is second only to 21-hydroxylase deficiency in terms of its frequency. As in 21-hydroxylase deficiency, the consequences depend on the severity of the deficiency in this enzyme as well as on involvement of more than one zone. In the zona glomerulosa, 11-hydroxylase is responsible for converting DOC into corticosterone, whereas in the zona fasciculata, the enzyme is responsible for converting 11-dexosycortisol (compound S) into cortisol (compound F). Thus, 11-hydroxylase deficiency can be perceived as Nature's metyrapone test, but on a permanent basis. All patients

TABLE 63
21-Hydroxylase Deficiency

Missing enzyme	21-Hydroxylase
Location	Zona fasciculata (ZF)
	Zona glomerulosa (ZG)
Products not formed as a consequence	11-Deoxycortisol, cortisol (ZF)
	DOC, corticosterone, aldosterone (ZG)
Precursors accumulated	17-α-OH-Progesterone (ZF)
	Progesterone (ZG)
Excess hormone synthesized	Androgens: dehydroepiandrosterone, androstenedione
Clinical effects	Lack of gluco- and mineralocorticoids
	Addisonian crisis
	Virilization

· TABLE 64
11-Hydroxylase Deficiency

Missing enzyme	11-Hydroxylase
Location	Zona fasciculata (ZF)
	Zona glomerulosa (ZG)
Products not	Cortisol (ZF)
formed as a	Corticosterone (ZG)
consequence	
Precursors accumulated	11-Deoxycortisol (ZF)
	11-Deoxycorticosterone (DOC) (ZG)
Excess hormone	Androgens:
synthesized	dehydroepiandrosterone,
	androstenedione
Clinical effects	Lack of cortisol
	Virilization
	Excess DOC

with 11-hydroxylase deficiency lack the enzyme in the zona fasciculata, and when the lack is severe and complete, the enzyme is also absent in the zona glomerulosa. Table 64 summarizes the constellation of features that lead to the expression of the syndrome. As in 21-hydroxylase deficiency, one layer (zona fasciculata) suffers from underproduction (of cortisol), and one layer (zona reticularis) has no choice but to hypersecrete androgens. One other important aspect relates to the zona glomerulosa. The product proximal to the block, DOC, possesses some mineralocorticoid activity, and therefore, when large amounts accumulate, the expression is mineralocorticoid excess. Thus, complete 11-hydroxylase defect is the only situation in which two zones (ZR, ZG) secrete excess hormones with biological activity (androgens and DOC) while another zone, (zona fasciculata) cannot produce its hormone, cortisol.

28.4.2. Clinical Features

The clinical features of 21- and 11-hydroxylase deficiencies should be viewed in the perspective of the hormonal excesses and hormonal deficiencies involved (Table 65).

The clinical effects of hyperandrogenism are described first, followed by

TABLE 65
21- and 11-Hydroxylase Deficiencies

Hormone	21 Block	11 Block
Glucocorticoids	↓	↓
Androgens	↑	↑
Mineralocorticoids	↓	↑ (DOC)

a description of the effects of under production of gluco- and mineralocorticoid hormones. Finally, the effects of excess secretion of DOC are outlined.

28.4.2.1. Androgen Excess

The hallmark of adrenogenital syndrome is androgen excess. This effect can be manifested at birth, during childhood, or in adult life. At birth, the hallmark is virilization of the female infant *in utero*. The effects of adrenal androgens on the developing external genitalia of the female fetus are mediated by the conversion of these androgens into testosterone and dihydrotestosterone. The latter compound virilizes the genital tubercle, resulting in clitoromegaly and partial or complete fusion of genital folds. In extreme cases the external genitalia can be completely masculinized, but in most cases the result is ambiguity of genitalia. In male infants the effects of virilization may not be noticeable but rarely may show macrosomia genitalia precox (enlarged phallic proportions).

During childhood, the excess androgens can cause precocious puberty in males and virilization in girls.

In adulthood, partial deficiencies of 21- or 11-hydroxylase express as hirsutism, infertility, and oligomenorrhea or amenorrhea. Thus, the effects of hyperandrogenism are identical in both 21- and 11-hydroxylase deficiencies.

28.4.2.2. Gluco- and Mineralocorticoid Deficiency

This can manifest at birth or, rarely, in childhood. In the complete form of 21-hydroxylase deficiency, the adrenal cortex cannot synthesize glucocorticoids or mineralocorticoids. The neonate, of either sex, rapidly develops vomiting, dehydration, hyponatremia, and hyperkalemia and dies of shock, the entire constellation being strikingly reminiscent of Addison's crisis. Unfortunately, the diagnosis can be missed in the male infant if adrenogenital syndrome (21-hydroxylase) is not kept in mind. In female infants, of course, the ambiguity of genitalia attracts attention. In childhood, especially in children with partial defects of 21-hydroxylase, adrenal insufficiency or crisis can be triggered by stress of infection.

Although glucocorticoid deficiency is a feature of both 21- and 11-hydroxylase deficiencies, hyponatremia, salt wasting, dehydration, and hyperkalemia are restricted to 21-hydroxylase deficiency. This is because in 11-hydroxylase deficiency, the accumulation of the precursor DOC protects against such an occurrence.

28.4.2.3. Mineralocorticoid Excess

This is limited to 11-hydroxylase (and the rare 17-hydroxylase) deficiency. As indicated above, the accumulation of the precursor DOC in patients with 11-hydroxylase deficiency leads to mineralocorticoid excess, resulting in hy-

TABLE 66
Comparative Features of 21- and 11-Hydroxylase Deficiencies

Features	21	11
Androgen excess		
At birth		
Ambiguity	+	+
Masculinization of female	+	+
Childhood		
Precocious puberty in boys	+	+
Virilization in girls	+	+
Adulthood		
Hirsutism	+	+
Amenorrhea	+	+
Infertility	+	+
Glucocorticoid deficiency	+	+
Mineralocorticoid secretion		
Deficiency (salt loss and dehydration)	+	−
Hypertension	−	+

pertension, hypokalemia, and alkalosis—a picture idential to primary aldosteronism.

Table 66 outlines the salient comparative clinical features of 21- and 11-hydroxylase deficiencies and is illustrative of the development of "simple virilizing," "salt losing," and "hypertensive" forms of adrenogenital syndromes.

TABLE 67
Stepwise Diagnostic Approach for Adrenogenital Syndrome

Step	Test	Purpose	Differential diagnosis
1	17-KS (in urine) or DHEA (in plasma)	To confirm adrenal hyperandrogenism	21-Hydroxylase deficiency 11-Hydroxylase deficiency Adrenal carcinoma
2	17-Hydroxyprogesterone	To show increase in the precursors proximal to the block	21-Hydroxylase deficiency 11-Hydroxylase deficiency Rarely, adrenal carcinoma
3	Dexamethasone suppression test	Suppressibility indicates ACTH dependence	21-Hydroxylase deficiency 11-Hydroxylase deficiency
4	Compound S (11-deoxycortisol) in plasma or 17-OHCS in urine	To separate 21 from 11 block	Elevation documents 11-block; decrease indicates 21-block

28.4.3. Diagnostic Studies

The hormal studies for adrenogenital syndrome caused by 21- and 11-hydroxylase deficiencies evolve through four diagnostic steps. The first step is the documentation of adrenal hyperandrogenism; this is done by demonstrating elevated DHEA in the plasma or elevated 17-ketosteroids in the urine. The second step, the confirmatory step, is demonstrating elevated precursor products; this is done by demonstrating an elevated plasma level of 17-α-hydroxyprogesterone, and exquisitely sensitive indicator of 21- to 11-hydroxylase deficiencies. The combination of elevated adrenal androgen and elevated 17-α-hydroxyprogesterone is virtually diagnostic of adrenogenital syndrome. However, rarely, such a combination may be encountered in adrenal carcinoma; the third step is demonstrating that the abnormalities are nonautonomous and ACTH dependent. Thus, the elevated androgens and 17-hydroxyprogesterone suppress in response to dexamethasone administration. Patients with adrenal carcinoma do not suppress to dexamethasone administration. The fourth step is delineation of the exact enzyme that is lacking. The major difference between 21- and 11-hydroxylase deficiency is in compound S levels. Compound S (11-deoxycortisol) levels are low in 21-hydroxylase deficiency, whereas these are elevated in 11-hydroxylase deficiency.

Table 67 illustrates the step-by-step approach to the diagnosis of adrenogenital syndrome caused by 21- or 11-hydroxylase deficiency.

28.4.4. Treatment

The disorder that originated from inadequate synthesis of cortisol can be arrested by supplementation of the glucocorticoid: 1 to 2 mg of dexamethasone administered at bedtime is effective in turning off ACTH and the attendant adverse effects that caused hyperfunction of zona reticularis. Dexamethasone therapy is associated with normalization of cortisol levels as well as a decrease in androgen and precursor levels. With institution of early therapy, menarche and fertility of these patients can be normally preserved or restored. During periods of stress, these patients would require supplementation of glucocorticoid therapy.

Hypofunction of the Adrenals

29.1. Introduction

Adrenal hypofunction exists in three forms: Addison's disease, a term used to describe primary adrenal failure, secondary hypoadrenalism, a consequence of pituitary ACTH deficiency, and selective hypoaldosteronism, which, as the term implies, reflects a breakdown in the mechanisms that mediate the synthesis and release of that mineralocorticoid. The hypoadrenalism caused by pituitary disease is discussed in Chapter 5. This chapter focuses on Addison's disease (usually resulting in "panhypoadrenalism") and selective hypoaldosteronism, in which the zona fasciculata and reticularis are structurally and functionally intact.

29.2. Addison's Disease

Addison's disease represents the classic endocrine disorder with the dual characteristics of being potentially fatal if unrecognized but completely and gratifyingly reversible with the simple replacement of cortisone.

29.2.1. Etiology

The causes for Addison's disease are outlined in Table 68.

The most common current etiology for Addison's disease is autoimmune adrenalitis, representing 66% of patients with primary adrenocortical failure. This disease develops as a result of the effect of autoantibodies directed against the patient's own adrenal cortices, leading to fibrosis and atrophy. Patients with autoimmune adrenalitis demonstrate a heightened susceptibility to de-

TABLE 68
Etiologies of Addison's Disease

Common	Less common	Rare
TB	Drug Heparin, Coumadin	Sarcoid Hemochromatosis Congenital Associated with leukodystrophy
Autoimmune	Sepsis Meningococcus Gram-negative Metastases Lung Breast Fungi Histoplasma Coccidia	

velop other autoimmunopathies such as pernicious anemia or collagen disease. But, more importantly, these patients are prone to develop failure of other endocrine glands (pluriglandular failure), also on an autoimmune basis. Thus, hypoparathyroidism, diabetes, hypothyroidism, and hypogonadism (particularly ovarian) are likely to be associated with or develop later in the patient with autoimmune adrenalitis.

Tuberculosis continues to remain an important etiology for primary adrenocortical failure. In most patients, a history of TB in the distant past is available. In some, active pulmonary TB is evident at the time when Addison's disease is diagnosed, and in others, adrenal involvement is part of miliary (disseminated) tuberculosis.

Metastatic disease to the adrenal, particularly from the lung, represents a common but least recognized etiology. Although autopsy studies reveal a high incidence of adrenal involvement in patients with lung cancer, it used to be thought that the clinical expression is disproportionately low. Careful testing of such patients has revealed an incidence higher than perceived before.

Less common causes are sarcoidoses, hemochromatosis, and sepsis. In infants, the Waterhouse–Freidrichson syndrome is a result of fulminant meningococcemia with adrenal hemorrhage, and in adults a similar entity can be encountered in *E. coli* (or other gram-negative) septicemia. Hemorrhage can also occur as a consequence of *anticoagulant* therapy. Fungal disease usually causes adrenal failure only when the disease is disseminated.

In clinical practice, the two most common etiologies of Addison's disease are autoimmune and TB. The differentiating features between the two conditions are discussed in Section 29.2.3.

29.2.2. Clinical Features

Addison's disease, in its early stages, is a disease that is insidious in onset and evolves gradually and imperceptibly. The classic picture, characterized by the triad of "typical pigmentary changes and wasting in a patient with a feeble pulse" are delayed features of chronically unrecognized disease. Today, no patient should be allowed to develop the classic changes described by Addison in the mid-1800s if the disease is suspected early.

The three major symptoms seen in nearly all patients with Addison's disease are weight loss, fatigue, and pigmentary changes. The three major signs seen in a majority of patients with Addison's disease are hypotension (often orthostatic), increased pigmentation, and objective muscle weakness. Table 69 outlines the possible differential diagnosis.

The pigmentation is generalized and characteristically involves the creases, knuckles, extensor surfaces, areola, scars, and to a lesser extent the mucous membrane. In some patients the pigmentation is barely noticeable ("lingering suntan"), but in others it is striking. The weight loss, weakness, and hypotension also depend on the severity of the disease, which is usually related to chronicity. Lack of axillary hair in the female is a strong sign for adrenocortical insufficiency of primary and pituitary etiologies.

The other symptoms encountered in Addison's disease include GI symptoms (diarrhea, lower abdominal cramps, nausea), depression, menstrual irregularities, impotence, and a tendency to decompensate under simple physical stress such as exercise.

Addison's disease can be the proverbial masquerader. The symptoms can be so nonspecific as to be passed off as nonsignificant. The presentations of Addison's disease can be so diverse and the recognition so difficult that the

TABLE 69
Major Symptoms and Signs of Addison's Disease

Symptom/sign	Reason	Differential diagnosis
1. Weight loss	Anorexia; loss of anabolic effects of adrenal steroids	Extensive: diabetes, hyperthyroidism, malabsorption, renal failure, chronic infection, and malignancy
2. Fatigue	Protein catabolism	Myopathy of any origin
3. Pigmentary changes	Excess β-lipotrophic hormone in response to low cortisol	Ectopic ACTH-secreting tumors, hemochromatosis, malnutrition
4. Orthostatic hypotension	Volume depletion, loss of Na, lack of aldosterone	Dehydration, drugs, dysautonomia, Shy-Drager's
5. Increased pigmentation	Same as 3	Same as 3
6. Muscle weakness	Protein catabolism, lack of anabolism	Myopathy

patient may have seen several specialists in widely different disciplines before the diagnosis is made. Thus, it is not uncommon for the chronically ill patient to have seen the gastroenterologist (for diarrhea), neurologist (for muscle weakness), hematologist (for anemia), cardiologist (for "dizzy spells"), psychiatrist (for depression), and dermatologist (for skin problems) before the entire picture is put together by the astute generalist and referred to the endocrinologist.

29.2.3. Diagnostic Studies

The hormonal evaluation of the patient with adrenocortical failure is detailed in Chapter 27. The following summary highlights some of those points:

1. The basal cortisol levels are of help only when very low. The diagnosis can be missed if basal cortisol levels are the only parameter used.
2. The same can be said for 24-hr urine 17-OHCS (metabolites of glucocorticoids) and urinary free cortisol.
3. The screening test (the rapid ACTH test) only determines if the patient is normal or not. A blunted or flat response is abnormal and is indicative of either primary or secondary (pituitary) hypoadrenalism.
4. The rapid ACTH test can be modified to provide better diagnostic yield. The three criteria to diagnose Addison's disease in the "modified" test are a low basal serum cortisol that repeatedly shows failure to increase following a bolus of intravenous ACTH (25 U or 2.5 mg), a low basal serum aldosterone that fails to rise after ACTH, and a low DHEA level that fails to respond to intravenous ACTH.
5. An elevated basal ACTH level in the plasma (>250 pg) coupled with a low cortisol is clearly diagnostic of primary adrenal failure. When this couplet of tests is clearly abnormal, no further test needs to be done. Unfortunately, the heterogeneity of circulating ACTH has hampered the establishment of a standardized radioimmunoassay.
6. The "gold standard" for establishing the diagnosis of Addison's disease continues to be the "standard ACTH test" (Section 27.3.1.2).

The routine tests are important in that hyponatremia and hyperkalemia are evident in 50–70% of patients with Addison's disease. A small-sized heart on X ray and/or calcifications of the adrenal may be helpful in suggesting the disease.

Once the diagnosis of Addison's disease is established, the etiology should be considered. The salient differences between the two common etiologies (TB, autoimmune) are outlined in Table 70.

29.2.4. Complications

The devastating complication of Addison's disease is the development of "Addisonian crisis." Crisis is often precipitated by stress (trauma, infection,

TABLE 70
Tuberculous versus Autoimmune Etiology

Features	TB	Autoimmune
Incidence	Decreasing (17–30%)	60%
History of TB (past or present)	Obtainable in 70–80%	
Duration of symptoms	Short (6–9 mo)	Longer (6 mo–2 yr)
Calcification of adrenals	30–50%	Rarely may be seen
Associated autoimmunopathy	—	40–70%
Medullary function (catecholamine response to posture)	Decreased	Intact
Genitourinary TB	30–40%	—

etc.) and is ushered in by gastrointestinal symptomology—diarrhea, vomiting, and abdominal cramps. These are rapidly followed by dehydration, hypotension, fever, hyponatremia, hyperkalemia, collapse, and death. Addison's crisis must be considered in every patient with volume depletion and dehydration without obvious cause.

29.2.5. Prognosis

The prognosis of treated Addison's disease is excellent. In fact, few diseases provide the opportunity to observe the drastic beneficial effect of simple treatment as Addison's disease does. The depressed, asthenic, cachectic patient too weak to do anything, living in fear of harboring a dreadful undiagnosed disease, is gradually metamorphosed with cortisone therapy into a healthy, happy, patient gaining weight, confidence, and hope. Such is the therapeutic triumph of proper diagnosis.

In patients with autoimmune adrenalitis, the follow-up should focus on detecting the development of coexistent endocrinopathies (Table 71).

29.2.6. Treatment

The treatment of Addison's disease is simply replacing the glucocorticoids and in some instances mineralocorticoids. The usual replacement dose is 25 mg of cortisone acetate in the morning and 12.5 mg in the evening orally or 20 mg hydrocortisone in the morning and 10 mg in the evening. This dose should be increased during periods of stress (cold, flu, etc.).

Mineralocorticoid replacement with fluorinef, 0.1 mg, is indicated in the presence of hypotension or hyperkalemia. The therapy is life long, and patients should be apprised of this fact to avoid the tendency to stop medication on their own when their general health improves considerably. Also, the

TABLE 71
Syndromes Associated with
Autoimmune Adrenalitis

1. COAP
   Candidiasis
   Ovarian failure
   Adrenal failure
   Parathyroid failure
2. HAM
   Hypoparathyroidism
   Adrenal failure
   Moniliasis
3. Schmidt
   Adrenal failure
   Thyroid failure
   Diabetes
4. Gonadal failure

patient should wear identification tags to indicate the diagnosis and the need for intravenous steroid therapy if found unconscious.

Adrenal crisis is treated by vigorous hydration with saline to replete the intravascular volume, intravenous hydrocortisone, 100 mg every 6 or 8 hr (300 to 400 mg/day), and DOC or fluorinef if hyperkalemia is significant.

29.3. Selective Hypoaldosteronism

As the term implies, selective (isolated) hypoaldosteronism involves deficient function of the zona glomerulosa with preservation of normal function in the rest of the adrenal.

29.3.1. Etiology

The abnormality in patients with selective hypoaldosteronism is physiological rather than structural. There are two mechanisms that could explain the hypoaldosteronism seen in this entity.

29.3.1.1. Hyporeninemic Hypoaldosteronism

The primary mechanism here is an inability of renin to respond to its provocative stimuli. The juxtaglomerular cells are unable to adequately generate the enzyme renin in response to posture, salt deprivation, or volume depletion. In the absence of renin, the angiotensins cannot be derived from renin substrate, and the absence of angiotensin II (A-II) deprives the zona glomerulosa of the single important physiological stimulus required to synthesize and release aldosterone. Thus, in this form of selective hypoaldosteronism, the fault lies in the failure of renin; the hypoaldosteronism can be viewed as "secondary hypoaldosteronism" acquired as a consequence of failed trophic signals.

The failure to generate renin by the juxtaglomerular apparatus is usually a result of mild renal disease involving the interstitium. Thus, hyporeninemic hypoaldosteronism is seen in association with several renal diseases such as diabetic nephropathy, the most frequent underlying disease, followed by analgesic nephropathy, lead nephropathy, etc. In addition to structural damage to the juxtaglomerular apparatus, neural mechanisms may also be involved in the impaired generation of renin. Since control of renin release is mediated by the autonomic nervous system, and since hyporeninemic hypoaldosteronism is encountered with a higher frequency in diabetics with autonomic neuropathy, the role of such neuropathy in causing impairment of renin release is a plausible hypothesis. Whatever the mechanism, the underlying abnormality in hyporeninemic hypoaldosteronism is a failure to adequately generate renin by the juxtaglomerular cells. The preservation of the ability of the zona glomerulosa to release aldosterone in response to direct stimuli (non-renin-mediated) such as infusions of ACTH or angiotensin II excludes structural problems within the adrenal gland.

29.3.1.2. Normoreninemic Hypoaldosteronism

The mechanism here may relate to the presence of intraadrenal defects within the zona glomerulosa. These patients demonstrate normal or near-normal renin dynamics but may suffer from failure of the adrenal cortex to respond to renin (target organ resistance). The possibility of decreased receptor affinity to angiotensin II, the possibility of an abnormal renin molecule, or the presence of enzymatic defects in the synthesis of aldosterone by the zona glomerulosa have all been postulated. The exact mechanism is far from clear.

29.3.2. Clinical Features

Many patients with selective hypoaldosteronism remain asymptomatic, and the diagnosis is suggested only by abnormal electrolytes. The symptoms, when present, are caused by hyponatremia and hyperkalemia. Thus, muscle weakness, orthostatic hypotension, cardiac arrhythmias, and CNS symptoms dominate the list of symptomology.

29.3.3. Diagnostic Studies

The biochemical hallmark of selective hypoaldosteronism is hyperkalemia disproportionately high to the degree of renal failure (the renal failure is mild, but the hyperkalemia is severe). Salt wasting is often evident in the urine. To this extent, the disorder resembles Addison's disease, which is also characterized by mineralocorticoid loss, hyponatremia, hyperkalemia, and salt loss.

The hormonal criteria for establishing the diagnosis of hyporeninemic hypoaldosteronism are:

1. Failure to generate renin (and aldosterone) in response to posture, salt deprivation, and volume depletion.
2. Preservation of cortisol response to ACTH.
3. Preservation of aldosterone response to non-renin-mediated direct stimuli such as infusions of ACTH or angiotensin II.

The demonstration of the last two criteria excludes Addison's disease and highlights the "isolated" and "selective" nature of the hypoaldosteronism.

29.3.4. Treatment

The treatment is simply replacing mineralocorticoid (0.1 mg/day). The normalization of serum K^+ level and improvement in the dizziness and orthostatic hypotension are evident within weeks after initiation of mineralocorticoid treatment.

30

Tumors of the Adrenal Glands

30.1. Introduction

Benign tumors of the adrenal cortex are frequently discovered as incidental findings during autopsy, indicating the asymptomatic nature of these tumors. Histologically, these benign tumors are adenomas, and although they are more often nonsecretory, they can potentially secrete hormones. When they do, a variety of hypersecretory syndromes result, depending on the site of origin of these adenomas. Thus, adenomas arising from the cells of zona glomerulosa secrete aldosterone, resulting in the clinical syndrome of primary aldosteronism (Conn's syndrome, Section 28.2). Adenomas that arise from cells of the zona fasciculata secrete glucocorticoids, resulting in the familiar expression of Cushing's syndrome (Section 28.3). Rarely, adenomas from the zona reticularis secrete androgens, resulting in hirsutism and even virilization. Adenomas arising from the adrenal medulla secrete catecholamines, resulting in the clinical expression of pheochromocytoma (Section 31.2). Benign, nonsecretory adenomas are seldom detected because of their asymptomatic nature. Benign, hypersecretory adenomas are treated by surgical removal of the tumor or the entire adrenal gland harboring the tumor.

Malignant adrenal tumors, particularly carcinoma of the adrenal cortex and paraganglionoma of the adrenal medulla, are devastating diseases. They strike younger patients, secrete a variety of hormones, progress relentlessly despite treatment, and widely disseminate to distant sites. Adrenal carcinoma, the prototype of malignant disease of the adrenal cortex, occurs much more frequently than it is recognized and merits discussion.

30.2. Carcinoma of Adrenal

Adrenal carcinoma can arise from any layer of the adrenal cortex, as indicated by its secretory versatility, but most commonly it arises from the zona reticularis or fasciculata. Malignant tissue studied by obtaining surgical or autopsy material invariably indicates involvement of more than one layer of the cortex, perhaps a reflection of extension to other areas of the cortex. Adrenal carcinoma occurs with a frequency of approximately 1 : 500,000. This malignancy can occur at any age, ranging from 5 months to 72 years, with a mean age of 37 years.

30.2.1. Clinical Features

There are four major presentations of adrenocortical carcinoma: clinically hyperfunctional tumors, nonfunctional tumors, clinically silent but biochemically functional tumors, and metastatic disease with an "occult" primary. Each of these presentations is important, and they underscore the heterogeneous nature of the manifestations of this deadly disease.

30.2.1. The Clinically Hyperfunctional Carcinoma

Contrary to the popular myth, only 25% of adrenal carcinomas are hypersecretory. The vast majority of adrenal carcinomas are nonsecretory. When the adrenal carcinoma hypersecretes, an array of fascinating syndromes may develop (Table 72). The two most important of these are the virilizing syndrome and Cushing's syndrome. It is important to recognize three aspects regarding the hypersecretion of androgens and glucocorticoids by the carcinoma of the adrenal. First, adrenal carcinomas seldom secrete excess glucocorticoids in the absence of concomitant hypersecretion of androgens. Second, isolated hypersecretion of androgens can occur for an extended period of time before the diagnosis of adrenal carcinoma can be established. Such instances of isolated hyperandrogenism could be mistaken for adrenogenital syndrome if suppression tests and computerized tomograms are not per-

TABLE 72
Hyperfunctioning Adrenal Carcinoma

Hormone secreted	Expression
Common	
Androgens	Hirsutism, virilization
Androgens with glucocorticoids	Cushing's with virilization
Estrogens	Feminization in males
	Precocious puberty in girls
Rare	
"Insulinlike" substance	Hypoglycemia
DOC or aldosterone	Hypertension, hypokalemia
Vasopressin	SIADH
Erythropoietin	Polycythemia

formed. Third, some patients with adrenal carcinoma demonstrate elevated levels of precursor products (17-α-hydroxyprogesterone or compound S), simulating adrenogenital syndrome even more closely. Thus, an important dictum to remember is that the diagnosis of adrenogenital syndrome rests on demonstrating suppression of these products to dexamethasone, a feature not observed in carcinoma.

The effects of hyperandrogenism in the prepubertal child depend on the sex. In boys, precocious puberty occurs, whereas in girls, virilization develops. The effect of androgen excess in adult females varies over a spectrum of clinical changes ranging from hirsutism to the development of clitoromegaly, recession of hair line, deepening of voice, increase in muscle mass, amenorrhea, and atrophy of the breasts. The effect of androgen excess in the adult male is negligible, although occasionally weight gain is a predominant complaint.

Since adrenal androgens are, at best, weak androgens, very large amounts are required to cause clinical effects. Further, when adrenal cells become malignant, there is some loss of the enzyme systems required for hormone synthesis. Therefore, it is not surprising that the tumor has to become quite large and often long standing before the clinical features are manifest. For the same reason, a palpable mass is found in nearly one-third of patients presenting with the hypersecretory variety of adrenal carcinoma.

In summary, the hypersecretory variety of adrenal carcinoma is characterized by the interesting clinical syndromes they produce, by their large size, and by the increase in circulating adrenal androgens.

30.2.1.2. The Nonfunctional Adrenal Carcinoma

These tumors are highly inefficient hormone secretors and present as an abdominal mass or with symptoms referable to metastatic events. As indicated above, the nonsecretory variety of adrenal carcinoma occurs more frequently than the secretory variety. The levels of adrenal hormones are normal in this entity, which can be diagnosed only by computerized tomography.

30.2.1.3. Clinically Silent but Biochemically Functional Adrenal Carcinoma

These tumors are characterized by the triad of an abdominal mass, an abundance of hormonal precursors in the urine or plasma, and no clinical evidence of hyperfunctional syndromes. The serum levels of 17-hydroxyprogesterone and 11-deoxycortisol are elevated.

30.2.1.4. Metastatic Disease

Adrenal carcinoma should be a consideration in patients presenting with metastases to the lungs or liver but with no obvious primary. All variants of adrenal carcinomas demonstrate a proclivity to disseminate to the lungs.

30.2.2. Diagnostic Studies

The two lines of diagnostic studies in the evaluation of adrenal carcinoma are hormonal tests and imaging studies.

30.2.2.1. Hormonal Tests

Elevated adrenal androgens (DHEA) and/or glucocorticoids are seen only in the hypersecretory adrenal carcinomas. In many instances, an increase in inactive precursors may be seen in the plasma or urine.

30.2.2.2. Imaging Studies

The advent of high-resolution computerized tomography has obviated the need for all other invasive (venography) and noninvasive ([^{131}I]iodocholesterol) imaging tests for the diagnosis of adrenal carcinoma. The CT scan not only effectively identifies the adrenal tumor but can also provide information regarding its malignant nature. Carcinomas can be identified by their irregular margin and infiltration into surrounding tissue. The yield with computerized tomography in delineating adrenal tumors is nearly 100%.

30.2.3. Prognosis

Adrenal carcinoma is a highly malignant disease. At the time of diagnosis, nearly 50% of patients already have metastases to the paraaortic nodes or distally. Distal metastases occur in the lungs, liver, and bones. In addition, adrenal carcinoma tends to be locally invasive, infiltrating the nearby blood vessels, particularly the inferior vena cava. Most patients with adrenal carcinoma die within 2 years of diagnosis.

30.2.4. Treatment

The two modes of treatment for adrenal carcinoma are surgery and chemotherapy. Surgical removal of the affected adrenal is the primary mode of therapy when the tumor is confined to the adrenal. Unfortunately, only 7% of patients with adrenal carcinoma demonstrate tumor confined to and contained within the adrenal gland. When the tumor is invasive, surgery is fraught with operative risk. When the cancer is disseminated, chemotherapy assumes primary importance. In such cases, the value of palliative adrenalectomy for "debulking" the tumor mass is debatable.

Chemotherapy with the drug o',p'-DDD has proved effective in the treatment of metastatic adrenal carcinoma. After an average course of 3 months, some improvement is seen in 35–60% of patients with metastatic adrenal carcinoma. In addition, to blocking synthesis of cortisol (and, in higher doses, synthesis of aldosterone), o',p'-DDD also alters mitochondrial morphology of adrenocortical cells. The dose of the drug ranges between 2 and 6 g a day and is attended by severe gastrointestinal reactions. The drug does prolong survival, and prolonged remission has been reported occasionally.

31

The Adrenal Medulla and Pheochromocytoma

31.1. Adrenal Medulla

The adrenal medulla synthesizes and releases catecholamines. Although this property is shared by sympathetic nervous tissue throughout the entire length of the sympathetic chain, the adrenal medulla differs in two important respects. First, the rate of production and release of catecholamines by the adrenal medulla are several hundredfold greater in comparison to the tissue of the sympathetic nervous system elsewhere. In this regard, the medulla can be regarded as a large "master ganglion" of the sympathetic system. Second, although norepinephrine can be secreted by the tissues of sympathetic nervous system as well as by the medulla, the enzymatic machinery required to produce epinephrine is possessed only by the adrenal medulla and the organ of Zuckerkandl, a structure composed of chromaffin-staining cells situated near the origin of the inferior mesenteric artery and often extending alongside the aorta until its bifurcation.

The cells of the adrenal medulla demonstrate unique staining properties. As early as 1860, Henle made the observation that cells of the adrenal medulla developed a reddish brown precipitate when treated with potassium dichromate. This "chromaffin reaction" is used even today to recognize cells of the sympathetic nervous system.

The synthetic products of the adrenal medulla are norepinephrine and epinephrine. These products, collectively called the catecholamines, are synthesized from the amino acid tyrosine. The adrenal medulla and sympathetic tissue belong to the APUD system (amino acid precursors uptake decarboxylation). Tyrosine is taken up by the medulla and, through the formation of dopa and dopamine, is converted to norepinephrine and epinephrine. The enzymes involved in the formation of the catecholamines are outlined in Figure 21.

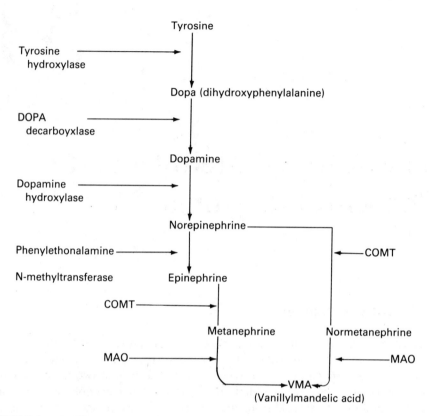

FIGURE 21. Synthesis and metabolism of catecholamines. COMT, catecholamine O'-methyl-transferase; MAO, monoamine oxidase.

Three important observations are clinically pertinent as they relate to catecholamine synthesis and metabolism. First, the enzyme phenylethanolamine N-methyltransferase is present only in the adrenal medulla and the organ of Zuckerkandl. Thus, elevation of epinephrine clearly indicates an origin from one of these structures. Second, both catecholamines are converted to their respective methylated compounds (normetanephrine and metanephrine) by the enzyme catecholamine O'-methyltransferase (COMT). These products are excreted in the urine. Third, these products are further inactivated by monoamine oxidase (MAO) into 3-methoxy-4-hydroxymandelic acid (VMA). With the above background, the colorful clinical picture of pheochromocytoma can be reviewed.

31.2. Pheochromocytoma

Pheochromocytoma, a tumor originating from the adrenal medulla or sympathetic tissue, is characterized by hypersecretion of catecholamines. The origin, clinical presentation, and biochemistry as well as the size, course, and associations of these tumors are incredibly heterogeneous. Thus, pheochromocytomas can arise from one or both adrenal medullas or may originate from the sympathetic ganglia anywhere in the body—in the mediastinum, at the carotid bifurcation, in the bladder, or in the organ of Zuckerkandl. The clinical presentation can range from being "classic textbook" type to being atypical enough to be missed by several physicians. The biochemical markers can readily be evident in some cases, but in others the pursuit of the diagnosis can become an exercise in frustration, requiring a plethora of provocative, dynamic maneuvers. The size of these tumors is also variable, ranging from tumors large enough to be visualized by nephrotomogram to those small enough to elude the most sophisticated high-resolution CT scanners. The course may be mild, so as to allow the patient several years before even the diagnosis is made, or it may be aggressive enough to kill the patient with an acute myocardial infarct or a cerebrovascular catastrophe. Finally, the associations of the pheochromocytoma can range from the mundane (*café-au-lait* spots and/or neurofibroma) to the exotic (multiple endocrine adenomatosis, type II). Thus, this tumor, fascinating as it is, represents a polymorphously perverse disorder.

31.2.1. Clinical Features

The peak incidence of pheochromocytoma is in the third and fourth decades, but it can occur at any age. The three facets of the clinical presentation of pheochromocytoma are hypertension, symptoms of sympathetic excess, and hypermetabolism.

31.2.1.1. Hypertension

The hypertension of pheochromocytoma is characteristically "paroxysmal" in a third of patients, "sustained" in a third, and "labile" with basally elevated pressure in the remaining third. Pheochromocytoma probably accounts for about 0.5% of patients with recently diagnosed hypertension. The hypertension can be unremarkable or may be characterized by paroxysms of marked elevation associated with headache, diaphoresis, and palpitations. The blood pressure during an acute paroxysm can become frightfully high (>300 mm) with the risk of imminent stroke. Pheochromocytoma is especially likely to be misued during pregnancy because of the unwarranted tendency to attribute accelerated hypertension to preeclampsia. One characteristic of the hypertension in pheochromocytoma is the tendency for postural drop; this is because of the concomitant presence of hypovolemia occasioned by catecholamine excess.

31.2.1.2. Sympathetic Excess

These symptoms include nervousness, palpitation, increased diaphoresis, and psychiatric disturbances. Pheochromocytoma should be always a consideration in patients with chronic anxiety, sinus tachycardia, supraventricular arrhythmias, and patients suspected of having hyperthyroidism but with normal thyroid indices.

31.2.1.3. Hypermetabolic Syndrome

Weight loss, increased appetite, and abnormal glucose levels seen in pheochromocytoma understandably lead to the erroneous diagnosis of "diabetes mellitus." The reason for glucose intolerance in pheochromocytoma is that catecholamine excess blunts the release of insulin from the pancreatic β cell.

31.2.1.4. Rare Features

These include sudden, unexplained postoperative shock, severe constipation, intestinal ileus, cardiomyopathy, polycythemia, and "fever of unexplained origin." Occasionally, a provocative history may be provided by the patient—an attack following cheese (tyramine) or a hot water shower with vigorous rubbing of the abdomen; micturition syncopy, a feature of bladder pheochromocytomas, also belongs in this category. Very rarely, Raynaud's phenomenon and even gangrene of the fingertips can result from vasospasm caused by catecholamines.

Thus, the presentations of pheochromocytoma can be classic enough to be diagnosed by history alone or may be confusing enough to lead the physician away from the etiology.

31.2.2. Diagnostic Studies

The three sets of tests involved in the diagnostic evaluation of pheochromocytoma are biochemical, dynamic, and localization (Table 73).

31.2.2.1. Biochemical Tests

In 80% to 90% of patients with pheochromocytoma, biochemical tests performed on the urine or blood provide ample evidence of catecholamine excess. Measurement of VMA (vanillylmandelic acid), methylated compounds (metanephrine and normetanephrine), and catecholamines in the urine are simple, excellent methods to establish catecholamine excess. The urine, for all these tests, need to be collected in special containers containing dilute hydrochloric acid.

Performed together, the VMA and metanephrine, normetanephrine assays establish the diagnosis of catecholamine excess in 80–90% of cases, underscoring the importance of these two tests as screening tests when pheochromocytoma is suspected. If these tests are normal but pheochromocytoma is still a consideration, the urine should be assayed for levels of catecholamines. The substances, drugs, and conditions that affect these three urinary tests are outlined in Table 74.

Measurement of plasma catecholamine level is useful mostly in a crisis situation. The pulsatile nature of catecholamines, the short half-life, and the

TABLE 73
Diagnostic Studies for
Pheochromocytoma

Biochemical
    24-hr urine VMA
    24-hr urine metanephrine
    24-hr urine catecholamines
    Plasma catecholamines
Dynamic tests
    Glucagon test
    Clonidine test
    Phentolamine test (in crisis)
Localization procedures
    CT scan
    Ultrasonography
    Arteriography
    Venography with venous catheter
      for catecholamines in the
      effluent
    $[^{131}I]$MIBG scan

myriad of physiological causes that affect plasma level of catecholamines have resulted in the placing of less reliance on plasma catecholamines than on urine assays. The measurement of basal catecholamines and the response to 0.3 mg of orally administered clonidine separates essential hypertensives from patients with pheochromocytoma with 95% accuracy. Nearly all patients with pheochromocytoma demonstrate postclonidine catecholamine levels above 500 pg/ml. However, the interpretation of the test heavily depends on the methodology, accuracy of sample collection, and the presence of other drugs, particularly propanolol in the circulation.

31.2.2.2. Dynamic (Pharmacological) Testing

These are less reliable than biochemical tests and are resorted to only in difficult cases. The major drawback of pharmacological tests is that they do

TABLE 74
Biochemical Tests in Pheochromocytoma

Test in 24-hr urine	Comment
VMA	Affected by diet high in vanillin Decreased by MAO inhibitors
Meta- and normetanephrines	Elevated by use of α-methyldopa, MAO inhibitors, and stress
Catecholamines	Elevated by use of nose drops, bronchodilators, and stress

not consistently identify the patients harboring a pheochromocytoma from those with essential hypertension.

Intravenous administration of glucagon elicits a prompt pressor response as well as a temporally related rise in plasma catecholamine levels in patients with pheochromocytoma, and supposedly such responses are not encountered in essential hypertensives.

Clonidine, when given to normal subjects or those with essential hypertension, results in a lowering of plasma catecholamines by inhibiting neurogenically mediated catecholamine release. In contrast, patients with pheochromocytoma do not show any alteration.

Both the glucagon provocative test and the clonidine suppression test suffer from a significant lack of sensitivity as well as specificity. The one pharmacological test that may provide exclusional information is the therapeutic use of phentolamine (Regitine®). The intravenous administration of phentolamine (a short-acting potent α blocker) causes a prompt decrease in the blood pressure of patients with pheochromocytoma (as well as some with essential hypertension). The value of the test should be viewed in the following perspective: in a patient presenting in hypertensive crisis, the failure of the blood pressure to decline following the intravenous use of 5 mg of phentolamine excludes pheochromocytoma, whereas a response could be indicative of either pheochromocytoma or essential hypertension.

Other tests using histamine, tyramine, or immersion of the hands in cold water (cold pressor tests) have all been abandoned.

31.2.2.3. Localization Tests

The use of high-resolution computerized tomography detects the tumor in 60–80% of instances. Very small tumors and extraadrenal tumors do not visualize well by CT. The combination of ultrasonography and CT imaging may improve the yield slightly. In patients with pheochromocytoma that fails to be visualized by computerized tomography, the only course in the past was to resort to invasive diagnostic tests such as transfemoral arteriography or venography with sequential sampling of the venous effluent from various levels of inferior vena cava and the adrenal veins. These invasive procedures require tremendous expertise and mandate adequate α blockage to avoid precipitating a crisis. The advent of a new isotopic imaging technique could obviate the need for invasive tests in the localization of the tumor. [^{131}I]*meta*-Iodobenzylguanidine (MIBG) is a radiopharmaceutical agent that enters adrenergic tissue and is concentrated in adrenergic vesicles. Tumor tissue, rich in these adrenergic vesicles, retains the radiopharmaceutical for a prolonged period and thus is visualized in delayed scans. The procedure can detect extraadrenal tumors and even the smallest adrenal tumors quite effectively.

31.2.3. Treatment

The treatment for pheochromocytoma is surgical removal of the tumor. Prior to surgery, medical preparation is absolutely necessary to avoid intraoperative or postoperative catecholamine crisis. This can be done by α blocking the patient with oral phenoxybenzamine, 20 to 40 mg a day for 4 weeks. After adequate α blockade, if necessary, a β blocker may be added. It should be noted that administering β blockers in the absence of α blockade could result in precipitous increases in the blood pressure. Before induction of anesthesia, 5 mg of phentolamine should be administered to prevent a rise in the blood pressure secondary to anesthetic. Thiopental and succinylcholine are used for induction, and nitrous oxide with meperidine or fentamyl can be used for anesthesia. Since a hypertensive crisis can occur while one is handling the tumor, phentolamine and nitroprusside drip should be on stand-by. Volume repletion should be ensured to avoid postoperative hypotension.

For malignant pheochromocytoma, therapy with α-methylparatyrosine (a tyrosine hydroxylase inhibitor) can be tried to decrease catecholamine secretion. Such therapy is, at best, palliative.

The features of pheochromocytomas associated with multiple endocrine adenomatosis II are described in Chapter 52.

Selected Readings

Aron, D. C., Tyrrell, J. B., Fitzgerald, P. A., et al.: Cushing's syndrome: Problems in diagnosis, Medicine 60:25, 1981.

Axelrod, L.: Glucocorticoid therapy, Medicine 55:39, 1976.

Bertagna, C., and Orth, D. N.: Clinical and laboratory findings and results of therapy in 58 patients with adrenocortical tumors admitted to a single medical center (1951–1978), Am. J. Med. 71:855, 1981.

Blankstein, J., Faiman, C., Reyes, F. I., et al.: Adult onset familial adrenal 21-hydroxylase deficiency, Am. J. Med. 68:441, 1980.

Bravo, E. L., and Gifford, R. W.: Current concepts: Pheochromocytoma: Diagnosis, localization and management, N. Engl. J. Med. 311:1298, 1984.

Cain, J. P.: The regulation of aldosterone secretion in primary aldosteronism, Am. J. Med. 53:627, 1972.

Chrousos, G. P., Loriaux, D. L., Mann, D. L., et al.: Late onset 21-hydroxylase deficiency mimicking idiopathic hirsutism or polycystic ovarian disease, Ann. Intern. Med. 96:143, 1982.

Conn, J. W.: Primary aldosteronism: A new clinical syndrome, J. Lab. Clin. Med. 45:6, 1955.

Cook, D. M., Kendall, J. W., and Jordan, R.: Cushing's syndrome. Current concepts of diagnosis and therapy, West. J. Med. 132:111, 1980.

Crapo, L.: Cushing's syndrome: A review of diagnostic tests, Metabolism 28:955, 1979.

Dluhy, R. G., Hiamathongkan, T., and Greenfield, M.: Rapid ACTH test with plasma aldosterone levels. Improved diagnostic discrimination, Ann. Intern. Med. 80:693, 1974.

Dunnick, N. R., Doppman, J. L., Gill, J. R., et al.: Localization of functional adrenal tumors by computed tomography and venous sampling, Radiology 142:429, 1982.

Dunnick, N. R., Heaston, D., Halvorsen, R., et al.: CT appearance of adrenal cortical carcinoma, J. Comput. Assist. Tomogr. 6:978, 1982.

Ganguly, A., Melada, G. A., Luetscher, J. A., et al.: Control of plasma aldosterone in primary aldosteronism: Distinction between adenoma and hyperplasia, J. Clin. Endocrinol. Metab. 37:765, 1973.

Gold, E. M.: The Cushing syndromes: Changing views of diagnosis and treatment, Ann. Intern. Med. 90:829, 1979.

Grim, C. E., and Weinberger, M. H.: Familial dexamethasone suppressible normokalemic hyperaldosteronism, Pediatrics 65:597, 1980.

Handwerger, S., and Silverstein, J.: Congenital adrenal hyperplasia, Urol. Clin. North Amer. 4:193, 1977.

Horton, R., and Finck, E.: Diagnosis and localization in primary aldosteronism, *Ann. Intern. Med.* **76:**885, 1972.

Hutter, A. M., and Kayhoe, D. E.: Adrenal cortical carcinoma. Clinical features of 138 patients, *Am. J. Med.* **41:**572, 1966.

Irvine, W. J., and Barnes, E. W.: Adrenocortical insufficiency, *Clin. Endocrinol. Metab.* **1:**549, 1972.

Jones, D. H., Allison, D. J., Hamilton, C. A., *et al.:* Selective venous sampling in the diagnosis and localization of pheochromocytoma, *Clin. Endocrinol.* **10:**179, 1979.

Keiser, H. R., Beaven, M. A., Doppman, J., *et al.:* Sipple syndrome, medullary thyroid carcinoma and parathyroid disease, *Ann. Intern. Med.* **78:**561, 1973.

Laursen, K., and Damgaard-Pedersen, K.: CT for pheochromocytoma diagnosis, *Am. J. Radiol.* **134:**277, 1980.

Lobo, R. A.: Adult manifestation of congenital adrenal hyperplasia due to incomplete 21-hydroxylase deficiency mimicking polycystic ovarian disease, *Am. J. Obstet. Gynecol.* **138:**720, 1980.

Lyons, D. F., Kem, D. C., Brown, R. D., *et al.:* Single dose captopril as a diagnostic test for primary aldosteronism, *J. Clin. Endocrinol. Metab.* **57:**892, 1983.

Melby, J. C.: Identifying the adrenal lesion in primary aldosteronism, *Ann. Intern. Med.* **76:**1039, 1972.

Michelis, M. F., and Murdaugh, H. V.: Selective hypoaldosteronism, *Am. J. Med.* **59:**1, 1975.

Mulrow, P. J.: Glucocorticoid suppressible hyperaldosteronism: A clue to the missing hormone, *N. Engl. J. Med.* **305:**1012, 1981.

Nerup, J.: Addison's disease—clinical studies. A report of 108 cases, *Acta Endocrinol.* **76:**127, 1974.

Orth, D. N.: The old and new in Cushing's syndrome, *N. Engl. J. Med.* **310:**649, 1984.

Orth, D. N., and Liddle, G. W.: Results of treatment in 108 patients with Cushing's syndrome, *N. Engl. J. Med.* **285:**243, 1971.

Schambelan, M., Stockigt, J. R., and Biglieri, E. G.: Isolated hypoaldosteronism in adults—a renin deficiency syndrome, *N. Engl. J. Med.* **287:**573, 1972.

Seidenwurm, D. J., Elmer, E. B., Kaplan, L. M., *et al.:* Metastases to the adrenal gland and the development of Addison's disease, *Cancer* **54:**552, 1984.

Sisson, J. C., Frager, M. S., Valk, T. W., *et al.:* Scintigraphic localization of pheochromocytoma, *N. Engl. J. Med.* **305:**12, 1981.

Streeten, D., Tomcyz, N., and Anderson, G. H.: Reliability of screening methods for the diagnosis of primary aldosteronism, *Am. J. Med.* **67:**403, 1979.

Valk, T. W., Frager, M. S., Gross, M. D., *et al.:* Spectrums of pheochromocytoma in multiple endocrine neoplasia, *Ann. Intern. Med.* **94:**762, 1981.

Weinberger, M. H., Grim, C. E., Hollifield, J. W., *et al.:* Primary aldosteronism—diagnosis, localization, and treatment, *Ann. Intern. Med.* **90:**386, 1979.

White, F. E., White, M. C., Drury, P. L., *et al.:* Value of computed tomography of the abdomen and chest in investigation of Cushing's syndrome, *Br. Med. J.* **284:**771, 1982.

The Testes

32

Anatomy of the Testes

The testes are oblong solid structures located in the scrotum. Each testis is an independent unit, performing two closely interrelated functions, androgen production and spermatogenesis. The testes measure 3.5 to 5 cm in their longest diameter. The embryology of testicular development is discussed in Chapter 42.

The testis is composed of two parts, the seminiferous tubules and the interstitium, which contains the all-important Leydig cells that secrete testosterone. Careful histological sections indicate that the seminiferous tubules lie embedded in the interstitium in close proximity to the Leydig cells, which are scattered throughout the interstitium.

The bulk of the testis is comprised by the seminiferous tubules. These are convoluted tubules characterized by an irregular pattern of anastomoses that end in individual ducts called the tubulus recti. The collective group of tubulus recti empty in the rete testis, which by a series of ducts is connected to the epididymal duct. The seminiferous tubule is lined by germinal epithelium, an extremely active layer directly envolved in spermatogenesis. The basement membrane of the seminiferous epithelium also contains large cells called *Sertoli* cells. These cells contain fingerlike projections that surround the germinal epithelial cells; the function of the germ cells is to produce sperm. The Sertoli cells provide nutrients to the germ cells, secrete a protein called androgen-binding protein (ABP) under the influenze of FSH (Chapter 33), and function as phagocytic cells.

The Leydig cells, scattered throughout the interstitium, are large cells that contain smooth endoplasmic reticulum in their cytoplasm. These organelles are actively involved in the synthesis of testosterone. After synthesis, the hormone is released into the interstitium.

The epididymis is a specialized structure located on the posterior surface of the testes. The epididymis terminates in the vas deferens, a long duct, approximately 20 inches long. The vas deferens traverses the inguinal canal as part of the spermatic cord and enters the pelvis, terminating in the ejaculatory duct. This structure also receives the ducts from the seminal vesicles.

The blood supply of the testes is derived from the internal spermatic arteries, which originate from the aorta at the level of the renal arteries. The venous return from the testes originates from a venous plexus called plexus pampiniformis. This plexus eventually forms a single vein, the testicular vein. On the right side this vein joins the inferior vena cava, whereas on the left side it drains into the left renal vein. The nerve supply to the testes is predominantly through the superior spermatic nerves, originating from the intermesenteric and renal part of celiac plexus.

33

Physiology of Testicular Function

The two principal functions of the testes are androgen production and spermatogenesis. The secretion, regulatory control, and action of testosterone are discussed first, followed by the control of spermatogenesis.

Testosterone, the most potent androgen, is secreted by the Leydig cells in the interstitium of the testes. The secretory activity of the Leydig cells assumes crucial importance during two periods of life. First, *in utero*, the fetal testes of the male fetus demonstrate intense secretory activity and secrete testosterone, the prohormone required to virilize the fetus into a male. Failure of this mechanism results in the birth of an infant with female external genitalia.

The second burst of secretory activity occurs during puberty, resulting in virilization of the boy into a "man" in the androgenic sense of that term. Failure of this mechanism results in sexual immaturity. During both of these crucial periods, the testes are stimulated by trophic hormones—in the fetal period, the stimulus is chorionic gonadotropin, and during puberty, the stimulus comes from the pituitary gonadrotropin luteinizing hormone (LH). The focus of discussion in this section is limited to testicular function in the postnatal life.

The secretory activity of the Leydig cells is in abeyance until the time of puberty. The reason for such dormancy is lack of adequate gonadotropins in the circulation, which are required to induce the receptor activity on the surface of Leydig cells. Puberty is preceded by a heightened sensitivity of the Leydig cell receptors to the action of pituitary LH. Under the trophic stimulus of LH, the secretory activity of the Leydig cells starts and, in the normal male, continues for the rest of life, showing a tendency to decelerate during "old age" (male climacteric). The exact mechanisms by which LH stimulates testosterone synthesis are not clear, but binding of LH to the receptors on the

Leydig cell surface and increased generation of cyclic AMP are important steps in the mediation of the action.

The biochemical steps involved in the synthesis of testosterone are strikingly similar to adrenal androgen synthesis. The starting point for synthesis is cholesterol. The first step, the formation of pregnenolone, is crucial and is felt to be the step that it intensely activated in response to stimulation by LH. The pregnenolone is directed into two pathways: the main pathway is conversion to progesterone, 17-α-hydroxyprogesterone, androstenedione, and testosterone; a minor pathway involves conversion to 17-α-hydroxypregnenolone, DHEA, and androstenediol, which is eventually converted into testosterone. This "minor" pathway in the testes becomes the "major" pathway in the adrenal, and vice versa (see Figure 22).

The testosterone concentration in the venous effluent of the spermatic vein is 10,000 to 60,000 ng/dl, whereas the concentration in the peripheral vein is 300–1000 ng/dl. There are three forms in which testosterone circulates in the plasma: 68% is bound to the testosterone-binding globulin (TeBG), also known as sex hormone-binding globulin (SHBG); 30% is albumin-bound; and 2% is free. The binding globulin is synthesized by liver and is altered in a variety of states such as liver disease, obesity, and thyroid disease. Physiologically, the portion of testosterone bound to the globulin dissociates poorly and is not free to enter the cells. Thus, the biologically active fractions are the albumin-bound hormone and the free hormone. It is the free fraction and possibly the albumin-bound fraction that exert negative feedback effects on the hypothalamic–pituitary unit.

The metabolic clearance of testosterone follows the following course:

1. Internalization of the hormone into the target cells. Inside the cell, testosterone undergoes 5-α reduction to become dihydrotestosterone.
2. Approximately 60% of testosterone is metabolized by liver into androsterone and etiocholanolone by reduction at the 5-α and 5-β po-

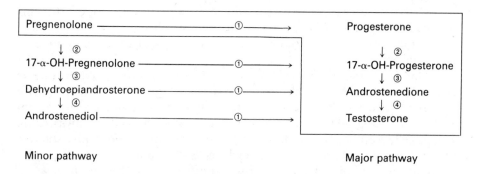

Minor pathway   Major pathway

FIGURE 22. Pathways for testosterone synthesis by the testes. Enzymes: (1) 3-β-hydroxysteroid dehydrogenase; (2) 17-α-hydroxylase; (3) 17,20-desmolase; (4) 17-β-hydroxysteroid dehydrogenase.

sitions respectively. This hepatic 5-α reduction is independent of the 5-α reduction that takes place in the target cells. A small proportion of the testosterone is conjugated by the liver into testosterone glucuronide.

3. Peripheral tissues convert testosterone into 17-β-estradiol by aromatization.

4. Approximately 8% of testosterone is converted to dehydroepiandrosterone (DHEA), a weak adrenal androgen.

In summary, the products of testosterone metabolism are of three varieties—a most active, powerful androgen (dihydrotestosterone), a host of "weak" androgens (androsterone, DHEA, and etiocholanolone), and estrogens (17-β-estradiol).

In addition to secreting testosterone, the Leydig cells secrete a very small amount of estrogen and estrone. Most of the estrogen in males is derived from peripheral conversion of testosterone; the contribution from synthesis by Leydig cells is very small. However, under unusual circumstances, the testes can secrete large amounts of estradiol. This is the case when the Leydig cells are chronically stimulated by HCG, which markedly increases aromatization within the testes and results in conversion of large amounts of testosterone in 17-β-estradiol within testicular tissue.

The relationship between testosterone and pituitary LH is a reciprocal one. Increasing testosterone concentrations in the plasma suppress the hypothalamic and pituitary components of gonadotropin release. This is exemplified by hormone data in normal males in whom testosterone administration causes a prompt decline in LH, as would be expected with protracted administration of testosterone. There is also a decline in FSH as a result of suppression of endogenous gonadotropin-releasing hormone by the hypothalamus. This is the reason for decreased fertility in subjects receiving chronic testosterone therapy.

Before outlining the multitude of important effects of testosterone, it is essential to outline the mechanism of testosterone action. The following steps are involved in the action of testosterone in peripheral target tissues:

1. The hormone enters the target cell.

2. Following entry, testosterone is converted to dihydrotestosterone (DHT) by a reduction reaction involving the enzyme 5-α reductase.

3. Both testosterone (T) and dihydrotestosterone (DHT) bind to high-affinity androgen-binding receptor proteins in the cytoplasm.

4. The hormone–receptor complex is transported to the nucleus of the cells, where it interacts with the acceptor sites in the nuclear chromatin.

5. The nuclear chromatin–hormone complex initiates transcription, resulting in the appearance of new messenger RNA and other proteins that effectively express hormone action.

Although testosterone serves as a prohormone for the formation of the much more potent dihydrotestosterone, the cytoplasm of adult target cells does possess receptors for binding of testosterone as well. This contrasts with the situation in the fetus, where the target tissue (genital tubercle, genital folds, and urogenital sinus, from which the phallus, scrotum, prostate, and male urethra are developed) contains receptors only for dihydrotestosterone.

The three major actions of testosterone are the following:

1. In the fetus, testosterone, by virtue of conversion to dihydrotestosterone, is exclusively responsible for virilizing the male fetus. In the absence of this hormone (or when complete resistance to its action occurs), the male fetus will not virilize, resulting in formation of female external genitalia (male pseudohermaphroditism).

2. Testosterone and dihydrotestosterone are responsible for pubertal virilization of boys, resulting in the development of secondary sexual characteristics. Thus, the pubertal hair growth in the face, the deepening of voice, the pubertal growth spurt, and the increase in muscle mass are stimulated by these androgens. Development of scrotal rugosity, scrotal pigmentation, and sexual hair on the scrotum, on the undersurface of the penis, and medial surface of the thighs are also stimulated by these hormones. The phallic growth to adult proportions, the development of male pubic hair pattern, and dense hair growth in the axilla, chest, and back are striking aspects of testosterone effects. The growth of the prostate during puberty is also mediated by testosterone. Thus, testosterone and dihydrotestosterone are the virilizing hormones of male puberty.

3. Testosterone also plays a permissive role in maintenance of normal spermatogenesis. It appears that for spermatogenesis to proceed normally, high intratesticular concentrations of the hormone are required.

Thus, testosterone and dihydrotestosterone are responsible for the formation of male genitalia, the development of "maleness" during puberty, and for proper spermatogenesis. The role of these hormones in the development of aggressive behavior, sexual arousal, and in preserving libido are less clearly defined. The bulk of evidence in subhuman primates indicates a role for the androgen in maintenance of aggressive and sexual behavior. The data in humans are strongly supportive but not conclusive.

The second function of the testes is spermatogenesis. Sperm production takes place in the seminiferous tubules, which constitute the bulk of testicular tissue. The process of spermatogenesis takes place in the germinal epithelium of the seminiferous tubules. Spermatozoa are derived from the immature *spermatogonia,* which divided to form *spermatocytes.* These spermatocytes immediately undergo meiotic (reduction) division to form the haploid cells called *spermatids.* Though a series of metamorphoses, the spermatids eventually become the motile, flagellated spermatozoa.

The hormonal control and regulation of spermatogenesis are not as clearly defined as the hormonal control of Leydig cell function. The old theory of dual hormonal controls (LH, FSH) for dual testicular functions (androgen production and spermatogenesis, respectively) is standard and is outlined first.

The recent developments that have modified this theory are subsequently outlined.

According to the standard theory, FSH is responsible for stimulating the immature, prepubertal testes and initiating spermatogenesis as well as maintaining it. The negative feedback between spermatogenesis and FSH is mediated by a protein called "inhibin" secreted by the Sertoli cells. When spermatogenesis fails, inhibin levels decline and signal FSH to be released in an effort to stimulate spermatogenesis. Thus, the standard theory is fairly simple: FSH stimulates spermatogenesis, and LH stimulates testosterone, which is required, in a permissive fashion, for FSH to stimulate spermatogenesis.

Many recent studies have modified the above theory to some extent. These studies in animal models suggest that although the induction and initiation of spermatogenesis ("the first wave") are clearly dependent on FSH, subsequent spermatogenesis can be maintained by testosterone *alone in the absence of FSH*. In other words, the immature prepubertal seminiferous tubules require FSH to initiate the process of spermatogenesis, but once this becomes established, the key factor that continues the process is high intratesticular concentrations of testosterone. This "new" theory proposed by several workers involves the following scheme:

1. Follicle-stimulating hormone stimulates the immature testes and induces the "first wave" of spermatogenesis. The role of FSH is transitory and obligatory in this regard.
2. The FSH stimulates the Sertoli cells to secrete a peptide called androgen-binding protein (ABP). This secretory process is mediated by stimulation of adenylate cyclase and generation of cyclic AMP.
3. The ABP binds testosterone avidly, thus increasing the local concentrations of testosterone to a remarkably high degree.
4. The ABP–testosterone complex passively diffuses into the germinal epithelium and reaches the nucleus, where testosterone probably initiates transcription and formation of new messenger RNA—a documented effect of the androgen in other target tissues.
5. The newly formed mRNA initiates spermatogenesis by effecting conversion of spermatogonia.

The current theory attaches importance to the concentrations of testosterone in the interstitum in maintenance of spermatogenesis once it has been initiated by FSH. Attractive as this theory is, it does not explain the indisputable finding that spermatogenesis declines when testosterone is administered to the normal male. Thus, the exact mechanisms involved in hormonal regulation of spermatogenesis are not completely clear.

34

Testing Testicular Function

34.1. Introduction

The two functions of the testes are testosterone production and spermatogenesis. Therefore, the indications for evaluating testicular function revolve
around symptoms relating to these two functions, i.e., hypoandrogenism and
infertility. The diagnostic tests outlined in this section not only include tests
that directly assess the two functions but also extend to involve a description
of tests that enter the workup of patients with hypoandrogenism. The tests
are discussed in the following manner. First, the tests that assess Leydig cell
function and spermatogenesis are discussed. Next, the tests to evaluate the
integrity of the hypothalamic–pituitary–gonadal axis are outlined. Third, the
tumescence studies, fourth, the chromosomal studies, and finally, the role of
testicular biopsy are discussed.

34.2. Assessment of Leydig Cell Function

The Leydig cells of the testes secrete testosterone, and, therefore, measurement of this hormone level in the serum provides a direct measure of
androgen production. Testosterone is the principal androgen secreted by the
Leydig cells under the trophic stimulation of leuteinizing hormone (LH) of
the pituitary. The normal range for testosterone in the plasma is 300–1000
ng/dl. The testosterone measured in the plasma measures the circulating
hormone bound to the globulin, testosterone-binding globulin (TeBG). The
importance of this protein is discussed in Chapter 33; by and large, the measurement of the TeBG-bound testosterone correlates well with the androgen
status of the patient and the free hormone concentrations. Occasionally, the
hormone levels may fluctuate considerably in the circulation, necessitating
multiple sampling at 15- to 20-min intervals and performing the assay in the
pooled sera. Most hypogonadal states characterized by sexual immaturity are
associated with grossly decreased serum testosterone level with one exception;

Reifenstein's syndrome is characterized by undervirilization with a normal or even slightly elevated serum testosterone level. In adult testicular failure, the decrease in testosterone level is less impressive.

34.3. Assessment of Adequacy of Spermatogenesis

Seminal fluid analysis is a simple and effective method for evaluating the adequacy of spermatogenesis. Indirectly, a completely normal seminal fluid analysis is indicative of the integrity of the entire hypothalamic–pituitary–testicular function; this is because proper spermatogenesis requires adequate functioning of FSH as well as some amount of testosterone and, therefore, adequate functioning of LH.

The seminal fluid should be collected in a clean, wide-mouthed container by masturbation after at least 2 to 3 days of sexual abstinence. Collection of the sample in condom sheaths is less desirable since some contain spermicides and because of the inevitable delay in transporting the sample to the laboratory. The parameters evaluated in the seminal fluid are the volume, the number of spermatozoa, the motility, the presence of abnormal forms or leukocytes, and the fructose content of the semen.

The normal volume of ejaculate is variable and ranges from 2.5 ml to 6 ml. The sperm count is also highly variable, with a wide range in normal fertile men; further, the sperm count can be impressively variable when performed at different times in the same person. The range of spermatozoa is between 80 to 120 million per milliliter. However, the criteria for abnormality, in terms of fertility potential, is a number below 20 million/ml on a persistent basis over a 2-month period. Motility of the sperm is evaluated by recording the percentage of actively motile spermatozoa in a drop of undiluted fluid. Abnormal motility is said to exist when fewer than 60% of the spermatozoa show less than grade 3 (highly active) motility. Abnormal forms, such as large oval heads, small oval heads, tapering heads, pyriform heads, etc., can be detected by microscopically evaluating the smear. These abnormal forms should not exceed 30–40% of the total sperm population. Also, in the same smear, the presence and number of leukocytes should be determined. A leukocyte count greater than 6×10^6 is indicative of genital tract infection. Absence of fructose in the seminal fluid is indicative of either congenital absence of both seminal vesicles or obstruction to vasa deferentia bilaterally.

34.4. The Hypothalamic–Pituitary Axis

Once defective hormone production or defective spermatogenesis has been documented, the next immediate step is to obtain levels of gonadotropins in the circulation. The purpose is to delineate if the testicular failure is primary or secondary; primary testicular failure results in elevation of LH and FSH, a physiological response of the normal pituitary to the negative feedback effect of declining testicular function, whereas these levels are low in, and causally related to, secondary testicular failure. The measurement of LH and FSH is enormously important, since all subsequent tests depend on whether the hypogonadism is hypergonadotrophic ($\uparrow$ LH,FSH) or hypogonadotrophic ($\downarrow$ LH,FSH).

In the patient with hypergonadotrophic hypogonadism, the hypothalamic–pituitary region has been completely exonerated, whereas in the hypogonadotrophic variety, this is where the problem lies. In such a patient (hypogonadism with decreased gonadotropin levels), the subsequent differentiation between a hypothalamic and a pituitary etiology may, theoretically, be made by administering synthetic LH-RH (leuteinizing hormone-releasing hormone). The patient with intrinsic pituitary disease should show no increase in LH and FSH following LH-RH, whereas the patient with hypothalamic disease should demonstrate a delayed rise following LH-RH, since the pituitary gonadotrophs are viable. In practice, however, the test does not consistently separate hypothalamic from pituitary forms by using a single bolus of synthetic LH-RH.

34.5. Nocturnal Penile Tumescence

Penile erection is a coordinated physiological process that involves the integreted participation of neurological, endocrine, and vascular processes. In normal males, there are one or more full-sized firm erections during REM sleep. Studies of nocturnal penile tumescence (NPT) in normal males indicate that during sleep there are four or five tumescent episodes lasting from 20 to as long as 40 min. Demonstration of a completely normal NPT study clearly excludes organic disease as a cause for erectile dysfunction and indicates normality of hormonal, neurological, and vascular mechanisms that mediate the erectile process. The difficulty is in obtaining NPT studies, which require the participation of a sleep laboratory and hence are not widely available. The expense of the study and the difficulties in interpreting borderline graphs also limit the use of the study.

Despite the above limitations, there are two indications for which the NPT study can be quite useful. First, in a patient who is thought to have psychogenic impotence, the demonstration of a normal NPT study supports the diagnosis, whereas an abnormal NPT study indicates coexistent organic etiology for impotence. Second, in the patient with erectile dysfunction and normal endocrine data, the NPT study is the next investigational avenue because an abnormal NPT study in a patient with normal hormone levels points to a vascular or neurological etiology for the erectile dysfunction.

34.6. Chromosomal Studies

Chromosomal abnormalities constitute a major etiology for primary hypogonadism. The indication to consider chromosomal disorders is the patient with the hypergonadotrophic variety of hypogonadism, i.e., low testosterone with elevated LH and FSH levels. The two studies available are buccal smear cytology and the standard karyotypic analysis. The buccal smear test is, at best, a screening procedure, whereas karyotype analysis is definitive.

The buccal smear cytology is performed by scraping the buccal mucosa and processing the material for cytology. The purpose is to search for "Barr bodies." In 1949, Barr and Betram demonstrated that the nuclei of the cells of female cats contained stainable chromatinlike material at the periphery of nuclei. These bodies, called "Barr bodies," represent the inactivated second X chromosome and are seen in at least 20% of the cells in the smear taken from scrapings of the buccal mucosa of karyotypic females but not karyotypic males. The presence of one Barr body indicates a sex chromosome constitution of two X chromosomes (normal female). This determination of "chromatin sex" is an easy method for predicting the number of X chromosomes. Normal males are "sex-chromatin negative" (since the chromosomal constitution is 46,XY), whereas normal females are "sex-chromatin positive" (since their chromosomal constitution is 46,XX). Patients with classic Klinefelter's syndrome, a disorder characterized by supernumerary X, are "sex-chromatin positive" even though the external genitalia and the gonads are of the male phenotype. When the patient's karyotype is XXXY, two Barr bodies are evident, and when the karyotype is XXXXY, three Barr bodies are seen; i.e., the number of Barr bodies seen is one less than the number of X chromosomes.

The buccal smear is an inexpensive simple screening test but provides insufficient information when the sample is poorly taken, prepared, or stained. Further, patients with Klinefelter mosaicism may be chromatin negative. The standard method for evaluating the karyotype is by performing a chromosomal study (karyotype analysis). Leukocytes cultured from blood are the usual source, but, less frequently, cultured skin fibroblasts or even gonadal tissue may be required. The advent of sophisticated staining techniques for identification of the chromosomes permits accurate karyotyping. Table 75 outlines the abnormal chromosomal constitution in various hypogonadal states.

A recent addition to karyotyping is the serotyping with assay for H-Y antigen. This antigen is the portion of Y antigen that is responsible for the differentiation and development of the fetal testes. All patients with testes

TABLE 75
Chromosomal Constitution in Male Hypogonadism

Condition	Karyotype
Classic Klinefelter's	47,XXY
Klinefelter mosaic	46,XY/47,XXY
Poly-X syndrome	48,XXXY; 49,XXXXY
Sex-reversal syndrome (de la Chapelle syndrome)	46,XX
Male Turner syndrome	45,XO/46,XY; 45,XO
Poly-Y syndrome	47,XYY

should be Y-chromosome positive and are H-Y antigen positive. There are some situations characterized by male hypogonadism, presence of testes, but absence of a Y chromosome in the karyotypic analysis. Classic examples of such a situation are hypogonadal males affected by the sex-reversal syndrome or the male Turner's syndrome. In such patients, the H-Y-positive serology is attestation to the fact that a Y chromosome was present in the early embryonic life and provided the necessary signals for the bipotential gonad to differentiate into a fetal testis.

34.7. Testicular Biopsy

With the rapid advances in chromosome analysis seen in the past decade, testicular biopsy is seldom required for the diagnosis of classic and nonclassic Klinefelter's syndromes. There are probably only two indications for which a testicular biopsy is required; both indications represent unique examples characterized by oligospermia or even aspermia in otherwise well-virilized, eugonadal males from the hormone standpoint. The first is bilateral obstruction to the vas deferens. These patients demonstrate normal FSH levels despite aspermia. This is because spermatogenesis is proceeding normally, but the spermatozoa are blocked by an "exit block" bilaterally. (The situation is analogous to the vasectomized male.) The fact that spermatogenesis is proceeding normally can be suspected on the basis of a normal (unelevated) FSH level but can be proven only with a testicular biopsy. The other condition in which a testicular biopsy has diagnostic value is in the *Sertoli cell only syndrome*. This syndrome resembles all other forms of selective seminiferous tubular failure, i.e., marked oligospermia, elevated FSH, normal testosterone, and normal LH. The characteristic biopsy appearance (loss of germinal epithelium of the seminiferous tubules, which are lined only by the Sertoli cells) differentiates this syndrome from other causes of selective seminiferous tubular failure.

Aside from these two examples, testicular biopsy is seldom indicated in the evaluation of male hypogonadism. Of course, the role of testicular biopsy in the evaluation of true hermaphroditism and testicular tumors is a well-established one.

35

Precocious Puberty in the Male

35.1. Introduction

Precocious male puberty refers to the development of pubertal virilization in boys under age 7 or 8 (isosexual precocious puberty).

The physiological changes of puberty normally start to develop between ages 10 and 14 in boys, with a mean age around 12.5. The spectrum of pubertal changes evolves gradually over a period of 3–5 years and occurs with considerable individual variability. The development of axillary hair, fine pubic hair, enlargement of the scrotum and the testes, facial hair growth, and enlargement of the phallus occur in most boys by the age of 15.

The quality of hair growth, first fine, long, and thin, gradually gives way to coarser, thicker, and curly hair in the axilla, face, and pubic region as well as over the scrotum. The pubertal growth spurt may occur before or during the development of pubertal virilization. Increased sabaceous gland secretion and acne with increased muscle mass usually occur towards the latter phase of puberty. The development of nocturnal erections can occur variably during middle, late, or even early puberty, but nocturnal emissions usually occur during late puberty.

When all the above changes start evolving between the age of 7 or 8, precocious puberty is said to exist. The onset of precocious puberty, in some instances, can occur as early as the second year of life.

35.2. Etiology

In contrast to precocious puberty in girls, the syndrome occurs less frequently in boys and is more often "nonidiopathic." The three main etiologies include central, adrenal, and testicular disorders resulting in precocious puberty.

Central precocious puberty is a result of premature activation of the hypothalamic–pituitary–testicular axis. The most important etiologies are tu-

mors, particularly pinealomas, hamartomas, and ependymomas of the suprasellar region. At least in some of these instances, elaboration of the hypothalamic peptide gonadotropin-releasing hormone has been documented to be
the mechanism of precocious puberty. Most of these tumors are malignant,
and nearly all are strategically located, resulting in obstruction to the CSF
flow, compression of the pituitary stalk, or visual field disturbances. Rarely,
the McCune–Albright syndrome (pigmentary lesions, precocious puberty, and
bone cysts) may underlie the etiology of central precocious puberty.

The two important adrenal disorders that result in precocious male puberty are adrenogenital syndrome and adrenocortical carcinoma. In the former, the reason for excess androgen synthesis is a block in adrenal steroidogenesis, and hence it is ACTH dependent; in adrenal carcinoma, the androgen
secretion is autonomous.

Testicular etiologies for precocious male puberty are rare. Tumors of
testes that secrete chorionic gonadotropin (teratoma or choriocarcinoma) are
rare examples of such a phenomenon.

35.3. Clinical Features

35.3.1. Precocious Pubertal Virilization

These changes, highly variable and individualized, are described earlier
in this chapter.

35.3.2. Pubertal Gynecomastia

Mild to even moderate gynecomostia can be noted as a result of conversion
of testosterone into estradiol.

35.3.3. Associated Changes

Depending on the etiology, other changes may be evident. The testes
may be small and prepubertal in size when an adrenal etiology underlies
virilization. (The adrenal androgens suppress pituitary gonadotropins, and,
therefore, the testes remain prepubertal despite evidence of virilization.) The
testes, in central precocious puberty are larger and may even attain adult size.
Unilateral masses in a testis should raise the suspicion of testicular tumor.

When central etiologies underlie the precocious puberty, a careful neurological examination may reveal field cuts in the visual field examination the
Perinaud's sign (limitation of upward gaze, a frequent finding in pinealomas)
or optic atrophy.

35.4. Diagnostic Studies

The diagnostic approach to precocious puberty should be taken in a
stepwise algorithmic manner.

1. Measurement of adrenal androgens. This can be achieved by measurement of urinary 17-ketosteroids or plasma dehydroepiandrosterone (DHEA). If these are elevated, the workup should be directed to exclude adrenogenital syndrome (Section 28.4) and adrenal carcinoma (Section 30.2). The diagnostic studies involved would be serum level of 17-α-hydroxyprogesterone, the dexamethasone suppression test and CT scan of adrenals.

2. If the adrenal androgen levels are normal, the serum testosterone should be measured. If elevated, a central or testicular etiology should be considered.

3. A CT scan of the brain, in particular of the sella and suprasellar area, should be obtained.

4. If the CT is negative, serum LH and FSH should be obtained. If these are in the adult male range, central etiology is diagnosed and, in the presence of a normal CT of brain, suggest the idiopathic variety. If the LH and FSH are low, a testicular etiology should be considered, and the tests planned would include HCG level in plasma and perhaps testicular biopsy to detect malignancy.

35.5. Treatment

The treatment depends on the underlying etiology. Precocious puberty caused by adrenogenital syndrome is tested by the use of dexamethasone. The treatment for adrenal carcinoma is discussed in Section 30.2.4. The CNS tumors that cause premature puberty are higly malignant and may be treated by surgery, radiation, or both. The same applies to testicular tumors.

36

Testicular Hypofunction

36.1. Introduction

In Chapters 33 and 34, the regulatory control of testicular function, the actions of testosterone, and the methods to evaluate adequacy of function are discussed. This chapter deals with the clinical syndromes that occur when testicular function fails. First, a general overview of the spectrum of testicular failure is provided, followed by a discussion of the significance of the physical findings common to several male hypogonadal states. This would facilitate the understanding of the specific hypogonadal syndromes that are discussed subsequently.

Testicular failure can occur during any stage of life. The condition can occur *in utero*, resulting in inadequate virilization of the male infant. This results in the birth of an undervirilized male infant or a "male" infant with female external genitalia (male pseudohermaphroditism). Male hypogonadism can occur after birth but before puberty, resulting in failure of pubertal virilization. This entity, called prepubertal hypogonadism, is a classic case in which the "boy" does not become a "man" in the androgenic sense of the term. The third entity is that in which gonadal failure occurs after adequate pubertal changes have occurred. This is referred to as postpubertal or adult testicular failure and could manifest as impotence, infertility, or both. Table 76 summarizes the mechanisms, examples, and presentations of these three types of hypogonadal states, providing a convenient classification for the spectrum of male hypogonadism.

Although the ultimate expression of testicular failure is lack of virilization or loss of it, the physical examination can provide several clues regarding the underlying etiology. In fact, there is a plethora of abnormal physical findings in the *in utero* and prepubertal varieties of male hypogonadism, whereas a paucity of abnormal physical findings characterize the patient with postpubertal (adult) testicular failure. This is not surprising, since the masculinization caused by testosterone would not be expected to disappear or to regress

TABLE 76
The Spectrum of Male Hypogonadism

Type	Age of onset	Presentation	Examples
In utero	Karyotypic male fetus affected before birth by hypogonadism	Undervirilization of male fetus or feminization of male fetus (male pseudohermaphroditism)	1. Swyer Syndrome 2. Enzyme defects in testosterone synthesis 3. 5-α-reductase deficiency 4. Reifenstein's syndrome 5. Testicular feminization
Prepubertal	After birth but before puberty	Phenotypic male who fails to develop pubertal virilization	1. Klinefelter's syndrome 2. "Functional prepubertal castrate" 3. Kallmann's syndrome 4. Hypopituitarism
Postpubertal	After normal puberty, in adult life (adult testicular failure)	Impotence or infertility in normally virilized male	1. Klinefelter's syndrome 2. Pituitary tumors (esp. prolactinoma) 3. Testicular damage from radiation, drugs, or trauma

rapidly when hormone deficiency occurrs in adulthood. The term "male hypogonadism" should be restricted to patients with sexual infantilism. The examination of the hypogonadal male can be more revealing than a battery of randomly performed laboratory tests. The following aspects are to be stressed in the clinical evaluation of patients with testicular hypofunction.

36.1.1. Drug History

A careful history may reveal the use or abuse of drugs that play a role in decreasing testosterone production, antagonizing its action, or interfering with ejaculation. Alcohol, marijuana, cocaine, spironolactone, cimetidine, chemotherapy, estrogen therapy, and α-methyldopa can all be involved in causing testicular or erectile dysfunction.

36.1.2. Hyposmia or Anosmia

When seen in conjunction with sexual infantilism, this symptom is pathognomonic of Kallmann's syndrome ("olfactogenital" syndrome).

36.1.3. Gynecomastia

This is an important accompaniment of diverse hypogonadal states, e.g., Klinefelter's syndrome, Reifenstein's syndrome, alcoholism, cirrhosis, feminizing (or HCG-producing) tumors, estrogen intake, and mild variants of true hermaphroditism.

36.1.4. "Eunuchoidal" Skeletal Proportions

When hypogonadism starts before puberty, the near total lack of testosterone (or estrogens) results in continued growth of the epiphyseal plates at the ends of the long bones. As a result of this failure of the epiphyses to close, an effect normally mediated by sex steroids, the skeletal proportions of patients with prepubertal hypogonadism demonstrate "eunuchoidal" proportions: span of outstretched arms greater than the height by at least 2 inches and the lower segment (symphysis pubis to feet) greater than the upper segment (crown to symphysis pubis). Such proportions merely point to the onset of the testicular failure well before the usual age for puberty. Lack of abnormal proportions attests to the presence of some amount of androgen to effect epiphyseal closure.

36.1.5. Hypospadias

Hypospadias of any degree or a poorly developed prostate gland in an undervirilized male should raise the possibility of Reifenstein's syndrome.

36.1.6. Subnormal Intelligence

Approximately 15% to 25% of patients with Klinefelter's syndrome show an IQ below 80 as well as personality disorders.

36.1.7. Somatic Stigmata

Brachydactyly (short metacarpal bone), webbing of the neck, and short stature in conjunction with sexual infantilism are indicative of Noonan's syndrome (male Turner's). Harelip, cleft palate, and facial asymmetry (along with dysosmia) are seen in Kallmann's syndrome.

36.1.8. Associated Endocrine Disorders

The presence of coexistent ACTH or TSH deficiency should indicate pituitary failure as the etiology for hypogonadism. There is a higher incidence of autoimmune thyroiditis in patients with Klinefelter's syndrome.

With the above overview, the five major syndromes of primary testicular failure can be reviewed. The term "primary" indicates that the problem is inherently testicular. The reader is referred to Chapter 43 for hypogonadism resulting from disorders of sexual differentiation and to Chapter 5 for hypogonadism resulting from hypothalamic–pituitary diseases. The five syndromes that are focused on in this chapter are Klinefelter's syndrome, Reifenstein's syndrome, the "vanishing testes" syndrome (anorchia), the "Sertoli cell only" syndrome, and the syndrome of adult testicular failure.

36.2. Klinefelter's Syndrome

Klinefelter's syndrome represents the most common cause of male hypogonadism. In fact, the incidence of chromatin-positive buccal smears in male neonates (indicating a supernumerary X, a feature of Klinefelter's) is approximately 0.2%. This, obviously, is a much higher number than the clinical incidence of Klinefelter's would lead us to believe. The discrepancy arises from the extreme heterogeneity in the expression of this disorder. At one end of the spectrum is the patient with classic Klinefelter's and sexual infantilism, whereas on the other extreme is the normally virilized patient with Klinefelter's complaining of infertility only. This heterogeneity of expression should be kept in mind in evaluating patients with Klinefelter's syndrome.

36.2.1. Etiology

The basic underlying defect in these patients is the presence of one or more supernumerary X chromosomes. The abnormality occurs during fertilization and is a consequence of dysjunction during the reduction division. Thus, the embryo is conferred with 47 chromosomes and a sex karyotype of XXY instead of 46 chromosomes and a normal male karyotype of XY. The extra X chromosome is possibly transmitted to the testicular progenitor cells during early testicular differentiation. Because of the presence of a normal Y, the fetal testes develop and secrete adequate amounts of hormone to virilize the fetus, which is born appearing as a perfectly normal male infant. The subsequent damage to the germinal epithelum and to the Leydig cells in extreme cases is believed to be secondary to the supernumerary X. The classic Klinefelter's karyotype is 47,XXY, with diverse variants complicating the picture. The three variants related to Klinefelter's syndrome are mosaicism, the poly-X syndromes, and the sex reversal syndrome. These are discussed under differential diagnosis (Section 36.2.4).

36.2.2. Clinical Features

These can be discussed in terms of the four major facets of the syndrome: hypogonadism, gynecomastia, abnormal skeletal proportions, and associated features.

36.2.2.1. Hypogonadism

As indicated above, the expression of hypogonadism can be quite variable. Although in extreme cases gross sexual infantilism may be manifested, the usual patient with Klinefelter's syndrome demonstrates some degree of virilization. In some instances, Klinefelter's patients may go through a normal puberty, enjoy satisfactory sexual activity, even father a child, and then, in their early 20s, may develop testicular failure. In other instances, the patient may be completely asymptomatic and normally virilized, seeking help as a couple for infertility. This wide variability in expression is typical for Klinefelter's syndrome.

The abnormalities in the secondary sexual characteristics depend on the degree of decreased testosterone. Thus, the lack of facial, axillary, or pubic hair is seen only when the defect is severe. The palpatory findings relating to the testes are characteristic in Klinefelter's syndrome. The small, firm testes are a result of the atrophied and hyalinized seminiferous tubules.

36.2.2.2. Gynecomastia

Gynecomastia is present in more than 80% of patients with Klinefelter's syndrome and is related to the degree of hypogonadism. The gynecomastia seen in these patients arises from an imbalance in the ratio of testosterone and estradiol levels.

36.2.2.3. Abnormal Skeletal Proportions

This finding, too, is related to the degree of androgen deficiency, with "eunuchoidal" proportions being encountered in the more severe forms of sexual retardation.

36.2.2.4. Associated Features

There are several clinical associations that may be encountered in patients with Klinefelter's syndrome. These include a higher incidence of subnormal intelligence, psychosocial problems, chronic obstructive lung disease, diabetes mellitus, autoimmune thyroiditis, and, most importantly, carcinoma of the breast.

36.2.3. Diagnostic Studies

36.2.3.1. Hormonal Dysfunction

Since Klinefelter's syndrome represents the prototype of "primary" testicular failure, the hormonal findings reveal the characteristic combination of target organ (testicular) hypofunction and trophic (pituitary) hormone compensatory drive. Thus, both components of testicular function (androgen production and spermatogenesis) demonstrate decreased function as evidenced by low testosterone levels in the plasma and oligospermia. As a result of the negative feedback effect, the corresponding pituitary trophic hormones, LH and FSH, respectively, are increased.

36.2.3.2. Karyotypic Analysis

The buccal smear may reveal the presence of a Barr body, indicative of the second X chromosome. The karyotype analysis performed on cultured skin fibroblasts or blood cells demonstrates the characteristic 47,XXY pattern in the case of classic Klinefelter's syndrome.

It must be pointed out that a testicular biopsy is rarely indicated today in the evaluation of Klinefelter's syndrome.

36.2.4. Differential Diagnosis

Klinefelter's syndrome with severe sexual infantilism needs to be differentiated from Kallmann's syndrome. The lack of olfactory dysfunction, the degree of gynecomastia, and the small, firm testes of Klinefelter's help to differentiate it from Kallmann's. Further, the gonadotropin levels clearly differentiate the two. Klinefelter's syndrome with bilateral cryptorchidism (seen in 5–10% of instances) may be difficult to distinguish from anorchia (the "vanishing testes" syndrome) on clinical grounds. The karyotypic analysis will clearly establish the diagnosis.

The distinction between milder degrees of Klinefelter's syndrome and other forms of adult testicular failure can be quite difficult and would require chromosomal studies and, rarely, testicular biopsy to obtain tissue for chromosomal studies.

Some variants of Klinefelter's syndrome are particularly relevant in terms of differential diagnosis. The Klinefelter mosaic syndrome is characterized by two cell lines, one with 46,XY and another with 47,XXY. These patients may be normally virilized and may seek help for oligospermia. A second variant, the poly-X syndrome, is characterized by several supernumerary X chromosomes, resulting in XXXY or XXXXY syndromes with and without mosaicism. These patients are more severely retarded, variably hypogonadal, and demonstrate skeletal abnormalities. The most fascinating variant of Klinefelter's syndrome is the sex-reversal syndrome described by de la Chapelle. These patients resemble Klinefelter's syndrome in every manner, clinically and hormonally, but the karyotype is that of a normal female, 46,XX. The presence of testes attests to the fact that the Y antigen must have been present during the embryologic development. These patients, it is believed, represent examples of the "lost Y chromosome," the loss of which occurred after it had initiated testicular differentiation. The residue of the Y chromosome in such patients is reflected in the serum by the positivity for H-Y antigen, that unique portion of Y responsible for testicular differentiation (Section 34.6).

36.2.5. Complications

The two important complications of Klinefelter's syndrome, aside from hypogonadism, are osteoporosis and the development of carcinoma of the male breast.

36.2.6. Treatment

The treatment of Klinefelter's syndrome is replacement testosterone therapy with deep intramuscular injections of testosterone enanthate or propionate, 200 mg every 3 to 4 weeks. The risk of hepatotoxicity is minimal, and the risk of prostatic cancer is negligible from this form of therapy.

36.3. Reifenstein's Syndrome

Reifenstein's syndrome is caused by partial resistance of the peripheral tissues to testosterone and dihydrotestosterone. The term "partial" is the key word here, because complete resistance to androgens results in testicular feminization syndrome, a disorder that occurs in patients who are phenotypic females with completely female external genitalia. Thus, both Reifenstein's syndrome and testicular feminization syndrome represent variable expressions of the same disorder, which has its origins during the intrauterine life of the male fetus; when the expression is incomplete, the result is an undervirilized male; when the expression is complete, the result is a well-feminized "male." Both represent disorders occurring in karyotypic males with normally developed functional testes. Both represent examples of target organ failure. The difference lies in the degree of resistance to androgens, Reifenstein's syndrome representing only partial resistance to androgen action.

The disorder starts *in utero* in the karyotypic male fetus in whom the formation of the testes, synthesis of testosterone, and conversion of testosterone into dihydrotestosterone have all progressed quite normally. The problem is in the expression of the hormonal action on fetal tissues that should normally become virilized. Since the defect is only partial (usually a decrease in the number of androgen-binding receptors in the cytoplasm), some virilization of the fetus does take place. The infant is born appearing almost like a normal male or with ambiguity in the genitalia. The pathognomonic clinical feature is hypospadias, a maldevelopment of the male urethra. When the degree of hypospadias is mild (first degree), the genitalia look "male," and the sex assignment is that of a male infant. If the hypospadias is extreme (third degree), a "pseudovagina" may be formed as a result of nonfusion of the genital folds, which resemble labial folds. In either event, testes are present in the folds or in a normally formed scrotum or in the inguinal canal.

As the child (usually reared as a boy) grows older and enters the pubertal phase, the peripheral tissue once again stubbornly resist virilization. However, under the stimulus of gonadotropins, the testes secrete more testosterone, which to some extent can "overcome" the partial block and result in some pubertal virilization. In spite of it all, the patient is, at best, only suboptimally virilized, resulting in an undervirilized adult phenotypic male.

Thus, it seems that both in fetal life and during puberty, suboptimal virilization because of partial resistance of peripheral tissues is the pathophysiology of Reifenstein's syndrome. The mechanism of resistance has been elucidated, and it is found to be a partial deficiency of the cytoplasmic receptor protein that is essential for transporting dihydrotestosterone to the binding sites in the nuclear chromatin of the target cells. The condition is familial, often inherited as an X-linked trait.

36.3.1. Clinical Features

The three facets of Reifenstein's syndrome are hypoandrogenism, feminization, and congenital developmental defects in the distal genitourinary tract.

36.3.1.1. Hypoandrogenism

At birth, the hypoandrogenism is reflected as hypospadias and suboptimal virilization of the genital tubercle, which forms the phallus.

During puberty, the hypoandrogenism is manifested by failure to completely undergo pubertal virilization. Thus, the male secondary sexual characteristics, although present, are suboptimal. Sparse body and facial hair, very little acne formation, and failure to increase the muscle mass are frequently observed. The testes are of normal size, but associated cryptorchidism can complicate the picture. The prostate gland is poorly developed, and, of course, hypospadias is always present.

36.3.1.2. Feminization

Gynecomastia is nearly always present and is caused by the high estradiol levels. The estradiol is derived from testosterone, which is usually slightly elevated because of the androgen resistance. Since there is no resistance to estrogens, the breast tissue hypertrophies.

36.3.1.3. Associated Congenital Anomalies

Hypospadias and poor development of the prostate are seen in the vast majority of patients with Reifenstein's syndrome.

The variability in the clinical expression of Reifenstein's syndrome is striking, ranging from normal-looking males with infertility and mild hypospadias to the classic form characterized by hypogonadism and gynecomastia.

36.3.2. Diagnostic Studies

36.3.2.1. Hormonal Studies

The testosterone level in patients with Reifenstein's syndrome is slightly elevated because of the peripheral resistance. The pituitary LH and FSH are variable, ranging from normal to high. The estradiol level is slightly higher than that in the normal male, reflecting increased conversion from testosterone.

36.3.2.2. Androgen Receptor Studies

These studies, performed on cultured fibroblasts, may reveal decreased binding of testosterone and dihydrotestosterone to cytoplasmic receptors.

36.3.3. Differential Diagnosis

The hypospadias is a characteristic hallmark of Reifenstein's syndrome. When this is mild (or missed), Reifenstein's syndrome should be differentiated from Klinefelter's syndrome, a distinction that can be readily made by measurement of testosterone level in plasma and by the karyotype analysis.

36.3.4. Treatment

The treatment is difficult, since the basic defect is peripheral resistance. However, with large doses of testosterone therapy, the resistance may be overcome and, at least in some cases, virilization achieved.

36.4. Anorchia—"Vanishing Testes" Syndrome

This entity, which results in one of the most florid expressions of sexual infantilism, is caused by "disappearance" (atrophy) of testicular tissue in the late intrauterine or neonatal period of life.

36.4.1. Etiology

The atrophy of testes takes place at a time after the male fetus has been adequately masculinized. This is supported by the clinical observation that at birth the baby is normally virilized, the only abnormality being an "empty scrotum"; this is often attributed to bilateral cryptorchidism. The assumption, therefore, is that some time after the 24th to 28th week of intrauterine life, after virilization has been achieved by the testes, these gonads undergo atrophy bilaterally. The reasons for this occurrence are not clear, but torsion of the testes during descent, perhaps because of a short vascular stalk, is one plausible hypothesis. Whatever the mechanism, when these children grow up, they develop extreme hypogonadism because of their complete lack of functional testes.

36.4.2. Clinical Features

The hallmark of the syndrome of anorchia is severe sexual immaturity coupled with no palpable testes in the scrotum or inguinal canal in a karyotypic male (46,XY).

The hypogonadism, as indicated above, is extremely severe, illustrating every feature of complete testosterone deficiency. The prepubertal phallic proportions, the nonpigmented scrotum, the complete lack of facial hair, the eunuchoidal skeletal proportions, the high-pitched voice, and the poorly developed muscle mass coupled with nonpalpable testes create a striking clinical picture. Palpation of the scrotum may reveal ill-defined tissue probably representing rudimentary vestiges of the Wolffian duct derivatives. Gynecomastia is usually absent or minimal because of the total lack of testosterone production.

36.4.3. Diagnostic Studies

36.4.3.1. Hormonal Studies

The hormonal studies of patients with anorchia are characteristic of primary testicular failure—extremely low testosterone level with elevated LH and FSH. These data are shared by other disorders that cause primary testicular failure such as Klinefelter's syndrome.

36.4.3.2. Testosterone Response to HCG

Since there is no viable testicular tissue, there is no increase in the testosterone level following the administration of human chorionic gonadotrophin (HCG). This test assumes particular importance in differentiating anorchia from a child with bilateral cryptorchidism before puberty.

36.4.4. Differential Diagnosis

At birth, the most important differential diagnosis of anorchia is bilateral cryptorchidism. It should be remembered that uncomplicated cryptorchidism does not result in hypogonadism. Therefore, in a hypogonadal adult with an "empty scrotum," there is no reason to consider bilateral cryptorchidism unless it is complicated by other hypogonadal states. The differential diagnosis between anorchia and bilateral cryptorchidism becomes relevant only in childhood (prepubertal period), before hypogonadism can be expressed. The distinction can be made by evaluating the testicular response to HCG. Even during the prepubertal period, the undescended testes respond by releasing testosterone following single or multiple doses of HCG, which stimulate the Leydig cells of the viable—but hidden—testicular tissue, but no such response is seen in anorchia.

36.4.5. Treatment

The treatment should focus on dual aspects of life-long treatment with testosterone, which effectively induces virilization, as well as scrotal implantation of prostheses that resemble testes.

36.5. The "Sertoli Cell Only" Syndrome

The "Sertoli cell only syndrome" is a primary testicular disorder characterized by a dissociation between Leydig cell function and spermatogenesis. The expression of this syndrome is infertility.

36.5.1. Etiology

Originally described in 1947 by Del Castillo, this syndrome is characterized by a failure of the germinal epithelium to develop properly. The testicular biopsy demonstrates a characteristic appearance highlighted by a total absence of germinal epithelium, with only Sertoli cells lining the seminiferous tubules (hence the imaginative term "Sertoli cell only" syndrome).

36.5.2. Clinical Features

The main feature of Sertoli cell only syndrome is infertility. There are no signs or symptoms of androgen deficiency. Thus, from the hormone standpoint, the syndrome is characterized by eugonadism and infertility. The physical examination may reveal testicles that may be smaller than normal, since the bulk of the testes is constituted by seminiferous tubules.

36.5.3. Diagnostic Studies

36.5.3.1. Seminal Fluid Analysis

The sperm count is always abnormal in the Sertoli cell only syndrome, revealing moderate to severe oligospermia.

36.5.3.2. Hormonal Studies

The FSH level is elevated, a feedback response to impaired spermatogenesis, but the testosterone and LH levels are normal, indicating adequate Leydig cell function.

36.5.3.3. The Testicular Biopsy

This reveals a characteristic absence of germinal epithelium in the seminiferous tubules, which are lined exclusively with Sertoli cells. The Leydig cells are normal.

36.5.4. Differential Diagnosis

The combination of infertility, oligospermia, and elevated FSH with normal testosterone and LH levels in a normally virilized male is not unique for the Sertoli cell only syndrome. The above constellation is shared by several disorders that result in selective seminiferous tubular failure, including the mosaic Klinefelter's syndrome. The definitive diagnosis of the Sertoli cell only syndrome can be established only by testicular biopsy.

36.5.5. Treatment

There is no treatment to improve spermatogenesis in patients with the Sertoli cell only syndrome.

36.6. Adult Testicular Failure

This syndrome comprises several conditions that result in testicular failure in a previously eugonadal, well-virilized male.

36.6.1. Etiology

The etiologies that result in adult testicular failure (postpubertal variety) may originate in the hypothalamic–pituitary area or primarily in the testes. Table 77 categorizes these causes.

36.6.2. Clinical Features

The clinical features of adult testicular failure evolve slowly and are characterized by varying degrees of hypoandrogenism and infertility. Thus, impotence is the presenting complaint in patients who are not concerned about fertility.

The physical findings are less dramatic in comparison to those seen in prepubertal testicular failure. This is because the effects of prior virilization

TABLE 77
Adult Testicular Failure

Site of lesion	Causes
Hypothalamus	1. Suprasellar tumors (craniopharyngioma of adulthood, dysgerminoma, etc.)
Pituitary	1. Pituitary tumors
	2. Prolactin excess
	3. Hypopituitarism from any cause (hemochromatosis)
Testicular	Klinefelter's
	Trauma: radiation drugs, chemicals, etc.
Miscellaneous	Estrogen excess
	HCG-producing tumors

do not simply regress with the advent of decreased androgen production. A decrease in the frequency of shaving, an appreciable decrease in the facial or pubic hair, and decrease in the size of the testes are the extent to which the physical features become impressive.

36.6.3. Diagnostic Studies

The abnormalities in laboratory studies depend on the extent to which the individual functions of the testes are impaired. Thus, in some patients seminiferous tubular failure predominates, whereas in others Leydig cell failure is the highlight of presentation. Hence, the diagnostic studies should focus on both aspects of testicular function.

36.6.3.1. Leydig Cell Function

Measurement of serum testosterone would reveal persistently low levels. (It should be noted that measurement of urinary 17-ketosteroids is not an index of androgen adequacy.)

36.6.3.2. Seminiferous Tubular Function

Seminal fluid analysis (when feasible) is the main index of spermatogenesis. Although most patients with decreased Leydig cell function also demonstrate oligospermia, the reverse is not true.

36.6.3.3. Pituitary Gonadotropins

In every patient with hypotestosteronemia or oligospermia, it is mandatory to measure the levels of LH and FSH in the plasma to delineate the source of the problem. The utility of these assays in the evaluation of the hypogonadal patient is discussed in Section 34.4.

36.6.3.4. Prolactin Level

Since hyperprolactinemia constitutes an important etiology of hypoandrogenism, this assay should be included in the diagnostic evaluation of hypotestosteronemia.

36.6.3.5. Additional Tests

Depending on the results of the LH and FSH, i.e., secondary or primary testicular failure, additional tests would be required. If the gonadotropin levels are low, a thorough functional and anatomic evaluation of the hypothalamic–pituitary region must be carried out, i.e., hormonal studies, CT scan, etc. If the gonadotropin levels are high, consideration should be given to performing a buccal smear for Barr bodies, chromosomal analysis, and per-

TABLE 78
Spectrum of Hypogonadism

	Disease	Karyotype	Clinical hallmarks	Lab	Comments
1.	Klinefelter's	XXY	Hypogonadism Small, firm testes Gynecomastia Skeletal proportions eunuchoidal	T ↓ FSH, LH ↑ Sperm count →	Associated diseases (thyroiditis DM, COPD, CA male breast); heterogeneous expression
2.	Reifenstein's	XY	Hypospadias Small, firm testes Gynecomastia marked Hypogonadism	T ↑ FSH, LH: N or ↑ Sperm count →	Partial androgen resistance; receptor studies can be performed, which would reveal decreased cytosol receptors to T
3.	Sex reversal syndrome	XX	Classic Klinefelter's type	T ↓ FSH, LH ↑ Sperm count →	H-Y antigen positive
4.	Anorchia	XY	"Vanishing testes" Gross hypogonadism Empty scrotum	T ↓ FSH, LH ↑ Azoospermia	
5.	Sertoli cell only syndrome	XY	Normally virilized male Oligospermia	T normal LH normal Sperm count → FSH ↑	DD is adult seminiferous tubular failure; testicular biopsy shows minimal germinal epithelium
6.	Kallmann's	XY	Hypogonadism, anosmia	T ↓ LH, FSH ↓	Isolated LH, FSH deficiency 2° to LH-LRH deficiency
7.	Hypopituitarism	XY	Hypogonadism Intra- or suprasellar lesions	T ↓ LH, FSH ↓	Usually 2° to tumors of the pituitary
8.	Noonan's (male Turner's)	XO/XY (mixed gonadal dysgenesis)	Somatic stigmata Short stature, small testes	T ↓ LH, FSH ↑	

haps a testicular biopsy. In addition, estrogen levels and HCG levels would be indicated when hyperestrogenism is evident.

36.6.4. Treatment

Although testosterone therapy is effective replacement therapy for all varieties of hypoandrogenism, specific treatment for the underlying etiology is required when applicable.

Table 78 provides a composite summary of various hypogonadal states, pointing out the salient clinical and laboratory features.

Selected Readings

Aiman, J., Griffin, A. E., Gazak, J. M., et al.: Androgen insensitivity as a cause of infertility in otherwise normal men, N. Engl. J. Med. **300**:223, 1979.

Bain, J.: Male hypogonadism, Compr. Ther. **9**:17, 1983.

Carlson, H. E.: Gynecomastia, N. Engl. J. Med. **303**:795, 1980.

Carter, J. N., Tyson, J. E., Tolis, G., et al.: Prolactin secreting tumors and hypogonadism in 22 men, N. Engl. J. Med. **299**:847, 1978.

Collins, E., and Turner, G.: The Noonan syndrome. A review of the clinical and genetic features of 27 cases, J. Pediatr. **83**:941, 1973.

de la Chapelle, A.: Analytic review: Nature and origin of males with XX sex chromosomes, Am. J. Hum. Genet. **24**:71, 1972.

Del Castillo, E. B., Trabucco, A., and De La Balze, F. A.: The syndrome produced by absence of the germinal epithelium without impairment of the Sertoli or Leydig cells, J. Clin. Endocrinol. **7**:493, 1947.

deMorsier, G., and Gauthier, G.: Olfacto-genital dysplasia, Pathol. Biol. **11**:1267, 1963.

Federman, D. D.: The assessment of organ function—the testes, N. Engl. J. Med. **285**:901, 1971.

Gordon, D. L., Krmpotic, E., Thumas, W., et al.: Pathologic testicular findings in Klinefelter's syndrome, Arch. Intern. Med. **130**:726, 1972.

Hainsworth, J. D., and Greco, F. A.: Testicular germ cell neoplasms, Am. J. Med. **75**:817, 1983.

Kallmann, R. J., Schoenfeld, W. A., and Barrera, S. E.: The genetic aspects of primary eunuchoidism, Am. J. Ment. Defic. **48**:203, 1944.

Klinefelter, H. F., Reifenstein, E. C., and Albright, F.: Syndrome characterized by gynecomastia, aspermatogenesis without a-Leydigism, and increased excretion of follicle stimulating hormone, J. Clin. Endocrinol. Metab. **2**:615, 1942.

Kolodny, H. D., Kim, S., Sherman, L., et al.: Anorchia. A variety of the "empty scrotum," J.A.M.A. **216**:479, 1971.

Loriaux, L., Menard, R., Taylor, A., et al.: Spironolactone and endocrine dysfunction (NIH conference), Ann. Intern. Med. **85**:630, 1976.

Males, J. L., Townsend, J. L., and Schneider, R. A.: Hypogonadotropic hypogonadism with anosmia—Kallmann's syndrome, Arch. Intern. Med. **131**:501, 1973.

Marshall, W. A., and Tanner, J. M.: Variation's in the pattern of pubertal changes in boys, Arch. Dis. Child. **45**:13, 1970.

McKendry, J. B. R., Collins, W. E., Silverman, M., et al.: Erectile impotence: A clinical challenge, Can. Med. Assoc. J. **128**:653, 1983.

Reifenstein, E. C., Jr.: Hereditary familial hypogonadism, Proc. Am. Fed. Clin. Res. **3**:86, 1947.

Sadeghi-Nejad, A., Kaplan, S., and Grumbach, M. M.: The effect of medroxyprogesterone acetate on adrenocortical function in children with precocious puberty, J. Pediatr. **78**:616, 1971.

Smals, A. G. H., Kloppenborg, P. W. C., and Benraad, T. J.: Body proportions and androgenicity in relation to plasma testosterone levels in Klinefelter's syndrome, Acta. Endocrinol. **77**:387, 1974.

Spark, R. F., White R. A., and Connolly, P. B.: Impotence is not always psychogenic. Newer insights into hypothalamic pituitary gonadal dysfunction, *J.A.M.A.* **243:**750, 1980.

Steinberger, E.: Hormonal control of mammalian spermatogenesis, *Physiol. Rev.* **51:**1, 1971.

Steinberger, E.: Disorders of testicular function (male hypogonadism), in DeGroot, L. J., Cahill, G. F., Odell, W. D., *et al.* (eds.): *Endocrinology, Vol. 3. New York, Grune and Stratton, 1979.*

Walsh, P. C.: A new cause of male infertility, *N. Engl. J. Med.* **300:**253, 1979.

Walsh, P. C., Swerdloff, R. S., Odell, W. D.: Feedback regulation of gonadotropin secretion in men, *J. Urol.* **110:**84, 1973.

Wang, C., Baker, H. W. G., Burger, H. G., *et al.:* Hormonal studies in Klinefelter's syndrome, *Clin. Endocrinol.* **4:**399, 1975.

Wasserman, M. D., Pollak, C. P., Spielman, A. J., *et al.:* Differential diagnosis of impotence: Measurement of nocturnal penile tumescence, *J.A.M.A.* **243:**2038, 1980.

Weiss, H. D.: The physiology of human penile erection, *Ann. Intern. Med.* **76:**793, 1972.

Wilson, J. D.: Recent studies on the mechanism of action of testosterone, *N. Engl. J. Med.* **287:**1284, 1972.

Wilson, J. D., Harrod, M. J., Goldstein, J. L., *et al.:* Familial incomplete male pseudohermaphroditism, type I, *N. Engl. J. Med.* **290:**1097, 1974.

VI

The Ovaries

37

Anatomy of the Ovaries

The ovaries are almond-shaped structures located in the pelvis and measure 2.5 cm in their longest diameter. The ovary is secured in position by several ligaments—the suspensory ligament that connects the ovary to the pelvic wall, the uteroovarian ligament that connects it to the uterus, and the mesovarium, which connects the ovary to the posterior surface of the broad ligament of the uterus.

The surface of the ovary is irregular, marked by "scars" from numerous previous ovulations. The bulk of the ovary is constituted by the stroma. The germinal epithelium lies superficial to the stroma, just beneath the surface of the ovary. The ovarian follicles are scattered throughout the stroma. Histologically, the follicles are surrounded by granulosa cells, which secrete estradiol. Several layers of granulosa cells are arranged in a concentric fashion around the mature follicles. The cells that are close to the follicles are called theca interna cells, and those that are peripheral, merging with the stroma, are called the theca externa cells. The theca cells primarily secrete androgens.

The blood supply to the ovaries is derived from the ovarian and uterine blood vessels that traverse in the mesovarium and enter the ovary at its hilum. The ovary is highly vascular. The medullary and cortical branches supply the entire ovary, with arborizations virtually supplying every follicle. The venous drainage is by the ovarian veins, which enter the inferior vena cava just below the entry of the renal veins.

38

Physiology of Ovarian Function

38.1. Introduction

The two functions of the ovaries are synthesis of estrogens and provision of mature ova for fertilization. There are several similarities between the ovaries and the testes, which also possess dual functions in terms of secreting androgens and spermatogenesis. The testes and ovaries originate from the same primitive bipotential gonad. The Leydig cells, seminiferous tubules, and the interstitium of the testes are represented by their counterparts in the ovary— the granulosa cells, primordial follicles, and the stroma, respectively. Both gonads depend on the pituitary gland for trophic control by the gonadotropins LH and FSH. To provide perspective in understanding ovarian function, this chapter focuses on the physiology of five phenomena:

1. Ovarian steroidogenesis (or formation of estradiol, progesterone, and androgens).
2. The process of follicular maturation and rupture (ovulation).
3. The hormonal basis for the normal menstrual cycle.
4. The role of gonadotropins in maintenance of ovarian function.
5. The feedback regulation of the hypothalamic pituitary unit by estrogens.

These five phenomena dominate understanding of the physiological principles that underlie ovarian function. Although they appear compartmentalized, these phenomena merge imperceptibly in a network of intricate and delicate events that characterize the reproductive years of the female. Hormonally, all these phenomena appear to be geared for one event—reproduction.

38.2. Ovarian Steroidogenesis

The ovaries secrete estrogens, progesterone, and, to a lesser extent, androgens. The granulosa cells are the primary source of estradiol secretion.

Estradiol can also be secreted by the corpus luteum. The primary source for progesterone production is the corpus luteum. The androgen secretion by the ovaries is carried out by the theca cells.

The *de novo* biosynthesis of estradiol by the granulosa cells involves biosynthetic pathways similar to the ones involved in testosterone synthesis by the testes and androgen synthesis by the adrenal cortex. Figure 23 outlines these steps.

The granulosa cells contain receptors for both FSH and LH. It is currently believed that both gonadotropins stimulate the granulosa cells to secrete estradiol, and the effect is mediated by adenylate cyclase stimulation and cyclic AMP generation. There is considerable experimental evidence that suggests that the theca cells are also capable of secreting estradiol under the stimulation of LH and FSH. The production rate of estradiol can be as high as 1 mg a day during the late follicular phase, a phase characterized by the most intense estradiol productivity.

The progesterone synthesis is exclusively a function of the luteinized granulosa cells and theca cells of the corpus luteum. The production rate of progesterone in the midluteal phase can approximate 25 mg per day, with plasma levels approaching 10 to 15 ng/ml.

The androgen secretion is carried out by the theca cells and the stromal cells, the activity of which can be augmented by administration of LH.

If the levels of estradiol are plotted by daily measurement of this hormone throughout the menstrual cycle, the following pattern emerges: the estradiol levels are low at the start of the cycle in the early follicular phase, gradually increasing to reach a peak at the late follicular phase. Following this peak, the estradiol levels slightly decline; in the midluteal phase a second rise, but of a lesser magnitude, is seen. The second rise reflects estradiol secretion by

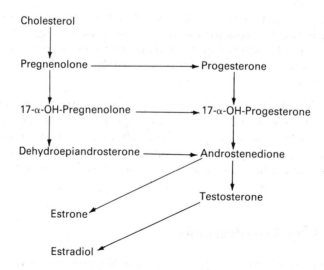

Figure 23. Ovarian steroidogenesis.

the corpus luteum. Towards the end of the cycle, the estradiol levels decrease and reach a nadir.

38.3. Follicular Maturation and Ovulation

Follicular maturation begins only after puberty. Prior to puberty, the ovary is filled with immature primary follicles containing oogonia that are not capable of cell division. The process of maturation is initiated by gonadotropins, in particular FSH, the follicle-stimulating hormone. (The situation is analogous to spermatogenesis, a process that requires FSH for initiation.) The maturation of the Graafian follicle not only depends on the availability of FSH but is also quite dependent on the intraovarian content of estradiol secreted by the granulosa cells of the follicle. Each month, one ovum is selected to "ovulate," although several follicles grow and mature. The mechanisms involved in such a highly selective process whereby only a single ovum undergoes ovulation while the rest undergo atresia are unknown. The established concepts in follicular maturation are these:

1. Pituitary gonadotropins are absolutely necessary for follicular maturation, since administration of estrogen alone to hypophysectomized women does not result in proper maturation.
2. Estradiol secreted by the granulosa cells is also crucial for follicular maturation.
3. The increase in the size of the follicle and the changes in cells that surround the follicle are dependent on estradiol concentrations. The follicle, which originally measures 50 μm enlarges about 400 times in size. The oocyte within the follicle also enlarges, and the surrounding granulosa cells proliferate and begin to secrete increasing concentrations of estradiol under the intense stimulation by FSH and LH. The stromal cells surrounding the follicles proliferate and become arranged in concentric layers around the follicle. The stromal cells close to the follicle are called theca interna cells, whereas the theca externa cells merge with the adjacent stroma.
4. By the time the follicle matures, the pituitary releases a surge of LH (and to a lesser extent FSH). Twenty-four hours after this surge, ovulation occurs, and the ovum is extruded from the follicle. The follicle emptied of the ovum becomes a sealed new structure called the corpus luteum. Following ovulation, the theca interna cells, the granulosa cells, and the theca externa cells undergo extreme mitosis with increased vascularity and fat content. This process, called "leutinization" of the granulosa cells and the theca interna cells, is mediated by LH (the luteinizing hormone). The corpus luteum secretes progesterone and to a lesser extent estradiol.

Thus, the hormonal highlights of ovulation are the surge of LH and FSH before ovulation and secretion of progesterone by the corpus luteum after ovulation.

38.4.   The Menstrual Cycle

The menstrual cycle is a constellation of cyclic hormonal events that occur on a monthly basis. The culmination of the events is the production of a single ovum for fertilization. If this goal is met, pregnancy ensues; if not menstruation occurs.

The menstrual cycle is divided into two phases: the early phase is follicular, since the major event in the first half of the cycle is maturation of the follicle; the latter phase is called the luteal phase, and the major happening during this phase is formation of the corpus luteum. The follicular and luteal phases are approximately 14 days each, being separated by the process of ovulation.

At the start of the cycle, immediately after the menses of the previous cycle, the estradiol levels are low. This stimulates the tonic part of the hypothalamus to secret gonadotropin-releasing hormone. As a result, the pituitary begins to gradually release FSH and LH. As the FSH and LH increase, the granulosa cells are stimulated by these hormones to synthesize and secrete estradiol. Under the combined influence of estradiol, LH, and FSH, the follicles undergo maturation. By the 14th day, the follicle has reached maturation, and the estradiol levels have reached their peak.

During this late follicular phase, the high concentrations of estradiol stimulate the cyclic hypothalamus. This is mediated by positive feedback in contrast to the tonic hypothalamus, which can be stimulated only by negative feedback. The cyclic hypothalamus, stimulated by estradiol, secretes gonadotropin-releasing hormone for a second time, resulting in a predominantly LH surge. This surge, 24 hr later, causes rupture of the mature follicle.

After ovulation, the estradiol concentrations decline gradually. The luteal phase is characterized by sustained secretion of progesterone. Toward the late luteal phase, estradiol is also secreted by the corpus luteum. If fertilization occurs, the corpus luteum persists; if not, it undergoes atrophy. The atrophy of the corpus luteum is accompanied by a drop in progesterone and estradiol levels. This flux in hormone levels results in withdrawal bleeding by the uterus.

38.5.   The Role of Gonadotropins

The role of gonadotropins in the maintenance of ovarian function extends in three directions: the first is estradiol synthesis, the second is in inducing ovulation, and the third is in maintenance of secretory function of the corpus luteum. Current evidence suggests that both hormones, LH and FSH, are required for all three functions. In the past it was considered that follicle maturation was mediated by FSH and ovulation by LH. Although this may still be predominantly so, studies using individual preparations of LH and FSH indicate that both gonadotropins work synergistically.

The secretion of estradiol by the granulosa cells clearly requires FSH and, to a lesser extent, LH. The midcyclic surge of LH (and to a less extent FSH) is crucial for ovulation. The maintenance of the corpus luteum is predominantly a function of LH.

38.6.   Feedback Regulation of LH and FSH

The reader is referred to Section 2.5 for the regulatory mechanisms that control LH and FSH in the female. The salient points are summarized here.

1. The female hypothalamus is unique in that physiologically it contains a tonic portion that responds to negative feedback by estradiol and a cyclic portion that responds to positive feedback by estradiol.
2. In the early follicular phase, the tonic hypothalamus responds to the low estradiol level and releases GnRH, which stimulates FSH and LH release.
3. In the late follicular phase, the estradiol levels at their peak stimulate the cyclic hypothalamus to release GnRH, which is the basis for the preovulatory LH surge.
4. Persistent administration of estrogens, as with oral contraceptives, leads to a sustained increase in estrogen levels, which suppress the hypothalamus and the pituitary.

The use of LH and FSH assays in evaluating ovarian function is discussed in Chapter 39.

39

Testing Ovarian Function

39.1. Introduction

The two aspects of ovarian function—estrogen production and follicular maturation leading to ovulation—are highly interdependent phenomena. Since follicular maturation critically depends on several hormonal factors, a crucial one being the local (intraovarian) concentration of estradiol, it is perhaps correct to perceive estrogen production as the primary function of the ovary. Without adequate estrogen synthesis, follicular maturation will not occur, nor will the hormonal stage be set for ovulation, i.e., rupture of the mature Graafian follicle. Thus, the tests that evaluate adequacy of ovarian function can be viewed in terms of tests that are aimed at evaluating estrogen synthesis by the granulosa cells of the ovaries, tests that evaluate if ovulation has occurred, tests that evaluate the hypothalamo–pituitary axis, tests that evaluate uterine responsiveness to the changing sex-steroid milieu, and tests that evaluate the entire female genital tract for patency and suitability for sperm viability (Table 79).

39.2. Tests for Estrogen Synthesis

39.2.1. 17-β-Estradiol

The direct method for evaluating the adequacy of estrogen secretion by the granulosa cells of the ovary is by measuring the circulating level of 17-β-estradiol in the serum. The level of 17-β-estradiol in the normal female varies considerably with the phase of the menstrual cycle, ranging from as low as 50 to as high as 700 pg/ml (in the follicular phase 50–100 pg/ml, in the midcycle 170–770 pg/ml, and in the luteal phase 200–300 pg/ml). Therefore, in a regularly menstruating female, some correlation is possible, but in the amenorrhic woman, the interpretation of a single value of 17-β-estradiol can become well nigh impossible. Indeed, this is the major limiting factor in inter-

TABLE 79
Testing Ovarian Function

Category	Tests
Tests for estrogen synthesis	Serum 17-β-estradiol level
Tests for ovulation	BBT
	Endometrial biopsy
	Serum progesterone
Tests for hypothalamic– pituitary disease	Basal LH, FSH
	LH-RH test
	Ancillary tests
Tests for uterine responsiveness	The progestin withdrawal tests
Tests that evaluate the entire genital tract	Tubal patency tests
	Postcoital test

pretation of values of the hormone in the range of 100–200 pg/ml. Although it is true that extremely hypogonadal females have circulating 17-β-estradiol levels below 50 pg/ml, the assay is hardly required in the presence of such overt hypogonadism. In situations in which one turns to the assay for help (for example, women with secondary amenorrhea), the results fall within ranges that are frustratingly difficult to interpret. It is for this reason that many clinicians resort to evaluating the "estrogen effect" rather than an estrogen level drawn during a single moment in time.

39.2.2. Vaginal Cytology

The epithelium of the vagina is responsive to estrogen. The vaginal epithelium of prepubertal girls and postmenopausal females shows the characteristic and extreme hypoestrogenic effect—nonkeratinized, relatively small, fragile epithelial cells, In contrast, the vaginal epithelium at the height of estrogen stimulation, as in during the late follicular or periovulatory phase of the menstrual cycle, shows cornified squamous epithelium staining pink with eosin and containing pyknotic nuclei. By carefully studying the vaginal smears, cytopathologists can provide a "maturation index" by comparing the superficial, transitional, and basal types of epithelial cells in the vaginal epithelial layer. In an expert's hands, the maturation index (or the karyopyknotic index) correlates with the estrogen status much more closely than a randomly obtained serum 17-β-estradiol level.

39.3. Tests for Ovulation

39.3.1. Basal Body Temperature

This method for detecting ovulation is based on the principle that ovulation, with the resultant increase in progesterone level, causes a slight increase in the basal body temperature (BBT) after ovulation. The patient is instructed to record her temperature carefully, with a special thermometer, every morning for a month or two. In the "classic" case of a normal ovulatory cycle, a biphasic BBT response is seen. The BBT demonstrates a sustained increase in temperature of 0.3 to 1.0°F or higher in the secretory (postovulatory) phase in comparison to the follicular (preovulatory phase). Careful retrospective analysis of the BBT charts reveals that the "exact" time of ovulation corresponds to the low-point day just before the first day of increased BBT. The reason for the sustained increase in BBT for 12 days after its initial rise is the maintenance of higher levels of progesterone by the corpus luteum following ovulation.

The demonstration of a characteristic dip (before ovulation) and sustained rise pattern in BBT (after ovulation) provides clear evidence of ovulation having occurred. When clearly positive, this simple test provides tremendous and far-reaching diagnostic information. It indicates sequentially adequacy of the hypothalamic gonadotropin-releasing hormone, intact FSH secretion by the pituitary, adequate estrogen synthesis by the granulosa cells to provoke a midcycle LH surge, and rupture of the Graafian follicle that has matured as a consequence of adequate local estradiol concentrations. No single test in endocrinology provides such a wealth of information as the simple recording of BBT to detect ovulation.

Unfortunately, the BBT helps only when it is characteristically positive. Approximately 20% of normally ovulating females may not show evidence of dip and sustained rise in BBT charts. The inference is twofold—if the BBT chart is clearly indicative of ovulation, the patient can be spared from an endometrial biopsy or measurement of progesterone level in the serum, but if the BBT is "negative," these tests should be performed before labeling the cycle anovulatory.

39.3.2. Endometrial Biopsy

This provides direct histological evidence of the "progesterone effect" on the endometrium. The demonstration of a "secretory" endometrium (exhausted secretory glands and compact stroma) is proof of ovulation having occurred; the timing of the endometrial biopsy is obviously crucial, since the secretory endometrium is at its best ("ripened") just before menstruation. The closer the study is timed to the onset of menses, the more rewarding is the secretory histology. It is best performed 12 hr after the onset of menses. The bleeding is not a histological deterrent for recognition of the characteristic secretory histology. This timing also obviates the risk of unintentionally disrupting early pregnancy. If the biopsy is to be performed in a patient with irregular cycles, she is asked to report as soon as menses have begun. In such a patient, demonstration of a secretory endometrium is indicative of the fact that she has ovulated, at least for that cycle. If, on the other hand, the endometrical biopsy is nonsecretory, the patient has had an anovulatory cycle with menstruation.

39.3.3. Serum Progesterone Level

After ovulation, the follicle is transformed into the corpus luteum and secretes progesterone. The secretion of progesterone continues for 12 days, during which time the hormone prepares the endometrium for possible implantation of the fertilized ovum. If pregnancy does not occur, the corpus luteum involutes, the serum progesterone precipitously drops, and the endometrium responds by withdrawal bleeding (menstruation). Thus, the hormonal hallmark of ovulation is increased progesterone in the serum. In a normally menstruating female with predictable cycles, the demonstration of even a single serum progesterone in excess of 5 ng/ml in the latter half of the menstrual cycle is proof of adequate luteal function and therefore, of ovulation. Unfortunately, the difficulty in determining the "latter half" of the cycle in a woman with amenorrhea and unpredictable cycles is obvious.

The indication for the above three tests is in the evaluation of infertility, where it is crucial to exclude anovulation as a cause.

39.4. Tests for the Hypothalamic–Pituitary Axis

39.4.1. Basal LH and FSH Levels

The measurement of a single basal level of LH or FSH is likely to be of value only in patients with intrinsic ovarian disease. In a patient with hypoestrogenism, the documentation of an elevated LH or FSH, even in a single basal sample, points to the ovaries as the site of disease. For example, in patients with Turner's syndrome, pure gonadal dysgenesis, premature ovarian failure, or during menopause, the demonstration of an elevated gonadotropin level documents intrinsic ovarian pathology regardless of etiology. Care should be taken in interpreting LH and FSH values because these hormones fluctuate widely during various phases of the menstrual cycle. An elevated LH or FSH has meaning only in the presence of a clinical or hormonally documented hypoestrogenic state.

Comparison of LH : FSH ratios in samples taken on multiple occasions may provide a clue for the diagnosis of polycystic ovary syndrome, a condition characterized by amenorrhea, hirsutism, anovulation, and persistently elevated LH : FSH ratios.

39.4.2. The LH-RH Test

The administration of a bolus of synthetic luteinizing hormone-releasing hormone to evaluate the reserve of gonadotropins is less useful than originally proposed for differentiating pituitary from hypothalamic disease. However, modifications of the test by using multiple doses of LH-RH for "priming" may be helpful in such delineation.

39.4.3. Ancillary Tests for Hypothalamic–Pituitary Disease

The two tests that are relevant are prolactin level in the serum and computerized tomography of the sellar and suprasellar region. Since hyperprolactinemia may be etiologically related in as many as a third of patients with secondary amenorrhea, the importance of screening with serum prolactin levels is underscored (Chapter 4). The value of computerized tomography in the evaluation of patients with pituitary disease is discussed in Chapter 7.

39.5. Tests for Uterine Responsiveness

The progestin withdrawal test, which has been in vogue for several years, is an attempt to evaluate the responsiveness of the uterus to fluxes in hormone milieu. If a patient demonstrates withdrawal bleeding following the administration of progestin orally (Provera®), this indicates:

1. The presence of functioning and responsive uterine endometrium.
2. The presence of adequate ovarian tissue to synthesize estrogens that have "primed" the endometrium to respond to progestin withdrawal.
3. Adequacy of FSH level to permit ovarian steroidogenesis.

Thus, the demonstration of withdrawal bleeding to progestin indicates reasonable integrity of the FSH–ovarian–uterine unit; the missing phenomenon of ovulation may be explained by postulating that estrogen production may have been adequate to prime the endometrium but suboptimal to provoke an LH surge required for ovulation.

The lack of response to progestin indicates either pregnancy or serious deficiency in secreting estrogen, the etiology of which could be hypothalamic, pituitary, or ovarian. When the progestin withdrawal test is negative, the test should be repeated after estrogen therapy. The demonstration of withdrawal bleeding after cyclic estrogen and progestin therapy is proof that endogenous estrogen secretion was inadequate to prime the uterine endometrium. If withdrawal bleeding fails to occur with cyclic estrogen and progestin therapy, this reflects uterine unresponsiveness because of local pathology.

In clinical practice, the progestin withdrawal test does not provide specific diagnostic information that would preclude the performance of other studies.

39.6. Evaluation of the Female Genital Tract

The focus on evaluation of the genital tract assumes importance in the workup of the infertile patient. The evaluation, in its simplest form, consists of a careful pelvic examination to exclude disorders in the outflow tract and abnormalities in the cervix and body of the uterus as well as the adenexa.

The assessment of tubal patency is crucial in the diagnostic and therapeutic approach to infertility. Tubal patency can be assessed by outlining the lower genital tract with contrast media, i.e., hysterosalpingography. This procedure has, in most institutions, supplanted the CO_2 insufflation test, which used to be done in the past by injecting CO_2 under pressure into the fallopian tubes and observing for shoulder pain.

The postcoital test is to evaluate the viability of the sperm in the cervical mucus. Since cervical factors (hostile mucus) constitute an important etiology of infertility, it is essential to evaluate if the spermatozoa are capable of surviving long enough to conduct their upward journey to fertilize the ovum. The test is done by analyzing the cervical mucus for the presence of motile spermatozoa 6 to 8 hr following coitus. The demonstration of more than 10 spermatozoa per HPF is good evidence for viability and excludes hostile mucus as a factor in infertility.

40

Precocious Puberty
in the Female

40.1. Introduction

Precocious puberty is arbitrarily defined as the development of pubertal feminization in a female child under age 8.

Normal puberty is an extremely complicated hormonal event that involves participation of the hypothalamus, the pituitary, and the ovaries in a strikingly synchronous fashion. The exact process that initiates puberty is not clear. The hypothalamic–pituitary unit of the prepubertal child is exquisitely sensitive to suppression by sex steroids. Administration of extremely small doses of ethinyl estradiol to prepubertal girls effectively causes suppression of the hypothalamic–pituitary unit. As puberty approaches, there is a decrease in the sensitivity of the hypothalamus to suppression by sex steroids. The hypothalamus, which is released from inhibition, secretes gonadotropin-releasing hormone. Very small amounts of GnRH are released in a pulsatile fashion. These pulses gradually sensitize the pituitary gland to stimulation by the hypothalamic peptide.

The pituitary gonadotrophs are gradually programmed, over a period of 2 to 3 years antedating actual puberty, to respond to various physiological stimuli, particularly sleep. The sleep-related LH response can be demonstrated several months prior to actual elevation of basal levels of LH during the day.

While the hypothalamus and the pituitary gonadotrophs are maturing, the ovaries begin to demonstrate restoration of sensitivity to stimulation by gonadotropins: FSH probably induces responsiveness of the gonad to LH by inducing new receptors to LH. Thus, a concerted drive by gonadotropin stimulation results in secretion of estradiol by the granulosa cells, resulting in feminization.

Staging of sexual maturation should take into account several aspects of pubertal feminization. The earliest changes of puberty are adrenarche (axillary and pubic hair growth) and/or the thelarche (breast development); one or both changes happen between 8.5 and 13 years in most girls. The interval between initial breast development and menarche is approximately 2 to 3.5 years, and the interval between adrenarche and menarche ranges from 1.5 to 6 years. In evaluating precocious puberty, the occurrence of both adrenarche and thelarche suggest early pubertal changes, and the combination of these changes with menarche, growth spurt, and psychological changes is indicative of advanced puberty. Thus, all facets of feminization should be considered in evaluating the child with early feminization.

40.2. Etiology

The most common variety of precocious puberty in girls is idiopathic and merely represents a premature maturation of the hypothalamic–pituitary–ovarian axis. This form of precocious puberty can also occur in McCune–Albright's syndrome as well as in certain CNS tumors.

Another variety of precocious puberty (pseudoprecocious puberty) is caused by estrogen-secreting tumors of the ovary or the adrenal cortex. The most important ovarian tumor is granulosa cell tumor, and the most important adrenal tumor that causes feminization is the rare but lethal adrenal carcinoma. These two varieties—central and periphral—of estrogen hypersecretion account for more than 90% of cases. Rarely, precocious puberty in girls can be caused by primary hypothyroidism (Section 15.3.5) or HCG-secreting tumors, particularly hepatocellular carcinoma.

40.3. Clinical Features

The obvious feature is premature feminization, consisting of the changes listed in the introduction of this chapter. Associated findings that may be seen in association with precocious puberty in the female are outlined in Table 80.

40.4. Diagnostic Studies

The diagnostic evaluation of the female child with precocious puberty should be approached in a step-by-step method, attempting to answer three questions.

1. Is the precocious puberty caused by central or peripheral mechanisms that result in hypersecretion of estradiol?
2. If a central mechanism is identified, is the etiology tumorous or nontumorous?

TABLE 80
Precocious Puberty in Girls

Physical finding	Significance
Headaches, visual field defects	Suprasellar tumor (pinealoma, hamartoma)
Pigmentation (cafe-au-lait spots)	McCune–Albright's syndrome
Abdominal mass	Adrenal carcinoma
Pelvic mass	Ovarian tumor (granulosa cell tumor)
Galactorrhea	Hypothyroidism with precocious puberty
Hepatomegaly	Hepatic malignancy secreting HCG

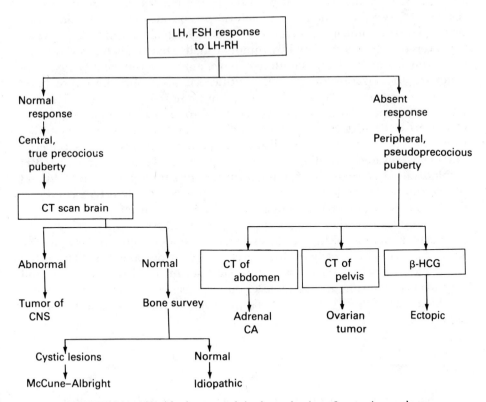

FIGURE 24. Algorithmic approach in the evaluation of precocious puberty.

3. If a peripheral mechanism is identified, does the problem lie in the ovary, in the adrenal, or elsewhere?

The single most important step in the evaluation of precocious puberty is to delineate if the precocious puberty is "true" (central) or "pseudo" (peripheral). This initial distinction can be made by applying the following physiological principle: when central mechanisms underlie the pathogenesis of precocious puberty, the hypothalamic–pituitary axis is normal but prematurely activated, whereas peripheral mechanisms that cause premature hypersecretion of estradiol result in suppression of the hypothalamic–pituitary axis. The laboratory distinction between the two can be made by two hormonal studies—first, by evaluating the response of LH and FSH to an intravenous bolus of LH-RH, and second, by the degree of estradiol elevation. Regarding the LH and FSH response to LH-RH, patients with central precocious puberty demonstrate a normal gonadotropin rise in response to LH-RH quite analogous to normal pubertal girls; on the contrary, patients with peripheral mechanisms (ovarian tumor, adrenal tumor, etc.) causing hyperestrogenism demonstrate a flat, absent response, since the gonadotropins are already suppressed. The absolute levels of estradiol in the plasma may also have some discriminatory value. The levels in central precocious puberty are only minimally elevated, comparable to the levels seen in normal pubertal girls, whereas the levels of estradiol secreted by tumors usually show marked elevation.

If the hormone data, as outlined above, indicate a central etiology, computerized tomography of the sella, suprasellar area, and the entire brain should be performed to exclude a tumor in these regions. If the CT scan is negative, a bone survey should be performed to search for cystic lesions that characterize the McCune–Albright syndromes and thyroid function studies to exclude primary hypothyroidism. The patient with precocious puberty, minimally elevated estradiol, normally responsive LH and FSH to LH-RH administration, normal CT of brain, normal bone survey, and normal thyroid profile can be concluded to have idiopathic precocious puberty, a condition that accounts for 90% of cases of precocious puberty in females.

If the hormone data suggest a peripheral mechanism, the tests planned should be aimed at excluding an estrogen-secreting tumor in the ovary or adrenal or a tumor elsewhere that secretes HCG ectopically; CT scans of the abdomen and pelvis, ultrasonography, and serum level of β-HCG are all helpful in recognizing the anatomic lesion responsible for precocious puberty.

Figure 24 outlines the algorithmic approach for the workup of precocious puberty.

40.5. Treatment

Therapy for precocious puberty is necessary in order to avoid psychological trauma, short stature as a result of early epiphyseal closure, and, in some cases, possible pregnancy. The treatment for tumor-related precocious puberty is ablation of tumor by surgery or radiation. The therapy for idio-pathic precocious puberty, the most common variety, is rather unsatisfactory. The mainstay of therapy has been the use of progestins to suppress the hypothalamic–pituitary axis. Recently, the use of LH-RH analogues that sup-press LH and FSH release when given as a long-acting preparation has been attended with successful results.

41

Ovarian Failure

41.1. Introduction

Ovarian failure may be defined as a failure in adequate synthesis of estrogens or in the proper formation and release of the ovum by the ovaries. The terms "primary" and "secondary" ovarian failure have multiple connotations, which can lead to some semantic confusion in usage. In one sense, "primary" ovarian failure indicates intrinsic ovarian pathology as opposed to "secondary" ovarian failure, where the hypothalamic–pituitary signals required for adequate ovarian function have failed. In another sense, "primary" ovarian failure may be taken to indicate the patient who has never been feminized (primary amenorrhea) as opposed to "secondary" ovarian failure, which, in this context, denotes the occurrence of gonadal failure after normal puberty regardless of etiology. In our discussion, the terms "primary" and "secondary" amenorrhea are used in this context, and the terms "intrinsic ovarian" and "hypothalamic–pituitary" disease are used to describe the conditions in their etiologic context.

The clinical presentations of patients with ovarian failure include the following: primary amenorrhea, sexual infantilism, infertility, and secondary amenorrhea.

These four symptoms illustrate the defects in the dual functions of the ovaries, steroidogenesis (feminization) and ovulation (fertility). Several syndromes of ovarian dysfunction overlap with syndromes resulting from disorders in sexual differentiation (Chapter 43) as well as disorders resulting from hypothalamic–pituitary disease (Chapter 5). This chapter focuses on the clinical syndromes that occur as a consequence of gonadal dysgenesis, the important conditions represented here being Turner's syndrome, the Turner variants, and the syndrome of gonadal dysgenesis ("pure gonadal dysgenesis"). Also, a general overview of secondary ovarian failure is provided in this chapter. The reader is referred to Section 5.5 for a discussion on Kallmann's syndrome and Chapter 43 for a detailed description of the several syndromes that arise as a result of disordered sexual differentiation in intrauterine life.

41.2. Turner's Syndrome

Turner's syndrome, the prototype of gonadal dysgenesis, is characterized in the classic form by the triad of sexual infantilism, short stature, and somatic abnormalities.

41.2.1. Etiology

Turner's syndrome is a chromosomal disorder that has its origins shortly after fertilization. The embryo, instead of becoming a normal female embryo (46,XX), suffers a dysjunctional defect during the critical phase of cell division. As a consequence, the embryo is conferred with a chromosomal constitution of 45,XO because of a missing second X chromosome. The effect of this abnormal chromosomal constitution is reflected in the development of the primitive bipotential gonad. At the tenth week of intrauterine life, the bipotential gonad normally differentiates into a testis if the Y chromosome is present or into an ovary if the Y is absent. In embryos with Turner constitution, the primitive gonad starts its development into an ovary. However, since a second X is needed for proper development of the fetal ovary, the gonad in Turner's syndrome becomes dysgenetic because of the lack of this important second X chromosome. Since the development of such a dysgenetic gonad precludes any androgen (or estrogen) synthesis, the internal and external genitalia develop along female lines, and the infant is born with female external genitalia. Table 81 illustrates these intrauterine events and their

TABLE 81
Turner's Syndrome

Feature	Comment	Embryological basis
Karyotype	45,XO	Dysjunctional defect after fertilization
Gonad	Dysgenetic	Lack of Y precludes formation of testes; lack of second X precludes formation of an ovary
Mullerian derivatives	Present but hypoplastic	Since there is no testis to secrete MIF
Wolffian derivatives	Atrophy	Since there is no testosterone
External genitalia anlagen	Female	Since there is no testosterone
Sex assignment at birth	Female	

embryological basis. The reader is also referred to Chapter 42 for the basics on normal sexual differentiation.

41.2.2. Clinical Features

The triad of classic Turner's syndrome is sexual infantilism, short stature, and somatic stigmata.

41.2.2.1. Sexual Infantilism

Patients with the classic 45,XO Turner's syndrome represent extreme examples of sexual retardation. At the time of puberty, the dysgenetic gonads fail to secrete any estrogens despite intense stimulation by the pituitary gonadotropins. The presenting symptomology is failure to undergo pubertal feminization and primary amenorrhea. The external genitalia are prepubertal, the uterus is hypoplastic, and the breasts are underdeveloped. These features of sexual infantilism are shared by other disorders such as Kallmann's syndrome (Section 5.5) and gonadal dysgenesis.

41.2.2.2. Short Stature

Short stature is a universal feature of the classic Turner's syndrome and is probably inherited as an expression of loss of the second X chromosome. Lack of growth hormone, or resistance to it, is not a feature of the growth retardation seen in association with the classic Turner's syndrome. It should be noted that usually, when the sex steroids are absent, epiphyseal growth continues and the hypogonadal patient is not short except in the case of Turner's syndrome.

41.2.2.3. The Somatic Anomalies

The most frequent somatic anomaly is webbing of the neck. The multitude of somatic anomalies that are encountered with variable frequency in patient's with Turner's syndrome are outlined in Table 82.

41.2.3. Diagnostic Studies

The diagnostic studies in patients with classic Turner's syndrome can be divided into hormonal, chromosomal, and laparoscopic.

41.2.3.1. Hormonal

The patient with classic Turner's syndrome represents the prototype of hormonal profile seen in patients with intrinsic ovarian failure—low estradiol coupled with markedly elevated FSH and LH (primary hypogonadism).

TABLE 82
Somatic Anomalies in Turner's Syndrome (45,XO)

Common
   Short stature (100%)
   Webbing of the neck, short neck (40%)
   Cubitus valgus
   Characteristic facies (micrognathia, low-set ears, fish-shaped
      mouth, ptosis)
   Shieldlike chest, microthelia
   Renal abnormalities (60%)
   Brachydactyly (50%)
Rare
   Puffiness of the dorsum of the hand; congenital lymphedema
      of feet, hands (30%)
   Excessive pigmented nevi
   Hearing loss (secondary to otitis media)
   Coarctation of aorta (20%)
   Intestinal telangiectasia
   Essential hypertension

41.2.3.2. Chromosomal

The buccal smear is chromatin negative since the second X chromosome is absent. The karyotype analysis would reveal 45 chromosomes including the unpaired X chromosome.

41.2.3.3. The Laparoscopic Features

Laparoscopy in patients with Turner's syndrome reveals bilateral "streak gonads," fibrous ridges that represent the ovarian tissue, with little or no evidence of primordial follicles.

41.2.4. Differential Diagnosis

Classic Turner's syndrome is unique, since no other entity presents with the triad of sexual infantilism, short stature, and characteristic somatic anomalies (Table 83).

Patients with variants of Turner's syndrome also present with varying degrees of sexual infantilism. Some of these patients are also short, but they differ from classic Turner's syndrome in that the somatic anomalies are generally absent. There are three variants of Turner's syndrome.

41.2.4.1. Mosaic Turner's Syndrome

These are patients with two cell lines—a normal 46,XX and an abnormal 45,XO cell line. Mosaic Turner patients are less severely sexually retarded

TABLE 83
Clinical Differential Diagnosis of Turner's Syndrome

Sexual infantilism	Turner's syndrome
	Turner variants
	Kallmann's syndrome
	Pituitary failure
	"Pure" gonadal dysgenesis
Sexual infantilism	Pituitary failure
with short stature	Turner's syndrome
	Turner variants
	Primary hypothyroidism
Sexual infantilism,	Turner's syndrome
short stature, and	Turner variants
somatic anomalies	(deletion of short arm, ring forms)

than those with classic Turner's syndrome. These patients, not infrequently, may even demonstrate evidence of primordial follicles in the rudimentary ovary, and some may periodically menstruate.

41.2.4.2. Abnormal Second X

These are patients with gonadal dysgenesis who do possess two X chromosomes but whose second X is qualitatively abnormal. Thus, deletions as well as isochromosomes of the short arm or the long arm of the second X chromosome can occur. Loss of the short arm is associated with short stature; therefore, short stature is encountered with sexual infantilism in Turner variants characterized by deletion of the short arm (Xp^-) or with isochromosome of the long arm (Xq^i). Conversely, deletion of the long arm (Xq^-) or isochromosome of the short arm (Xp^i) is associated with sexual infantilism with normal stature.

41.2.4.3. Ring Forms

The ring form of the second X chromosome represents loss of both short arms and results in severe sexual infantilism and short stature.

It is important to recognize that the buccal smear may reveal a positive Barr body in some of the Turner variants.

41.2.5. Treatment

The treatment for Turner's syndrome and its variants is estrogen replacement. Adequate feminization can be achieved by the use of estrogen replacement therapy. The concomitant use of progestins coupled in a cyclic fashion at the end of the "cycle" affords protection against the development of endometrial carcinoma.

41.3.   Pure Gonadal Dysgenesis

This disorder, also resulting from gonadal dysgenesis during intrauterine life, represents an important etiology for hypogonadism in the phenotypic female. Pure gonadal dysgenesis is of two types based on the chromosomal constitution—46,XY gonadal dysgenesis and 46,XX gonadal dysgenesis. Regardless of the karyotype, these patients are phenotypic females.

41.3.1.   Etiology

The mechanism of both pure XY gonadal dysgenesis (Swyer's syndrome) and pure XX gonadal dysgenesis is based on a single intrauterine mishap; the primitive gonad, instead of becoming a normal testis or a normal ovary, becomes a dysgenetic gonad. These patients with 46,XY or 46,XX gonadal dysgenesis, instead of developing into, respectively, a normal male or a normal female as originally intended, develop into phenotypic female infants at birth and hypogonadal females in adulthood. To this extent, these disorders resemble Turner's syndrome, another instance typified by the maldevelopment of a primitive gonad into a dysgenetic one. But, unlike Turner's syndrome, pure gonadal dysgenesis is not associated with short stature or somatic anomalies, and unlike Turner's, these patients have 46 chromosomes with a normal pair of male or female chromosomes (XY or XX).

The basic reason why a normal karyotypic embryo should suffer an experiment of nature is not entirely clear. In the 46,XY pure gonadal dysgenesis, it is believed that even though a Y chromosome is present, it fails to induce the differentiation of the primitive bipotential gonad into a testis (Chapter 42). As for XX pure gonadal dysgenesis, it has been proposed that the presence of a mutant gene on one of the pairs of autosomes can profoundly impair

TABLE 84
Pure Gonadal Dysgenesis

Feature	Comment	Embryological basis
Karyotype	46,XY (Swyer's)	Normal male karyotype
	46,XX	Normal female karyotype
Gonad	Dysgenetic	The primitive bipotential fails to differentiate into testis or ovary
Mullerian derivatives	Present and hypoplastic	Since there is no MIF
Wolffian derivatives	Atrophy	Since there is no testosterone
Ext. genitalia anlagen	Female	Since there is no testosterone
Sex assignment at birth	Female	

the differentiation of the primitive gonad into the ovary. The possibility of abnormal receptors in the primitive gonad cannot be ruled out at the present time as a mechanism to explain the lack of differentiation in both varieties of pure gonadal dysgenesis.

Whatever the mechanism, the failure of the primitive gonad to differentiate into a normal testis or ovary results in dysgenetic gonad (fibrous streak) that can secrete neither androgens nor estrogens. As a consequence, the Mullerian derivatives persist, the Wolffian derivatives atrophy, and the urogenital sinus and the genital tubercle develop along female lines. The baby is born with female external genitalia and is assigned a female sex. Table 84 illustrates these intrauterine events and their embryological basis. A comparison of Table 81 and Table 84 reveals that the only embryological difference between Turner's syndrome and pure gonadal dysgenesis lies in the chromosomosomal constitution. Of course, the clinical expression differs in that the stigmata that usually accompany Turner's syndrome are absent in 46,XY or 46,XX gonadal dysgenesis.

41.3.2. Clinical Features

The highlight of pure gonadal dysgenesis, regardless of the karyotype, is extreme sexual infantilism, which becomes obvious during puberty—an event that never arrives for these patients. The skeletal proportions are eunuchoidal, and these patients are tall or of normal height. The lack of breast development, the prepubertal external genitalia, the shallow vagina, and the hypoplastic uterus are attestations to remarkably absent pubertal feminization, since the streak gonad cannot secrete estrogens.

41.3.3. Diagnostic Studies

The hormonal and laparoscopic features of pure gonadal dysgenesis are identical to those seen in Turner's syndrome and reflect a low estradiol level coupled with high FSH and LH levels and laparoscopy revealing "streak gonads" consisting mostly of fibrous tissue with no primordial follicles.

41.3.4. Differential Diagnosis

The three clinical disorders characterized by extreme sexual infantilism are Turner's syndrome, pure gonadal dysgenesis, and Kallmann's syndrome. Table 85 outlines the clinical hallmarks and laboratory highlights for each of these entities.

41.3.5. Treatment

The treatment of pure gonadal dysgenesis is life-long therapy with combined estrogen–progestin replacement. The one important complication of 46,XY pure gonadal dysgenesis is development of gonadoblastoma, a highly

TABLE 85
Differential Diagnosis of the Three Major Etiologies for Sexual Infantilism

Condition	Clinical hallmark	Laboratory feature	Confirmatory test
Turner's syndrome	Short stature Somatic anomalies	↑ LH, FSH	Karyotype 45,XO
Pure gonadal dysgenesis	Normal stature	↑ LH, FSH	Karyotype 46,XX or 46,XY
Kallmann's syndrome	Normal or tall stature Anosmia	↓ LH, FSH	CT to exclude pituitary tumor

malignant germ cell tumor, in the dysgenetic gonad. This appears not to be a risk for XX gonadal dysgenesis. The presence of a Y chromosome confers a high risk for malignancy in the dysgenetic gonad. Therefore, gonadectomy is recommended in the setting of 46,XY gonadal dysgenesis.

41.4. Secondary Ovarian Failure

Secondary ovarian failure is the term used to indicate the occurrence of ovarian failure in adult life following the establishment of normal ovarian function. The term, in this context, is used regardless of the etiology.

There are four major mechanisms for adult ovarian failure: intrinsic ovarian pathology, pituitary–hypothalamic disease, androgen excess, and systemic disease. The symptoms of secondary ovarian failure are often the same regardless of etiology and consist of oligomenorrhea, amenorrhea, or infertility.

Intrinsic ovarian disease as a cause of ovarian failure can occur from several etiologies. Repeated pelvic inflammatory disease, autoimmune ovarian failure, the "resistant ovaries syndrome," and premature menopause represent a few examples. Decreasing menses and infertility are the major presenting symptoms. The physical examination is unremarkable, with no obvious clinical evidence of hypoestrogenism. The laboratory studies indicate minimal estrogen effect in vaginal cytology, low 17-β-estradiol in plasma, elevated LH and FSH, and no evidence of ovulation as a consequence of the intrinsic ovarian disease.

Pituitary hypothalamic disease is an extremely important category of causes for adult ovarian failure. The decline in ovarian function here is secondary to deficient trophic drive from the pituitary gonadotropins, LH and FSH. The cause for hypothalamic pituitary failure is discussed in Chapter 5. Briefly, the four major etiologies are tumors of the pituitary and suprasellar area, Sheehan's syndrome, idiopathic hypothalamic amenorrhea, and microprolactinomas. The clinical expression is highly variable, ranging from oligomenorrhea or amenorrhea to complete lack of estrogens, resulting in atrophy of breasts. The laboratory profile includes low estradiol coupled with low LH and FSH and little or no withdrawal bleeding to progesterone administration. All indices of ovulation are generally absent; prolactin levels and computerized tomography are mandatory in all such patients.

Androgen excess as a cause for declining ovarian function is classically seen in patients with virilizing tumors (of the adrenal or ovaries), the adrenogenital syndrome, and the polycystic ovary syndrome. On physical examination, the hallmarks are hirsutism or virilization coupled with amenorrhea. Laboratory tests reveal markedly elevated androgens of either adrenal (DHEA) or ovarian (testosterone) origin. The subsequent workup is highly variable, depending on the type of androgen excess. If adrenal androgens are elevated, the tests include 17-α-hydroxyprogesterone measurement in the serum (to screen for adrenogenital syndrome), ultrasonography of pelvis (to evaluate ovarian disease), and CT scan of abdomen (to exclude adrenal tumors). If the testosterone levels are markedly elevated, a predominant ovarian disorder is to be suspected and investigated by CT scan, laparoscopy, etc.

Systemic diseases, both endocrine and nonendocrine, can result in ovarian dysfunction. Thus, Cushing's syndrome, Addison's disease, hypothyroidism, hyperthyroidism, diabetes mellitus, etc. can all be associated with oligomenorrhea or amenorrhea. Nonendocrine disorders, particulary chronic renal disease, hepatic disease, chronic inflammatory bowel disease, steatorrhea, cardiopulmonary disease, malignancy, obesity, and lupus, can all be associated with varying degrees of decreased ovarian function. The ovarian dysfunction is clearly overshadowed by the effects of the primary disease, which is usually chronic and severe. Diagnostic workup for ovarian dysfunction should be deferred until the underlying systemic disease is controlled, if possible. The mechanism of gonadal dysfunction in these situations is far from clear.

Selected Readings

Barr, M. L., and Bertram, E. G.: A morphological distinction between neurons of the male and female and the behavior of the nucleolar satellite during acceleration of nucleoprotein synthesis, *Nature* **163**:676, 1949.

Bell, J., Spitz, A., Slonim, A., *et al.*: Heterogeneity of gonadotropin response to LHRH in hypogonadotropic hypogonadism, *J. Clin. Endocrinol. Metab.* **36**:791, 1973.

Bohnet, H. G., and Dahlen, H. G.: Hyperprolactinemic anovulatory syndrome, *J. Clin. Endocrinol. Metab.* **42**:132, 1975.

Boyar, R. M., Finkelstein, J. W., David, R., *et al.*: Twenty-four hour patterns of plasma LH and FSH in sexual precocity, *N. Engl. J. Med.* **289**:282, 1973.

Brosnan, P. G., Lewandowski, C., Toguri, A. G., *et al.*: A new familial syndrome of 46 XY gonadal dysgenesis with anomalies of ectodermal and mesodermal structures, *J. Pediatr.* **97**:586, 1980.

Casper, R. F., Sheehan, K. L., and Yen, S. S. C.: Gonadotropin–estradiol responses to a superactive LHRH agonist in women, *J. Clin. Endocrinol. Metab.* **50**:179, 1980.

Comite, F., Cutler, G. B., Rivier, J., *et al.*: Short term treatment of idiopathic precocious puberty with a long acting analogue of luteinizing hormone releasing hormone, *N. Engl. J. Med.* **305**:1546, 1981.

Conte, F. A., Grumbach, M. M., Kaplan, S. L., *et al.*: Correlation of LRH induced LH and FSH release from infancy to 19 years with the changing pattern of gonadotropin secretion in agonadal patients, *J. Clin. Endocrinol. Metab.* **50:**163, 1980.

Conte, F. A., Grumbach, M. M., and Kaplan, S. L.: A diphasic pattern of gonadotropin secretion in patients with the syndrome of gonadal dysgenesis, *J. Clin. Endocrinol. Metab.* **40:**670, 1975.

Gemzell, C. A.: Induction of ovulation, *Acta Obstet. Gynecol. Scand.* [*Suppl*] **47:**1, 1975.

Hall, R., and Warrick, C.: Hypersecretion of hypothalamic releasing hormones. A possible explanation of the endocrine manifestations of polyostotic fibrous dysplasia, *Lancet* **1:**1313, 1972.

Harden, D. G.: The chromosomes in a case of pure gonadal dysgenesis, *Br. Med. J.* **2:**1285, 1959.

Herman, S., Lovet, J. P., and Ross, G. T.: Interaction of estrogen and gonadotropins on follicular atresia, *Endocrinology* **96:**1145, 1975.

Israel, R., Mishell, D. R., Stone, S. C., *et al.*: Single luteal phase serum progesterone essay as an indicator of ovulation, *Am. J. Obstet. Gynecol.* **112:**1043, 1972.

Jenkins, J. S., Gilbert, C. J., and Ang, V.: Hypothalamic pituitary function in patients with craniopharyngioma, *J. Clin. Endocrinol. Metab.* **43:**394, 1976.

Jette, N. T., and Glass, R. H.: Prognostic value of the post coital test, *Fertil. Steril.* **23:**27, 1972.

Jones, G. S., and Madrigel-Castro, V.: Hormonal findings in association with abnormal corpus luteum function in the human. The luteal phase defect, *Fertil. Steril.* **21:**1, 1971.

Judd, H. L., Scully, R. E., Atkins, L., *et al.*: Pure gonadal dysgenesis with progressive hirsuitism. Demonstration of testosterone production by gonadal streaks, *N. Engl. J. Med.* **282:**881, 1970.

Kallmann, F., Schoenfeld, W. A., and Barrera, S. E.: The genetic aspects of primary eunuchoidism, *Am. J. Ment. Defic.* **48:**203, 1944.

Kemmann, E., and Jones, J. R.: Hyperprolactinemia and primary amenorrhea, *Obstet. Gynecol.* **54:**692, 1979.

Keye, W. R., Jr., and Jaffe, R. B.: Strength–duration characteristics of estrogen effects on gonadotropin response to GnRH in women I. Effects of varying duration of estradiol administration, *J. Clin. Endocrinol. Metab.* **41:**1003, 1975.

Levine, L. S.: Treatment of Turner's syndrome with estrogen, *Pediatrics* **62:**1178, 1979.

Marshall, W. A., and Tanner, J. M.: Variations in patterns of pubertal changes in girls, *Arch. Dis. Child.* **44:**291, 1969.

McDonough, P. G., Byrd, J. R., Tho, P. T., *et al.*: Phenotypic and cytogenetic findings in 82 patients with ovarian failure—changing trends, *Fertil. Steril.* **28:**638, 1977.

Moghissi, K.: Accuracy of basal body temperature for ovulation detection, *Fertil. Steril.* **27:**207, 1976.

Schally, A. V., Arimura, A., Baba, Y., *et al.*: Isolation and properties of the FSH and LH-releasing hormone, *Biochem. Biophys. Res. Commun.* **43:**393, 1971.

Soules, M. R., and Hammond, C. B.: Female Kallmann's syndrome: Evidence of hypothalamic LHRH deficiency, *Fertil. Steril.* **33:**82, 1980.

Speroff, L., and Vande Wiele, R. L.: Regulation of the human menstrual cycle, *Am. J. Obstet. Gynecol.* **109:**234, 1971.

Sprong, J. W., and Archer, D. F.: Relationship of serum progesterone and endometrial histology in infertile women, *Fertil. Steril.* **27:**205, 1976.

Taymor, M. L.: The use of LHRH in gynecological endocrinology, *Fertil. Steril.* **25:**992, 1975.

Turner, H. H.: A syndrome of infantilism, congenital webbed neck, and cubitus valgus, *Endocrinology* **23:**566, 1938.

Wachtel, S. S.: The dysgenetic gonad—aberrant testicular differentiation, *Biol. Reprod.* **22:**1, 1980.

Wahby, O., and Sobrero, A. M.: Hysterosalpinography in relation to pregnancy and its outcome in infertile women, *Fertil. Steril.* **17:**520, 1966.

Wertelecki, W., Fraumenir, J. F., and Mulvihill, J. J.: Nongonadal neoplasia in Turner's syndrome, *Cancer* **26:**485, 1970.

Wilson, J. D.: Sexual differentiation. *Annu. Rev. Physiol.* **40:**279, 1978.

Young, J. R., and Jaffe, R. B.: Strength–duration characteristics of estrogen effects on gonadotropin response to GnRH women II. Effects of varying concentrations of estradiol, *J. Clin. Endocrinol. Metab.* **42:**432, 1976.

VII

Disorders of Sexual Differentiation

42

Embryology of Sexual Differentiation

42.1. Introduction

The disorders of sexual differentiation consist of a group of diverse disorders. They occur as a consequence of failure in the generation of the normal signals required for proper differentiation. In some instances, these disorders can be recognized at birth, but in many instances they manifest at the time of puberty with hypogonadism. To understand the varied mechanisms that underlie this fascinating group of disorders, it is essential to review the basic principles involved in the normal differentiation of the fetus into the male or female infant.

Sexual differentiation is a coordinated process involving the sequential interaction of several hormonal and nonhormonal factors. Sexual differentiation can be perceived from three points of view; in order of appearance, these are the karyotypic sex, the gonadal sex, and the phenotypic sex. The karyotypic sex refers to the chromosomal constitution conferred at the time of fertilization of the ovum by the sperm. The term gonadal sex refers to the development of a normal testis or ovary from the same primitive bipotential gonad. The term phenotypic sex refers to the development of male or female external genitalia with their appropriate accessory organs. Each of these processes is reviewed individually in terms of the factors involved in proper differentiation. At the end of the chapter, an overview of the defects that can occur at each stage is provided to facilitate classification of these disorders.

42.2. Karyotypic (Genetic) Sex

The karyotypic sex of the embryo is established at the time of fertilization. A heterogametic complement (XY) confers a male karyotype to the embryo, whereas a homogametic complement (XX) confers a female karyotype. The factors that determine the derivation of XY or an XX constitution are not clear.

42.3. Gonadal Sex

The primitive gonads, in embryos of both sexes, are bipotential. Around the 40th day, the bipotential gonad starts differentiating into a testis or an ovary, a process that is not hormone dependent. The crucial determinant of gonadal differentiation is the presence or absence of a Y chromosome. In the presence of a Y, the primitive bipotential gonad develops into a fetal testis, and in its absence, the primitive bipotential gonad develops into a fetal ovary, providing a second X chromosome is present. Recent studies indicate that the differentiation of the primitive bipotential gonad into a testis does not require the entire Y but requires an important portion of the Y called the H-Y antigen. This is a cell surface antigen that probably binds to surface receptors on the primitive gonad to induce differentiation into a testis.

The development of the primitive gonad into the fetal testis is achieved by growth and proliferation of the cortical portion destined to become the testis and atrophy of the medullary portion, which in the absence of Y is destined to become an ovary. The exact mechanism that directs atrophy of the ovarian elements of the primitive gonads is unknown. By the tenth week of intrauterine life, the primitive bipotential gonad, in the male, develops into a normal fetal testes complete with the necessary secretory apparatus.

The development of the primitive gonad into the fetal ovary is achieved by growth and proliferation of the medullary portion of the gonad, destined to become the ovary. For proper differentiation, two factors are needed—the lack of Y and the presence of a normal second X. Thus, in an embryo of 46,XX, the primitive gonad progressively differentiates into a fetal ovary by the end of the tenth week.

42.4. Phenotypic Sex

The differentiation of the internal accessory organs and the external genitalia into their respective sex organs is referred to as the phenotypic sex. Fetuses of both sexes possess both Wolffian (male) and Mullerian (female) ducts. Therefore, for proper differentiation, if the Wolffian ducts develop, then the Mullerian ducts should involute, and vice versa.

In the male fetus, the Wolffian duct develops into epididymis, vas deferens, seminal vesicles, and ejaculatory duct, and the Mullerian duct derivatives atrophy. These dual phenomena are secondary to two substances secreted by the fetal testes, testosterone and a peptide called Mullerian involutional factor (MIF). The Wolffian ducts, which possess receptors for testosterone, differentiate under this hormonal influence into the male accessory organs, whereas the Mullerian ducts, under the influence of MIF, undergo atrophy.

In the female, the Mullerian duct develops into the uterus, fallopian tube, and upper vagina, the only determinant required being the obligatory lack of MIF. The Wolffian ducts will undergo atrophy because of the lack of testosterone.

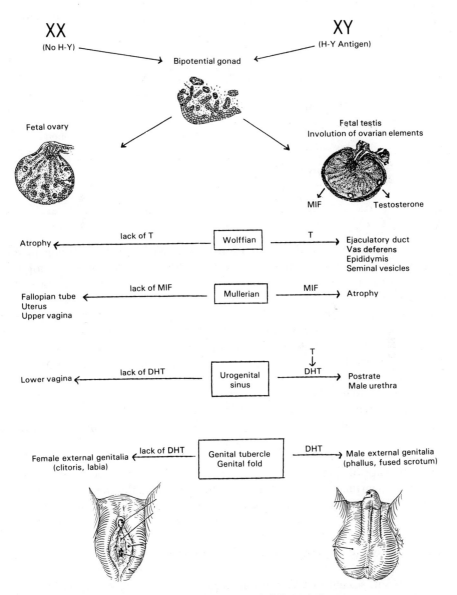

FIGURE 25. Normal sexual differentiation.

TABLE 86
Normal Sexual Differentiation

Developing organ	Determining factor	Male embryo	Female embryo
Gonad bipotential up to 40 days	H-Y antigen	Testes	Ovary (requires XX)
Mullerian duct anlage	Mullerian duct involutional factor	Involutes	Uterus, fallopian tube, upper vagina
Wolffian duct anlage	Testosterone	Epidydimis, vas, seminal vesicles, ejaculatory duct	Regresses
Urogenital	DHT (not testosterone) Androgen receptors	Prostate and male urethra	Lower vagina
Genital tubercle	DHT Androgen receptors	Penis	Clitoris
Genital swelling	DHT Androgen receptors	Scrotum (fused)	Labia major

Subsequent to the differentiation of the Wolffian and Mullerian duct systems, the next important structure to undergo differentiation is the urogenital sinus. This common structure is the same in both sexes. In the male, the urogenital sinus will develop into the prostate and the male urethra, whereas in the female it becomes the lower vagina. The deciding factor here is the availability of dihydrotestosterone (DHT), a potent androgen derived from reduction of testosterone by the enzyme 5-α-reductase in target tissues. When this hormone is available, and the receptor action of the androgen is expressed, the urogenital sinus develops along male lines. The urogenital sinus of the female fetus, in whom no testosterone is available for conversion into DHT, does not undergo such virilization.

Following the differentiation of the urogenital sinus, the final sequential step is differentiation of genital tubercle and genital folds. These structures, in the presence of DHT, differentiate into the penis and scrotum, whereas in the absence of DHT, or when receptors for DHT are lacking, these structures fail to virilize and therefore develop along female lines. Figure 25 and Table 86 summarize the embryological events of sexual differentiation.

42.5. Deviations from Normal Development

Errors in sexual differentiation can occur anywhere along the line. The classification provided in Table 87 is based on sequential errors in the process of normal differentiation. Chromosomal errors such as 45,XO (Turner's) syndrome and its variants are discussed in Section 41.2. Failure in proper differentiation of the primitive bipotential gonad into a testis or ovary (pure gonadal dysgenesis) is discussed in Section 41.3. Reifenstein syndrome is discussed in Section 36.3.

The terms true and pseudohermaphroditism deserve clarification. When gonads of both sexes are present in the same individual, the term "true hermaphroditism" is applicable. Pseudohermaphroditism refers to a discordance between the karyotypic sex and phenotypic sex. The term "male pseudohermaphroditism" is used to describe the karyotypic male with testes and female external genitalia. The term female pseudohermaphroditism is used to describe the karyotypic female with ovaries and male external genitalia.

Male pseudohermaphroditism is caused by inadequate virilization of the karyotypic male fetus. Failure of virilization of the male fetus can occur through several mechanisms:

1. Failure of the primitive bipotential gonad to differentiate into a testis (Swyer's syndrome).
2. Failure of the normally formed testes to secrete testosterone (enzymatic blocks in steroidogenesis).

TABLE 87
Classification of Disorders in Sexual Differentiation

Disorder	Syndrome	Physiological basis
1. Karyotypic abnormality 45,XO	Turner's	Lack of second X results in dysgenetic gonad
2. Falure of primitive gonad to differentiate	46,XY pure gonadal dysgenesis	The primitive gonad is not induced to become testis and becomes dysgenetic
	46,XX pure gonadal dysgenesis	The primitive gonad is not induced to become ovary and becomes dysgenetic
3. Persistence of ovarian elements in fetal testes	True hermaphrodite	Although the primitive gonad is induced to become testis, the ovarian part fails to regress
4. Failure to synthesize testosterone	Male pseudohermaphrodite	Enzymes needed to synthesize testosterone are absent
5. Failure of T → DHT conversion	Male pseudohermaphrodite	Deficiency of 5-α-reductase in target cells precludes formation of DHT
6. Target organ resistance	Male pseudohermaphrodite: partial, Reifenstein; complete, testicular feminization	Partial or complete lack of receptors to T or DHT

3. Failure of conversion of testosterone into dihydrotestosterone (5-α-reductase deficiency).
4. Failure of dihydrotesterone to express its action because of target organ resistance (testicular feminization syndrome when complete, Reifenstein's syndrome when partial).

Female pseudohermaphroditism is caused by inappropriate virilization of the karyotypic female fetus. Such virilization occurs when excess of dihydrotesterone is present in the fetus. The classic example of such an occurence is the complete form of adrenogenital syndrome, a condition characterized by excess adrenal androgens that serve as substrates for testosterone and dihydrotestosterone. The adrenogenital syndrome is discussed in Section 28.4.

True hermaphroditism occurs when the ovarian elements persists along with testicular elements, both tissues functional and capable of hormone secretion. The disorders in the differentiation of the karyotypic male constitute the bulk of errors in sexual differentiation and are described in Chapter 43.

43

Syndromes of Disordered Sexual Differentiation

43.1. Introduction

As indicated in Chapter 42, most disorders of sexual differentiation are a result of failure of adequate virilization of the karyotypic male fetus and consist of the following:

1. Swyer's syndrome.
2. True hermaphroditism.
3. Defective steroidogenesis.
4. 5-α-Reductase deficiency.
5. Testicular feminization syndrome.

43.2. Swyer's Syndrome

Swyer's syndrome, 46,XY pure gonadal dysgenesis, is described in Section 41.3 under the syndromes of pure gonadal dysgenesis. The salient features of this entity are outlined in Table 84. Briefly, the disorder is a result of failure of the primitive bipotential gonad to differentiate into the testis despite the chromosomosal constitution of XY. Since a second X chromosome is not present, the gonad, which can develop into neither a testis nor an ovary, becomes a dysgenetic gonad.

The Wolffian ducts fail to differentiate into male accessory organs because no testosterone is secreted, but the Mullerian ducts develop into a hypoplastic uterus since MIF is not secreted by the dysgenetic gonad. The external genitalia develop along female lines since no androgen is secreted. The net result is a karyotypic male infant born with female external genitalia (male pseudohermaphroditism).

43.2.1. Clinical Features

The infant, who is assigned a female sex at birth, is reared as a girl with strong female gender identity. At puberty, since there is no viable ovary, feminization fails to occur, and therefore sexual infantilism prevails. On physical examination, the external genitalia are prepubertal, and a hypoplastic uterus is present. The gonadal tissue is represented by a fibrous ridge.

43.2.2. Diagnostic Studies

Characteristically, LH and FSH are elevated in Swyer's syndrome. The diagnosis can be confirmed by the karyotype study (46,XY) and the laparoscopic findings of a streak gonad.

43.2.3. Treatment

Because of the increased risk of gonadoblastoma developing in the dysgenetic gonad, gonadectomy is recommended, followed by estrogen replacement for feminization.

43.3. True Hermaphroditism

True hermaphroditism is the combined occurrence of testicular and ovarian tissue in the same patient, often in the same gonad (ovotestis).

43.3.1. Etiology

The hallmark of true hermaphroditism is the persistence of ovarian tissue in a gonad containing testicular tissue. The chromosomal constitution must contain a Y chromosome (or an H-Y antigen) for testicular induction to take place. The reason for the failure of the ovarian portion of the bipotential gonad to regress is not known. The development of the Wolffian and Mullerian systems and that of the urogenital sinus is extremely bizarre and quite variable, depending on the availability of androgen (testicular preponderance). Thus, various combinations such as a hemiuterus on one side with seminal vesicles on the other side can occur. Similarly, the degree of virilization of the external genitalia can also be quite variable, ranging from near-male appearance with hypospadias to gross ambiguity.

43.3.2. Clinical Features

Most patients with true hermaphroditism are assigned a male sex at birth and are reared as males. Considerable ambiguity exists in these patients regarding gender identification. During puberty, the hallmark of true hermaphroditism is the occurrence of pubertal feminization and virilization. The ovotestes are just as responsive as the normal gonad to stimulation by pituitary gonadotropins, but unlike the normal gonad, they secrete both estrogens and androgens. The relative preponderance depends on the amount of testicular tissue that is present. Gynecomastia with suboptimal pubertal virilization is the most common presentation. A less frequently encountered presentation is gynecomastia in a reasonably virilized male. Hypospadias is extremely common. The gonad may be present in the abdomen, inguinal region, or even in the scrotum. The diagnosis of true hermaphroditism is clinically apparent by the triad of ambiguous genitalia coupled with virilization with simultaneous feminization.

43.3.3. Diagnostic Studies

The diagnostic studies in patients with true hermaphroditism fall under three categories: hormonal, chromosomal, and histological.

43.3.3.1. Hormonal Studies

The pubertal or postpubertal patient with true hermaphroditism will demonstrate significant hyperestrogenemia; the testosterone levels can be in the normal or below normal range of postpubertal males. Occasionally, the ovarian elements may contain primordial follicles that "ripen" under the influence of gonadotropins, resulting in cyclic elevations of progesterone in the serum.

43.3.3.2. Chromosomal Studies

The chromosomal pattern of true hermaphrodites is quite varied: 46,XY and 46,XX/XY mosaicism are the most frequently seen karyotypes. Occasionally, 46,XX karyotype may be seen; the paradox of testicular tissue being present in the absence of a Y chromosome is explained by the fact that the H-Y antigen is positive in most of these patients.

43.3.3.3. Histological Studies

The diagnostic confirmation for true hermaphrodism is obtained by tissue diagnosis; gonadal biopsy will disclose the presence of both testicular and ovarian elements.

43.3.4. Treatment

The treatment for true hermaphroditism is not simple. These patients, representing a cruel misadventure of nature, suffer enormous psychological turmoil. In the lucky few who have a strong gender identity and an established sexual preference, the treatment consists of removing both gonads and initiating replacement therapy of their choice. Plastic surgery for correction of the external genitalia as well as for the gynecomastia is an integral part of treatment. In the unlucky majority of true hermaphrodites with ambiguous gender identification and even more ambiguous genitalia that defy any reconstruction, the choices and options are few. These patients, with no recourse to psychological, anatomic, or hormonal "cures," live unhappy lives and often die from malignant transformation of the gonad, especially if intraabdominal.

43.4. Defective Steroidogenesis

These are patients with defects in testosterone synthesis by the fetal testes. When the defect is complete, testosterone cannot be formed at all, a situation analogous to the testes not being present.

43.4.1. Etiology

The reason for failure to secrete testosterone is the lack of the necessary enzymes involved in steroidogenesis. The enzyme block can occur during any step in the synthesis of testosterone. Regardless of where the block is, if the block is complete, no testosterone can be formed by the fetal testes. Since the fetal tissues have receptors only for dihydrotesterone, which is derived from testosterone, no other androgen can substitute for lack of testosterone.

The embryological consequences that occur from lack of testosterone are straightforward: the Wolffian ducts, urogenital sinus, and genital tubercle all develop along female lines since no testosterone is available. However, since the testes do secrete Mullerian involutional factor (MIF), the Mullerian ducts involute, resulting in nondevelopment of the uterus. At birth, the karyotypic male fetus is born as an infant with female genitalia.

43.4.2. Clinical Features

The baby is raised as a female with strong female gender identification. Depending on the site of block in hormone production, at puberty two distinct syndromes may develop. If the block is proximal, this precludes formation of any androgen or estrogen, and the presentation is hypogonadism. If the block is distal, there is accumulation of androgen precursors proximal to the block, which results in pubertal or postpubertal virilization.

43.4.2.1. Proximal Blocks

This primarily involves the enzyme 17-α-hydroxylase. At puberty, because of total lack of the enzyme, there is failure to secrete any sex steroid. The presentation is characterized by a phenotypic female with primary amenorrhea, sexual infantilism, and absent uterus. The testes may be evident as masses in the inguinal region but more often are intraabdominal.

43.4.2.2. Distal Blocks

This primarily involves the enzyme 17-β-hydroxysteroid dehydrogenase, which normally converts androstenedione into testosterone. During puberty, under the influence of pituitary gonadotropins, the testes are stimulated to secrete, but because of the enzyme block, the process is stymied. The result is an accumulation of the precursor products proximal to the block. These precursors are weak androgens that, in large amounts, can result in virilization of the adult, as opposed to the fetal tissues where dihydrotestosterone is the only virilizing hormone. The clinical presentation is characterized by a phenotypic female with primary amenorrhea, sexual infantilism, absent uterus, and evidence of pubertal or postpubertal virilization.

43.4.3. Diagnostic Studies

The hormonal profile of patients with proximal blocks consists of low estradiol, low testosterone, and elevated gonadotropins. The condition should be differentiated from other etiologies of sexual infantilism, particularly Turner's variants and pure gonadal dysgenesis. The absence of the uterus helps to distinguish it from these entities.

The hormonal profile for patients with distal blocks consists of low estradiol, low testosterone, elevated precursor androgens, and elevated LH and FSH. This condition needs to be differentiated from the various virilizing syndromes—adrenogenital syndrome, adrenal carcinoma, etc.

43.4.4. Treatment

Since these patients are phenotypic females with strong female gender identification, the treatment consists of locating the testes and removing them. These gonads, usually intraabdominal, serve no purpose and potentially are at high risk for developing malignancy. Following gonadectomy, these patients should be placed on replacement estrogen therapy for feminization.

43.5. 5-α-Reductase Deficiency

5-α-Reductase deficiency is a form of male pseudohermaphroditism resulting in nonconversion of testosterone into DHT. The condition is familial, inherited as an autosomal recessive trait.

43.5.1. Etiology

The total lack of the enzyme 5-α-reductase in target tissues is the underlying defect in this disorder. Consequently, only the Wolffian ducts develop, since this anlage requires only testosterone and not DHT. The urogenital sinus, genital tubercle, folds, and swellings, which depend on DHT for proper virilization, develop along female lines since DHT cannot be formed peripherally. Consequently, at birth the child is unambiguously female.

43.5.2. Clinical Features

The child with 5-α-reductase is raised as a female with strong female gender identification. During puberty, however, remarkable changes begin to occur. The testis secretes testosterone, which causes virilization in spite of not being able to be converted to DHT. Phallic enlargement, muscular development, and the growth of facial and pubic hair are similar to the normal male puberty. The paradox of embryonal nonvirilization but pubertal virilization in patients with 5-α-reductase deficiency may relate to several factors— differential response in tissues, quantitatively high levels of hormone, unidentified molecular change with age, etc. Whatever the reason, gradually over a period of years, the "female" child undergoes pubertal virilization. More importantly, in spite of having been raised as girls, many patients have a reversal of gender identity. It is remarkable that a patient with 5-α-reductase deficiency enters puberty as a girl and exits as a young man.

43.5.3. Diagnostic Studies

The hormonal studies in patients with 5-α-reductase deficiency are characterized by an elevation in testosterone level and a decrease or total absence of dihydrotestosterone level. The confirmatory test for 5-α-reductase deficiency is demonstration of partial or complete lack of the enzyme 5-α-reductase in cultured skin fibroblasts.

43.5.4. Treatment

The only treatment required for this syndrome is plastic surgery and reconstruction of external genitalia.

43.6. Testicular Feminization Syndrome

The testicular feminization syndrome (TFS) is the prototype of male pseudohermaphroditism and is a result of complete peripheral androgen resistance. As a consequence, the karyotypic male fetus fails to undergo virilization.

43.6.1. Etiology

The primary defect in testicular feminization syndrome is a quantitative or qualitative abnormality of the cytoplasmic receptors for testosterone and dihydrotestosterone in all peripheral tissues. To cause virilization of the fetus, testosterone needs to be converted into dihydrotestosterone, which binds to high-affinity androgen receptor proteins in the cytoplasm. The hormone–receptor complex is transported to the nucleus of the cell, where it interacts with acceptor sites to increase transcription, with the resultant appearance of new messenger RNAs and proteins that effect the hormone's action. The basic defect in TFS is either absent cytosol receptors for T and DHT or an extremely low number of receptors or structurally abnormal (thermolabile) low-affinity receptors. As a result of this target organ resistance, the Wolffian duct, urogenital sinus, genital tubercle, and genital folds fail to virilize and develop along female lines. The Mullerian duct, however, atrophies, since the production of MIF by the testes as well as its actions are normal. The karyotypic male fetus is thus born with female external genitalia. Testicular feminization is familial; the gene for this condition is X-linked.

43.6.2. Clinical Features

The infant, assigned a female sex, is reared as a girl and identifies strongly with that gender. The only clue for the presence of testicular feminization may come accidentally, when inguinal testes may be discovered during surgery for "hernia," a not infrequent occurrence in these patients. The prepubertal life of these girls is otherwise normal until they enter puberty.

The following sequence of phenomena occurs during the pubertal phase of patients with testicular feminization:

1. At puberty, under the influence of LH, the testes secrete testosterone. Since there is peripheral resistance to the hormone action, there is no pubertal virilization.
2. The increased testosterone serves as a precursor for estradiol conversion, and hence, more estradiol is formed from testosterone. In addition, there is an increased secretion of estrogens directly by the chronically stimulated Leydig cells.
3. Since the pituitary is also resistant to the suppressive effects of testosterone, there is continued increased LH production, which in turn leads to intense stimulation of the Leydig cells. Consequently, more testosterone is synthesized, with more conversion into estradiol.
4. Since there is no peripheral resistance to estrogens, the patient becomes well feminized. The combination of the increment in the estrogens, to which the tissues are responsive, and the resistance to androgens is the reason for the remarkably well-developed breasts and well-feminized external genitalia in the presence of functioning testes.
5. Since there is no uterus, the only complaint by these patients is primary amenorrhea.

The triad to suspect the disorder is primary amenorrhea in a well-feminized female with no uterus. Patients with testicular feminization syndrome have little or no axillary hair and fail to develop acne during puberty.

43.6.3. Diagnostic Studies

The three categories of studies in patients with testicular feminization are hormonal, chromosomal, and receptor studies.

43.6.3.1. Hormone Studies

The testosterone level in patients with testicular feminization syndrome is strikingly elevated, often higher than that of normal males. The estradiol levels also exceed those seen in normal males but are slightly lower than the range seen in normal females in the late follicular phase.

43.6.3.2. Chromosomal Studies

The karyotype of patients with testicular feminization is that of a normal male (46,XY). The buccal smear is chromatin negative like that of a normal male.

43.6.3.3. Receptor Studies

These are seldom required but are quite illustrative of the basic problem in testicular feminization syndrome, showing little or no binding of testosterone to cytoplasmic androgen-binding receptors of peripheral cells.

It is of interest that normal female relatives of patients with the testicular feminization syndrome may reveal abnormalities in androgen receptors in the cultured fibroblasts of the genital skin. This establishes the presence of XX female heterozygotes in the sibship of pedigrees of patients with testicular feminization syndrome.

The only other condition that resembles testicular feminization is Mullerian agenesis. (The difference between the two can be established by the level of circulating testosterone and the karyotype.)

43.6.4. Treatment

The treatment of testicular feminization is gonadectomy after puberty. The reason for removal of the gonads is the increased risk of gonadal tumors developing in the intraabdominal testes. After gonadectomy, estrogen replacement should be provided for maintenance therapy. Occasionally, the vagina may require nonsurgical dilatation.

The five syndromes described above are all characterized by failure of the karyotypic male embryo to develop normally into a phenotypic male infant. Table 88 provides a composite of these five entities, illustrating the similarities and differences that prevail among this group as a whole and individually.

TABLE 88
Disorders of Sexual Differentiation

Features	Swyer	True hermaphroditism	Dyshormonogenesis	5-α-Reductase deficiency	Testicular feminization
Karyotype	46,XY	46,XY or XX/XY	46,XY	46,XY	46,XY
Defect	Failure to induce testicular differentiation	Persistence of ovarian tissue	Failure to secrete testosterone	Failure in conversion of T → DHT	Complete peripheral resistance
Gonad	Dysgenetic streak	Ovotestis	Testis	Testis	Testis
Wolffian ducts	Involuted	Variably present	Involuted	Developed	Involuted
Mullerian ducts	Present	Variable	Involuted	Involuted	Involuted
Genital tubercle, folds	Nonvirilized	Variably virilized	Nonvirilized	Nonvirilized	Nonvirilized
Sex assigned at birth	Female	Female/male	Female	Female	Female
Pubertal phenomena	Hypogonadism	Feminization with virilization	Hypogonadism or virilization	Virilization without feminization	Feminization
Uterus	Present	Variable	Absent	Absent	Absent
Gender identification	Female	Ambiguous	Female	Female with reversal at puberty	Female
Risk of malignancy of gonad	High	High	High	None	High

Selected Readings

Amrhein, J. A., Klingensmith, G. J., Walsh, P., *et al.*: Partial androgen insensitivity—Reifenstein's syndrome revisited, *N. Engl. J. Med.* **297:**350, 1977.

Boyar, R. M., Moore, F. J., Rosner, W., *et al.*: Studies of gonadotropin gonadal dynamics in patients with androgen insensitivity, *J. Clin. Endocrinol. Metab.* **47:**116, 1978.

French, F. S., Van Wyk, J. S. D., Baggett, B., *et al.*: Further evidence of a target organ defect in the syndrome of testicular feminization, *J. Clin. Endocrinol. Metab.* **26:**493, 1966.

Griffin, J. E.: Testicular feminization associated with a thermolabile androgen receptor in cultured fibroblasts, *J. Clin. Invest.* **64:**1624, 1979.

Griffin, J. E., and Wilson, J. D.: The syndromes of androgen resistance, *N. Engl. J. Med.* **302:**198, 1980.

Griffin, J. E., Punyashthiti, and Wilson, J. D.: Dihydrotestosterone binding by cultured human fibroblasts; Comparison of cells from control subjects and from patients with hereditary male pseudohermaphroditism due to androgen resistance, *J. Clin. Invest.* **57:**1342, 1976.

Imperato McGinley, J., Peterson, R. E., Gautier, T., *et al.*: Androgens and the evolution of male gender identity among male pseudohermaphrodites with 5-alpha reductase deficiency, *N. Engl. J. Med.* **300:**1233, 1979.

Keenan, B. S., Meyer, W. J., Hadjian, A. J., *et al.*: Syndrome of androgen insensitivity in man; absence of 5-alpha dihydrotestosterone binding protein in skin fibroblasts, *J. Clin. Endocrinol. Metab.* **38:**1143, 1974.

Lyon, M. F., and Hawkes, S. G.: X-linked gene for testicular feminization in the mouse, *Nature* **227:**1217, 1970.

Money, J., and Ehrhardt, A. A.: Fetal feminization induced by androgen insensitivity in the testicular feminization syndrome. Effect on marriage and maternalism, *John Hopkins Med. J.* **123:**105, 1968.

O'Connell, M. J., and Ramsey, H. E.: Testicular feminization syndrome in three sibs: Emphasis on gonadal neoplasia, *Am. J. Med. Sci.* **265:**321, 1973.

Ohno, S., Nagai, Y., Ciccarese, S., *et al.*: Testis organizing H-Y antigen and the primary sex determining mechanism in mammals, *Recent Prog. Horm. Res.* **35:**449, 1979.

Oshima, H., and Troen, P.: Endocrine and environmental influences on sexual roles, *Am. J. Med.* **70:**1, 1981.

Peterson, R. E., Imperato McGinley, J., Gautier, T., *et al.*: Male pseudohermaphroditism due to steroid 5-alpha reductase deficiency, *Am. J. Med.* **62:**170, 1977.

Reifenstein, E. C.: Hereditary familial hypogonadism, *Proc. Am. Fed. Clin. Res.* **3:**86, 1947.

Siiteri, P. K., and Wilson, J. D.: Testosterone formation and metabolism during male sexual differentiation in the human embryo, *J. Clin. Endocrinol. Metab.* **38:**113, 1974.

Swyer, G. I. M.: Male pseudohermaphroditism: A hitherto undescribed form, *Br. Med. J.* **2:**709, 1955.

Van Niekerk, W. A.: True hermaphroditism. An analytical review with a report of 3 new cases, *Am. J. Obstet. Gynecol.* **126:**890, 1976.

Wachtel, S. S.: Immunogenetic aspects of abnormal sexual differentiation, *Cell* **16:**691, 1979.

Walsh, P. C., Madden, J. D., Harrod, M. J., *et al.*: Familial incomplete male pseudohermaphroditism, Type II, *N. Engl. J. Med.* **291:**944, 1974.

Wilson, J. D.: Sexual differentiation, *Annu. Rev. Physiol.* **40:**279, 1978.

Wilson, J. D., Harrod, M. J., Goldstein, J. L., *et al.*: Familial incomplete pseudohermaphroditism, Type I, *N. Engl. J. Med.* **290:**1097, 1974.

VIII

Diabetes and Glucose Intolerance

44

Physiology
The Synthesis, Release, and Actions of Insulin

44.1. Synthesis of Insulin

Insulin, the secretory product of the β cell, is derived from a single-chain precursor proinsulin. This precursor is a 9000-dalton polypeptide with very little biological activity and is synthesized in the rough endoplasmic reticulum. Proinsulin is cleaved, yielding, in equimolar proportions, insulin and the connecting peptide (C-peptide). This proinsulin cleavage requires trypsinlike proteases and carboxypeptidases and takes place in the Golgi appartus. The next step following the cleavage is the active processing of the newly formed insulin and C-peptide into β secretory granules. Electron microscopic and autoradiographic studies indicate that the secretory granule formation occurs with the Golgi apparatus. The earliest change involves the formation of "progranules" consisting of condensed vacuoles; after a series of biochemical changes, the progranules "mature" into insulin-secretory granules, which consist of a dense central crystalline inclusion containing zinc. The C-peptide released during the cleavage process is represented within the granules as a clear space surrounding the dense insulin crystal. The mature secretory granule within the cytoplasm is released from the β cell by a process of exocytosis.

The β cell responds to a variety of physiological stimuli, the most dominant one being glucose. The insulin-releasing effects of other physiological stimuli such as amino acids, fatty acids, and ketone bodies depend on the presence of substimulatory levels of glucose (glucose-dependent stimuli). The β-cytotrophic effect of these fuels is mediated by the presence of fuel receptors (glucoreceptors or amino acid receptors) located in the cell membrane of the β cell. These receptors are exquisitely sensitive to changes in the circulating levels of metabolic fuels, particularly glucose. Stimulus recognition may also be mediated by the events connected with the metabolism of the particular fuel. For instance, in the case of glucose, the glycolytic metabolites may be the factors involved in the triggering of the glucose-mediated insulin release.

Since glucose is the predominant regulator of insulin release, several important aspects of this phenomenon bear emphasis.

1. The glucose-mediated insulin release occurs as a consequence of combination of glucose with highly specific receptors on the cell membrane, the glucose–receptor complex activating the process of insulin release.

2. The intracellular metabolism of glucose within the β cell may also serve as the signal for the release of insulin. The intracellular channeling of glucose into the Krebs cycle, the pentose phosphate shunt, or the glycolytic pathway may result in metabolites, energy, or ions that mediate the release of insulin. When phosphorylation of glucose is blocked by mannoheptulose, insulin release is promptly inhibited, implying an important role for the intracellular metabolism of glucose in mediation of insulin release.

3. Intracellular increase in cyclic AMP concentrations within the β cell also provokes insulin release. Evidence for cyclic AMP mediation is particularly striking in peptide-hormone-mediated insulin release as opposed to substrate- (or fuel)-mediated insulin release. For instance, the β-cytotrophic effects of various hormones such as pancreatic glucagon, secretin, enteroglucagon, gastric inhibitory polypeptide (GIP), and pancreozymin are mediated by cyclic AMP generation within the β cells. It is not completely clear if glucose-mediated release is cyclic AMP related.

4. The relationship of serum glucose concentrations to the rate of insulin release by the pancreatic β cell is sigmoidal. The maximal response of the β cell occurs with blood glucose levels in the range of 300 to 500 mg/dl.

5. The glucose-mediated insulin release is calcium dependent. Evidence from *in vitro* studies supports the notion that exclusion of calcium from the perfusate results in marked blunting of insulin release to a variety of provocative stimuli.

6. The insulin release in response to glucose administered orally is much greater than that to intravenously administered glucose. The reason for this phenomenon is that the absorption of glucose by the gastrointestinal tract enhances the release of several gut hormones (particularly gastric inhibitory polypeptide) that possess β-cytotrophic activity.

7. Insulin secretion and release in response to a constant glucose stimulus follows a characteristic biphasic response. This consists of a rapid early insulin peak (beginning within 1 min and lasting for about 5 to 10 min) and a second more slowly rising peak. It is believed that

insulin exists in two pools within the β cells. The first phase of insulin release is release of hormone from the labile pool of the storage compartment, whereas the second phase represents release of hormone from a slowly discharging pool of the storage compartment.

8. Neural control of glucose-mediated insulin release can be modified by the autonomic nervous system. Stimulation of the parasympathetic system results in enhancement of glucose-mediated insulin release. α-Adrenergic stimulation results in blunting of glucose-mediated insulin release, whereas β-adrenergic stimulation potentiates it. Infusion of catecholamines is attended by a marked attenuation of insulin response to a variety of β-cytotrophic stimuli including glucose.

9. The glucose-mediated insulin release can be enhanced by sulfonylurea. The glucose-sensing ability of the glucoreceptors on the β-cell membrane is probably accentuated by these drugs. Alternatively, it is not clear if sulfonylureas modify the postreceptor actions involved in the glucose-mediated insulin release.

10. The circulating glucose concentration regulates insulin release by a linear mechanism; i.e., hyperglycemia stimulates and hypoglycemia suppresses insulin release. The circulating glucose concentration regulates glucagon release by a reciprocal mechanism; i.e., hypoglycemia stimulates and hyperglycemia suppresses glucagon release. Thus, insulin may be regarded as the "hormone of feasting," and glucagon can be perceived as the "hormone of fasting." Physiologically this see-saw mechanism preserves glucose homeostasis. In the fed state, insulin is required to facilitate glucose transport into cells for energy derivation. In the fasted state, glucagon is required to maintain euglycemia and prevent hypoglycemia by virtue of its glycogenolytic and neoglucogenic potential.

44.2. Metabolic Clearance of Insulin

The half-life of circulating insulin is short, approximately 3 to 5 min. The liver and the kidneys represent the two major sites for uptake and degradation of insulin. Insulinase and transhydrogenase are the two enzyme systems involved in the degradation of insulin.

All three peptides—proinsulin, insulin, and C-peptide—are secreted into the portal circulation and must pass through the liver before entering the peripheral circulation. During peak secretion, insulin and C-peptide are present in equimolar concentrations in the portal blood, confirming that insulin and C-peptide are released in equimolar concentrations by the β cell in response to glucose. However, because of major differences in the metabolic clearance of insulin and C-peptide, this relationship is not maintained in the peripheral circulation. The clearance of insulin is much faster than that of C-peptide.

44.3. Actions of Insulin

The regulatory mechanisms of the body are such that hormonal factors work in concert to ensure an adequate supply of fuel to various tissues in the fed and in the fasted state. The actions of insulin are called on in the fed (postabsorptive) state to promote glucose uptake by cells for energy purposes and to divert fuel to storage sites in the liver, fat depots, and muscle. The actions of glucagon are diametrically opposite and are therefore called on in the fasted state. The homeostatic adjustments of the fasted state are outlined in Chapter 51. Only the actions of insulin are focused on in this chapter. Table 89 compares the actions of glucagon and insulin on various metabolic systems.

The four main actions of insulin are as follows:

1. Insulin promotes glucose transport and utilization by all peripheral cells.
2. Insulin inhibits hepatic glycogenolysis.
3. Insulin also inhibits hepatic gluconeogenesis.
4. Insulin is a powerful inhibitor of lipolysis and ketogenesis.

Insulin promotes uptake of glucose by peripheral tissues and facilitates the intracellular processes whereby energy is derived from glucose. When insulin is lacking, or when there is resistance to its action, glucose uptake and utilization by peripheral tissues is impaired, resulting in accumulation of glucose in the blood (hyperglycemia).

The role of insulin on hepatic glycogen metabolism is in the direction of converting the liver from a glucose-producing organ to a glucose-consuming organ. Insulin inhibits hepatic glycogenolysis probably by reducing cyclic AMP concentrations within the hepatocytes. This leads to a reduction in the activity of cyclic-AMP-dependent protein kinases and phosphorylases. In addition to inhibiting glycogenolysis, insulin effectively inhibits the output of glucose from the liver. Small increments in plasma insulin are capable of effectively inhibiting hepatic glucose production. The third effect of insulin in this metabolic

TABLE 89
Comparison of the Actions of Insulin and Glucagon

Metabolic system	Action of insulin	Action of glucagon
Hepatic glycogenolysis	Inhibition	Stimulation
Hepatic gluconeogenesis	Inhibition	Stimulation
Lipolysis	Inhibition	Stimulation
Hepatic ketogenesis	Inhibition	Stimulation
Lipogenesis	Stimulation	Inhibition
Glucose transport and utilization	Stimulation	Inhibition

system is its ability to inhibit glycogen synthesis. This effect, however, is closely related to circulating glucose concentration.

The bulk of *in vitro* evidence favors the notion that insulin has an inhibitory action on gluconeogenesis. Gluconeogenesis is a process whereby glucose is synthesized from amino acids. Insulin can inhibit glucagon-induced or catecholamine-induced gluconeogenesis, probably by its ability to lower cyclic AMP levels. In addition, insulin reduces the availability of the supply of gluconeogenic substrates to the liver, particularly glycerol. Finally, insulin may also impair the uptake of amino acids by liver.

Insulin is intensely antilipolytic. Lipolysis is a process whereby stored fat is broken down into mono- and diglyceride with release of free fatty acid and glycerol into the circulation. The process of lipolysis is normally mediated by an enzyme called hormone-dependent lipoprotein lipase located in the adipocyte membrane. Insulin inhibits this enzyme, whereas glucagon and catecholamines stimulate this lipase. In addition to its antilipolytic activity, insulin promotes storage of dietary triglyceride as depot fat, an important reason for weight gain in overinsulinized patients.

The role of insulin on hepatic ketogenesis is also inhibitory in nature. Insulin inhibits ketogenesis by two mechanisms—first, by preventing lipolysis and thereby decreasing the availability of the supply of ketogenic substrates (free fatty acids), and second, by a direct inhibitory effect of oxidation of free fatty acids into ketone bodies. Excess insulin stimulates triglyceride synthesis from free fatty acids by the hepatocytes.

The sum total of the effects of insulin is to maintain glucose homeostasis within a narrow range despite the great variability in consumption of glucose. In concert with glucagon, insulin prevents the development of hyperglycemia or hypoglycemia during wide variations in fuel availability. Lack of insulin results in poor peripheral utilization of glucose, hyperglycemia, lipolysis, ketogenesis, glycogenolysis, and increased hepatic glucose output.

The molecular basis for the action of insulin is discussed in Chapter 45.

45

The Definition, Classification, and Etiology of Diabetes

45.1. Definition

The term "diabetes mellitus" actually denotes a heterogeneous syndrome characterized by chronic hyperglycemia and often associated with specific microvascular and macrovascular complications. Conceptually, diabetes should be viewed as an entity embracing a wide variety of causes of disturbed glucose tolerance. In this sense, "diabetes" should be viewed as an expression of several unrelated disorders rather than a single disease, analogous to hypertension, anemia, or arthritis. Once this heterogeneity is accepted, it becomes easier to view the disorder as the "the diabetic syndrome" and not as a single disease.

45.2. Classification

The categorization of diabetes into various classes defies a simple classification since the diabetic syndrome is extremely heterogenous. The basic classification of all diabetics into insulin dependent (IDDM) and non-insulin dependent (NIDDM), while having some merit, is hardly watertight because of the presence of an intermediary group of patients who are neither "insulin dependent" nor "independent" but rather insulin requiring. The classification of diabetes into "juvenile" and "adult onset" based on age is hardly valid, since the "maturity"-onset type of diabetes can occur in the young (MODY). The classification of diabetes into "ketosis-prone" and "ketosis-resistant" diabetes also falls short of clarity, since several patients presumed to be ketosis resistant can and do develop ketosis under certain circumstances. Classifying diabetes into "brittle" and "stable" diabetes is extremely nebulous, since this may reflect nothing more than the therapeutic endeavors directed in control of the disease. The conventional classification of diabetes into prediabetes, latent diabetes, chemical diabetes, and overt diabetes is strictly based on chemical testing with the glucose tolerance test, a diagnostic procedure that has come under attack in recent years. The classification of diabetics into obese and thin diabetics is nothing more than a classification based on physiognomy. Clearly then, the diabetic syndrome hardly yields itself to simple categorization. Table 90 outlines a simple classification that, although hardly complete, provides a clinical basis of classification of this syndrome into four subclasses—overt diabetes, secondary diabetes, gestational diabetes, and impaired glucose tolerance.

Despite the accepted heterogeneity of the diabetic syndrome in clinical practice, overt diabetes is customarily viewed as two distinct disorders—insulin dependent and non-insulin dependent. Table 91 outlines the characteristics of these two disorders, with frequent exceptions to these general rules. In general, IDDM typically occurs in younger people, often occurring with an explosive, abrupt onset. The term "insulin dependent" highlights the fact that when insulin is withheld, ketoacidosis develops rapidly. In contrast, NIDDM generally occurs in older (>40 years of age) patients who are often but not invariably obese. The onset of NIDDM is gradual. The term "noninsulin dependent" denotes that these patients do not lapse into ketoacidosis when insulin is withheld. However, such an occurrence may develop during periods of stress or infection. In between these two major groups there is another clinical group characterized by non-insulin dependence in terms of development of ketoacidosis but requiring insulin for control of hyperglycemia. This group, simply referred to as insulin-requiring diabetes, may merely represent another facet of NIDDM.

TABLE 90
Classification of the Diabetic Syndrome

Overt diabetes
  Insulin-dependent diabetes (IDDM, type I)
  Non-insulin-dependent diabetes (NIDDM,
      type II)
  Obese
  Nonobese
  Insulin-"requiring" diabetes
Secondary diabetes
  Hormonal
    Acromegaly, Cushing's,
      pheochromocytoma,
      primary aldosteronism, glucagonoma,
      etc.
  Pancreatic disease
    Hemochromatosis
    Chronic pancreatitis
  Insulin receptor abnormalities
  Drug induced (steroids, etc.)
Gestational diabetes
Impaired glucose tolerance

TABLE 91
Characteristics of the Two Major Clinical Types of Diabetes

Feature	IDDM	NIDDM
Synonyms, current and past	Type I "Juvenile onset"	Type II "Adult or maturity onset"
	Ketosis prone "Brittle"	Ketosis resistant "Stable"
Onset	Usually abrupt	Gradual
Age	Usually young but can occur at any age	Usually older but can occur in the young (MODY)
Ketosis	Ketosis prone	Not ketosis prone except under stress, infection, etc.
Insulin level	Insulinopenic	Normal or hyperinsulinemic
Genetic basis	Genetic determinants (HLA) play a role	Strong familial pattern
Islet cell antibodies	Frequently present	Not present

45.3. Etiology

The etiology of diabetes is multifaceted. Since the diabetic syndrome is heterogeneous and represents the final expression of several possible unrelated conditions, it is not surprising that widely diverse etiologies underlie the expression of the disorder (Table 92).

45.3.1. Etiology of IDDM

The etiology of type I (IDDM) diabetes has been unraveled in the recent years by way of an explosive amount of information developing in leaps and bounds. The bulk of evidence supports the notion that type I diabetes is an autoimmune disorder. This is supported by the following lines of evidence:

1. The association of IDDM with several autoimmune diseases is a well-noted observation. Table 93 outlines the disorders that have been reported to occur with a greater frequency in patients with IDDM. In addition to the familial aggregation of several autoimmune disorders in type I diabetes, there is an increased prevalence of antithyroid, and antiadrenal, and gastric parietal cell antibodies. More importantly, the clinical association of pluriglandular failure involving parathyroids and adrenals invokes the presence of cytodestructive antibodies in the circulation of these patients. The recent demonstration of increased titers of islet cell antibodies in type I diabetics further supports an antigen–antibody reaction in the islet cells with "insulitis" and destruction of the β cells.

TABLE 92
Etiology/Mechanisms in Various Diabetic States

Condition	Etiology/mechanism
Overt diabetes	
IDDM	Autoimmune
	Genetic diathesis (HLA B-8, B-15, DR3, DR4)
NIDDM	Insulin resistance
	β-Cell insensitivity
	Genetic diathesis
Secondary diabetes	
Acromegaly	Peripheral resistance to insulin imposed by growth hormone
Cushing's	Glycogenolytic and gluconeogenic effects of glucocorticoids
	Peripheral antagonism to insulin posed by glucocorticoids
Pheochromocytoma	Catecholamines inhibit insulin release
	Catecholamines promote glycogenolysis
Primary aldosteronism	Chronic hypokalemia inhibits insulin release
Glucagonoma	Glucogen excess promotes marked glycogenolysis and gluconeogenesis
Hemochromatosis	Pancreatic destruction by infiltration with hemosiderin
Chronic pancreatitis	Pancreatic fibrosis as a sequel to repeated episodes of inflammation
Insulin receptor abnormalities	
Obesity	Down-regulation of receptors
Insulin resistance with acanthosis	Increase in circulating antireceptor antibodies that block binding of insulin to receptors
Gestational	Diabetogenic effect of estrogen, progesterone, and human placental lactogen secreted by the placenta

2. Abnormalities in cell-mediated immunity (CMI) have been demonstrated in several type I diabetics. Leukocyte migration inhibiton, a crude test for detecting CMI, has been found to be positive in a large number of type I diabetics. Attempts to characterize specific T-cell subpopulations that are cytotoxic to the β cells are under way.

3. A genetic diathesis has always been cited to explain the familial aggregation of type I diabetes. This disease demonstrates a complex association with the HLA system. It appears that type I diabetes is closely linked to the HLA types B8, B15, DR3, and DR4. The genetics of type I diabetes and its relationship to HLA genotype are best studied in families with two or more affected children. Analysis of HLA haplotypes in type I diabetic sibling pairs is indicative of identical HLA type in 60% of the pairs studied. Although this emphasizes that the

TABLE 93
Autoimmune Diseases
Associated with IDDM

Rheumatoid arthritis
Pernicious anemia
Graves' hyperthyroidism
Hashimoto's thyroiditis
Addison's disease
Vitiligo
Myasthenia gravis
Collagen vascular disease

susceptibility to develop the disease may be HLA linked, most genetic studies of type I diabetes have failed to establish clearly the mode of inheritance of this disease.

Although the aforementioned facts suggest that type I diabetes mellitus is an autoimmune disease occurring in susceptible populations with a certain haplotype distribution, research in another direction has fostered evidence to link this disease with a viral etiology. Postmortem studies of children dying from fulminant viral infections of an assorted nature indicate heavy pancreatic involvement, especially with Coxsackie B virus. Similarly, viral cytopathology in the islets has also been documented in people dying from cytomegalovirus infection. It is estimated, based on postmortem studies, that pancreatic involvement with virus injury to the β cells is encountered in approximately 11% of patients dying from viral disease. However, premortem studies of children affected by and recovered from diverse viral illnesses (mumps, rubella, Coxsackie, etc.) have failed to demonstrate a close correlation between epidemics of these illnesses and the incidence of diabetes developing. Several isolated cases have been reported in the literature of children who developed diabetes following a documented episode of Coxsackie B viral infection. The most that can be said of the viral connection is that certain viruses are clearly β cytotropic, capable of causing extensive β-cell destruction, and that documented cases continue to be reported in the literature in which type I diabetes developed after a viral infection. It is generally agreed that the viral etiology can not and does not explain all.

In summary, the development of type I diabetes is based on an autoimmune process that results in β-cell destruction in genetically predisposed individuals. The resultant syndrome that evolves rapidly is characterized by lack of insulin (insulinopenia) and normal or even accentuated receptor sensitivity.

45.3.2. Etiology of NIDDM

Although the etiology of type I diabetes is only partly unraveled, the etiology of type II diabetes continues to be as baffling as ever. The etiology of NIDDM should be viewed in terms of three perspectives: insulin receptor function in NIDDM, insulin reserve in NIDDM, and the genetics of that disease.

45.3.2.1. Insulin Receptors in NIDDM

The role of the insulin receptor in the pathogenesis of NIDDM is discussed first. The "receptor connection" emerges from the observations that more than 80% of NIDDM are obese and that nearly all obese people have varying degrees of receptor insensitivity to the action of insulin. It is a well-established fact that obesity is the most frequent cause of "down-regulation" of insulin receptors. Several lines of clinical and experimental evidence support the notion that obesity results in insulin resistance. Various animal studies have shown that when animals are rendered obese, this state is associated with a diminished effect of exogenously administered insulin. This effect is contemporaneously associated with fasting hyperglycemia and fasting hyperinsulinemia—a classic combination of target organ insensitivity. Further, the pancreatic β-cell response to glucose loading is also accentuated. This triad of phenomena—diminished glucose-lowering effect of administered insulin, fasting hyperglycemia with hyperinsulinemia, and an exaggerated β-cell response to an oral glucose load have all been shown to characterize obese subjects. The reversibility of the down-regulated receptors with weight reduction has also been documented in animals and humans.

45.3.2.1a. Nature of Receptor Problem in NIDDM. As to the specific nature of the defect in receptor function, it is essential that the action of insulin on target tissue be briefly reviewed. In overall terms, the regulation of glucose metabolism by insulin at a cellular level is mediated by a series of steps: receptor binding, stimulation of effector systems, stimulation of glucose transport, and enhancement of intracellular glucose metabolism. The exact elucidation of the action of insulin has been hampered, in part, by the failure to reproduce the hormone's action in a cell-free system. Another difficulty in understanding the mechanism of action is the pleiotropic effects of the hormone, which can, theoretically, be mediated by diverse mechanisms. The first step of insulin action (i.e., binding) is the least controversial. This can be studied effectively by evaluating binding of the hormone to monocytes, adipocytes, hepatocytes, and skeletal muscle cells. The ability of any of these cells to bind exogenously administered radiolabeled insulin correlates closely to the ability to bind endogenous insulin. Since insulin binding is the first step, an impairment in this early step must necessarily blunt or impair the subsequent stages.

Following binding, the action of insulin has to be mediated by a messenger system. The quest to identify the exact messenger that mediates the hormone action remains unfulfilled. The three contenders, cyclic AMP, cyclic GMP, and intracellular calcium, have been discarded as putative mediators of insulin action. In this regard, it should be noted that some of the actions of insulin—particularly its antilipolytic effect—are mediated via a reduction in cyclic AMP levels. The glucose-lowering effect, however, is mediated by neither a decrease nor an increase in cyclic AMP level in the target cell. Although insulin can and does stimulate a specific membrane-bound phosphodiesterase (that degrades cyclic AMP) in certain cell systems, this probably has no role in explaining the action of insulin.

Cyclic GMP, another high-energy cyclic nucleotide, has been shown to increase following the addition of insulin to slices of liver or fat tissue. However, no correlation has been found between the degree of elevation of cyclic GMP and the effect of hormone (such as lipolysis).

Following the discarding of cyclic nucleotides as possible messengers for the action of insulin, attention focused on calcium as the intracellular mediator of insulin action. This is supported by several observations: insulin action is blunted in calcium-free cell systems; elevation of cytosolic calcium (with procaine) mimics the antilipolytic action of insulin; insulin may increase cytosolic concentrations of calcium by inhibiting calcium binding to the plasma membranes of liver and fat cells. Yet, the consensus is that calcium is at best a facilitator and not the sole mediator of the action of insulin.

If cyclic AMP, cyclic GMP, and calcium are not the mediator, what then mediates the effect of insulin? Based on extremely elegant *in vitro* studies, the existence of other peptide messengers has been postulated. The isolation of such a factor(s) that inhibits cyclic-AMP-dependent protein kinase (thereby opposing the action of hormones such as epinephrine or glucagon, which raise cyclic AMP) has added strong support to the idea of peptide messenger mediation. This factor is acid and heat stable and has been isolated from rat muscle. Partly purified by preparative paper chromatography and by gel filtration, it appears that this messenger may contain more than one mediator of insulin action. (The situation is strikingly analogous to the somatomedins generated by growth hormone.) The "insulin-generated mediators" have been shown to inhibit lipolysis, stimulate glycogen synthetase, and activate pyruvate dehydrogenase, an important enzyme in glycolysis (Embden–Meyerhoff pathway). All three of the above actions are hallmarks of insulin effects.

45.3.2.1b. Decreased Receptor Binding of Insulin in NIDDM. Returning to the "insulin resistance" seen in obesity (and in type II NIDDM), the nature of receptor insensitivity is clearly heterogeneous. Several studies have demonstrated a decrease in the specific equilibrium insulin binding to circulating monocytes and fat cells of obese type II diabetics. Further characterization has resulted in the notion that the diminished binding seen in these patients results from a decrease in the number of insulin receptors. Down-regulation of receptors can be a consequence of several phenomena, the two most important ones being obesity and hyperinsulinemia. Attractive as the theory of decreased binding is, not all patients with obesity or NIDDM demonstrate the phenomenon of decreased binding. Several studies have demonstrated normal (and even increased) insulin binding to cells of obese patients with NIDDM. More importantly, the correlation between insulin binding to cell membrane and its effectiveness in mediating its effect have not been shown to be logarithmic. Thus, reduction in binding does not completely explain the degree of impairment in metabolic responsiveness. Therefore, alterations in postreceptor events in insulin-sensitive cells must play a role in insulin resistance.

 45.3.2.1c. Receptor Insensitivity and NIDDM. There are two major theories that are in vogue to explain the insulin resistance associated with obesity and the development of diabetes. Figure 26 illustrates the first theory, which supposes that obesity *per se* induces insulin resistance by decreasing receptor sensitivity, which sequentially results in hyperinsulinemia and eventual β-cell exhaustion. Figure 27 illustrates the other viewpoint, which supposes that dietary factors, particularly fat calories, increase β-cell mass and cause hyperinsulinemia; the receptor insensitivity is secondary and is a protective mechanism against the development of hypoglycemia.

 Regardless of whether the insulin resistance is primary or secondary, it

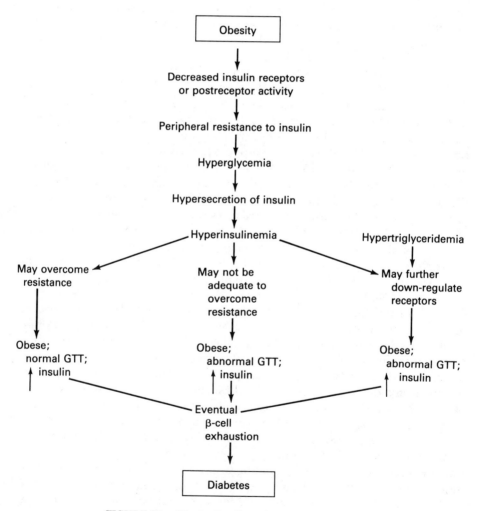

FIGURE 26. Obesity, insulin resistance, and diabetes.

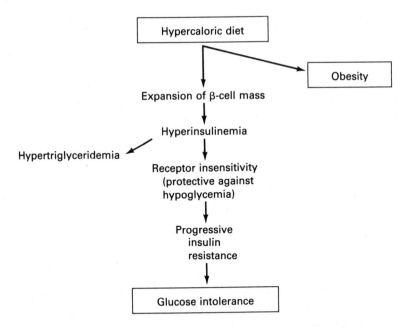

FIGURE 27. Dietary factors, hyperinsulinemia, and insulin resistance.

is irrefutable that when obesity is associated with NIDDM, the insulin resistance can cause or contribute to the glucose intolerance. Yet not all cases of NIDDM can be explained on this simplistic hypothesis. A small but significant number of patients with NIDDM are not obese, not hyperinsulinemic, and fail to show any problems with their receptors. Further, even in the obese population of patients, only 50% to 60% of subjects may show hyperinsulinemia, glucose intolerance, and receptor (or postreceptor) defects. Finally, even in patients with obesity and overt NIDDM, a subclass of patients with normal receptor sensitivity (and nonhyperinsulinism) does exist. Therefore, type II diabetes mellitus in and of itself is a heterogeneous disorder. When obesity is associated with type II DM (as it is in nearly 80% of instances), the explanations based on receptor insensitivity and hyperinsulinemia make sense. Clearly, other mechanisms must operate in the others.

45.3.2.2. Insulin Secretion in NIDDM

There is a wealth of information in the literature regarding the secretory patterns of insulin in patients with NIDDM. Since many patients with NIDDM are also obese, the effects of obesity on insulin secretion should be considered in interpreting insulin response data.

Obesity is associated with an increase in the fasting immunoreactive insulin (IRI) levels as well as a hypersecretory response to a glucose load. For comparable fasting blood glucose levels, the obese person secretes more insulin than the lean counterpart. This is because the obese subject has to overcome the receptor resistance induced by the decreased number of insulin receptors very often associated with the obese state.

In obese patients with mild NIDDM, the fasting insulin levels are usually elevated, but the β-cell response to a glucose load is variable. In many, the secretory response of the β cell is characterized by sluggishness or delay in the initial phase of response followed by a significantly increased insulin response late in the course after the administration of oral glucose. This "reactive" or "compensatory" hyperinsulinemia may account for the reactive hypoglycemia encountered in some patients with NIDDM 3 hr after a meal.

There is considerable evidence to imply that the "glucose-sensing" mechanism of the β cells of patients with NIDDM may be blunted. These patients often reveal a brisk and immediate insulin response to other secretagogues such as tolbutamide or glucagon. In fact, it is well established that the sluggish initial response of the β cell to glucose can be improved by prior treatment with theophylline or growth hormone. All this evidence, of course, points to the fact that the glucose-sensing receptors on the surface of the β cell may not be optimally receptive in responding to a glycemic challenge. This observation places NIDDM in the realm of a disorder characterized by "dual receptor insensitivity"—one at the periphery (insulin receptor) and one centrally at the level of the β cell (glucose receptor). It is postulated that the common link to both is poor "glucose penetrance"; i.e., the ability of the β cell to respond to a glycemic stimulus also depends on insulin, the hormone regulating glucose penetrance into all cells. A unifying defect occurring globally, in peripheral tissues as well as the β cell, may result in "insulin insensitivity" at the periphery associated with an impairment in the ability of the β cell to secrete insulin effectively in response to a glucose challenge.

With advanced NIDDM, the more severe the degree of glucose intolerance (as judged by the fasting and postprandial blood sugars), the lower is the insulin response during glucose testing. This situation is seen regardless of whether the patient is obese or not; but, on an average, for comparable degrees of hyperglycemia, the plasma insulin levels are higher in the obese than in the nonobese.

In summary, the fasting insulin levels in patients with NIDDM tend to be high, more so when obesity is associated with NIDDM. The insulin secretory response in mild NIDDM is characterized by a sluggish initial phase followed by an overdrive; the insulin secretory response in advanced NIDDM is characterized by a blunting of release that is proportional to the degree of abnormality in the glucose tolerance.

45.3.2.3. Genetic Predisposition to NIDDM

The diathesis for NIDDM is clearly inherited, much more so than for IDDM. Studies of monozygotic twins indicate 100% concordance in identical twins, in contrast to IDDM, which only shows 50% concordance of inheritance. Yet the familial aggregation of NIDDM does not follow a single mode of inheritance. The exception to this is those patients with maturity-onset diabetes of the young (MODY). These patients (also referred to as Mason-type diabetics) clearly demonstrate an autosomal dominant pattern of inheritance. As the name implies, the diabetes in these youngsters behaves more like NIDDM; yet the mode of inheritance is clearly different. In most studies, 85% of patients with MODY have a diabetic parent, 50–55% of the siblings tested show glucose intolerance or overt diabetes, and in 40–50% of instances three generations of vertical transmission of the disease can be demonstrated. The reason for the lack of a clear-cut inheritance pattern for NIDDM is probably genetic heterogeneity. A burgeoning amount of literature exists in regard to inheritance of NIDDM, and the answer is far from clear. The genetics of diabetes has taken one giant leap forward with the discovery of the "insulin gene," which has been localized to the short arm of the 11th chromosome. "Fragment length polymorphism" of the insulin gene has been described in populations of patients with NIDDM but not with IDDM. If confirmed, as expected, this gene marker for NIDDM would permit studying transmission of a disease that has eluded geneticists for half a century.

In summary, NIDDM is etiologically related to insulin resistance caused by binding of insulin to receptors or impairment in postreceptor events. In addition, abnormal glucose sensing by the pancreas with an impairment in insulin secretion to glycemic stimulus plays a major role. These events are woven intricately in a genetic background that may be closely linked to polymorphism of the insulin gene.

46

The Clinical Features of Diabetes

46.1. Introduction

The symptoms of diabetes mellitus are highly variable, extending over a wide spectrum of presentations. On one end, the disease may remain asymptomatic and be detected during routine screening; at the other end of the spectrum, the disease can cause diverse symptoms involving several organ systems with acute or chronic decompensation.

The classic triad of polyuria, polydipsia, and polyphagia coupled with weight loss is seen with uncontrolled diabetes, particularly when insulin dependent. The polyuria is a reflection of osmotic diuresis induced by glucose, and the increased thirst (polydipsia) is a physiological response to hyperosmolarity of the plasma. The weight loss results from enhanced lipolysis and the negative nitrogen balance from protein catabolism. The increased appetite (polyphagia) is a compensatory response to the catabolic process. The above constellation, in its extreme form, is seen in diabetic ketoacidosis (DKA); the clinical features of DKA are discussed in Section 48.2.

The symptoms and signs of nondecompensated diabetes mellitus depend, to a large extent, on the presence and severity of chronic complications of the disease. These symptoms can be viewed in terms of the organ systems involved by diabetes mellitus, which encroaches on practically every discipline in medicine.

46.2. Constitutional Symptoms of Diabetes

The constitutional symptoms of diabetes are the most frequent ones experienced by diabetics. Fatigue, lack of energy, the lack of a sense of well-being, and malaise are particularly common during periods of suboptimal glycemic control.

Weight loss is an important symptom in diabetics. The most common reason for weight loss is uncontrolled or poorly controlled diabetes. Less frequent reasons for weight loss in diabetics include gastroenteropathy, diabetic cachexia, the development of renal failure, associated endocrinopathy, or carcinomatosis. Weight loss of diabetic gastroenteropathy is a reflection of malabsorption resulting from steatorrhea or diarrhea. Diabetic cachexia (neuropathic cachexia) is particularly seen in males and is characterized by the triad of profound weight loss despite mild hyperglycemia, anorexia, and sensory neuropathy. Chronic renal failure resulting from nephropathy is a frequent cause of weight loss; the factors contributing to the weight loss in this entity are anorexia, limitation of anabolic processes, and increased catabolism of muscle protein. The association of autoimmune adrenal insufficiency and insulin-dependent diabetes is a well-recognized one and an important cause for weight loss in the diabetic. Finally, there is a higher incidence of pancreatic adenocarcinoma in diabetics than in the general population; therefore, this condition should be suspected when unexplained weight loss occurs in the diabetic.

46.3. Gastrointestinal Symptoms

The gastrointestinal tract is heavily involved in the diabetic, giving rise to several symptoms such as anorexia, vomiting, abdominal pain, dysphagia, diarrhea, or constipation (Table 94).

Diabetes can involve virtually every part of the gastrointestinal tract, with symptoms occurring as a consequence of involvement of the esophagus, stomach, small and large intestines, liver, gallbladder, and pancreas.

Esophageal symptoms are relatively infrequent in diabetics. Rarely, dysphagia can occur as a result of motility disturbances. Abnormal esophageal

TABLE 94
Gastrointestinal Symptoms in Diabetics

Symptom	Cause
Anorexia	Ketoacidosis (from the anorectic effect of ketones)
	Diabetic neuropathic cachexia
Vomiting	Ketoacidosis
	Gastroparesis
Diarrhea	Diabetic enteropathy (autonomic)
	Steatorrhea ("blind loop")
	Concomitant adult celiac disease
Dysphagia	Esophageal dysmotility
Abdominal pain	Ketoacidosis
	Mesenteric vascular occlusion
	"Abdominal angina"
Constipation	Autonomic neuropathy (colonic dysmotility)

manometry has been described in symptomatic as well as asymptomatic diabetics. Considered to be a result of autonomic neuropathy, the motility disturbances consist of poor peristalsis and occasionally uncoordinated movements similar to diffuse esophageal spasm.

The gastric involvement of diabetes is referred to as "diabetic gastroparesis." The underlying abnormality, characterized by poor contraction of the gastroduodenal sphincter, delayed emptying, and dilatation of the stomach, is caused by autonomic neuropathy. Recurrent vomiting is the major symptom. Mild gastroparesis can be accentuated during diabetic ketoacidosis with intensified vomiting and even aspiration. The prolonged gastric emptying time can be improved by the use metaclopramide, a dopamine antagonist.

The involvement of small intestines by diabetes can be via several mechanisms. The most impressive manifestation is "diabetic diarrhea." This is usually seen in conjunction with sensory or autonomic neuropathy and can be quite distressing.

Several general comments can be made about "diabetic diarrhea" (enteropathy).

1. It occurs mostly in insulin-dependent diabetics, often young and male and with signs of peripheral neuropathy.
2. Other features of autonomic neuropathy (orthostatic hypotension, impotence, and bladder dysfunction) are generally present.
3. The classic history is intermittent diarrhea, often consisting of painless passage of brown, watery, homogeneous stool without blood or pus. The episodes vary in severity and are usually characterized by nocturnal exacerbation, often with fecal incontinence. The usual history is that between the episodes of enteropathy the patient is asymptomatic. The episodes usually last for several days to weeks, only occasionally extending for months. The diarrhea can occasionally become intractable.
4. Steatorrhea (fat malabsorption) is less common that diarrhea but can be associated with diabetic diarrhea. This is usually a result of hypomotility of the gut leading to stasis and bacterial overgrowth.

Other causes for diarrhea in the diabetic include steatorrhea secondary to bacterial proliferation or concomitant adult celiac diseases, a disorder occuring with a higher frequency in diabetics.

Severe constipation in diabetics represents a manifestation of poor peristalsis secondary to autonomic dysfunction. Diminished gastrocolic reflex as well as decreased responsiveness to electric stimulation have been observed in diabetics.

Hepatic involvement in diabetes is particularly evident during DKA. Decompensated diabetes is associated with increased fat accumulation in the liver. Acute fatty liver with distension of the Glisson's capsule can result in pain in the right upper quadrant. Right upper quadrant pain in the diabetic is more often caused by acute or chronic cholelithiasis because of a higher incidence of gallstone formation in diabetics. More importantly, diabetics tend to develop acalculous cholecystitis and a dreaded variant of cholecystitis called emphysematous cholecystitis.

As indicated earlier, pancreatic adenocarcinoma tends to occur more frequently in diabetics than in the general population. The reason for this is not clear.

46.4. Diabetes and the Eyes

Ocular symptoms are frequent in chronic diabetes. Transient blurring of vision is often encountered during hyperglycemia and may be related to edema of the lens. Sudden loss of vision in diabetics can be a result of several entities such as macular edema, vitreous hemorrhage, vascular occlusion, and retinal detachment. Gradual loss of vision in the diabetic can occur from the development of glaucoma, cataracts, vitreous opacities, and progressive proliferative retinopathy. Diabetic retinopathy is described in Section 49.2.

Ptosis of the upper eyelid in the diabetic is often a consequence of neuropathies of diabetes. The sudden development of pain, chemosis, and ptosis with fever in an ill diabetic should raise the concern of mucormycosis-related cavernous sinus thrombosis.

46.5. Genitourinary Symptoms in Diabetes

Genitourinary symptoms are extremely common in diabetics. The frequent occurrence of polyuria has been already alluded to. Urinary frequency in the diabetic can be indicative of a lower urinary tract infection, bladder dysfunction secondary to diabetic autonomic neuropathy, or severe polyuria. Urinary tract infections represent the most common infections in the diabetic.

Vaginal itching caused by candidal vaginitis occurs in diabetics with such frequency that it is axiomatic to screen for diabetes in every woman with vaginal candidiasis, especially when recurrent.

Erectile dysfunction in diabetic males is more common than is perceived. Approximately 40% of diabetic males demonstrate some degree of erectile dysfunction. The three reasons for erectile dysfunction in the diabetic are autonomic neuropathy, vascular compromise from atherosclerosis (Lerische's syndrome), and psychological impotence from depression associated with a chronic disease.

In summary, the three important genitourinary symptoms seen in diabetics are frequency of micturition, vaginal itching, and impotence in males.

46.6. Diabetes and Neurological Symptoms

The neurological manifestations of diabetes are outlined in Section 49.4. The major symptoms of sensory neuropathy are parasthesias such as tingling, numbness, and pain; the main symptom of motor neuropathy is muscle weakness; and the main symptoms of autonomic neuropathy are bladder dysfunction (incontinence or retention of urine), constipation, impotence, diarrhea, and dizziness from orthostatic hypotension. The classification, symptomology, and clinical characteristics of diabetes neuropathy are described in Section 49.4.

46.7. Cardiovascular Features in Diabetes

The cardiovascular manifestations associated with diabetes are threefold: a high incidence of hypertension, atherosclerotic heart disease, and intractable orthostatic (postural) hypotension. As a group, diabetics tend to suffer from a higher incidence of hypertension. This is a major contributory factor in the development of rapidly progressive renal failure in the diabetic. Coronary heart disease occurs two- to fourfold more frequently in diabetics, and when it does, it is characterized by "silent" myocardial infarction or atypical chest pain. Also, the mortality rate in diabetics with coronary heart disease is greater than in nondiabetics. Orthostatic hypotension in diabetics results from the loss of compensatory responses that normally occur when an upright posture is assumed.

46.8. The Skin and Diabetes

The skin manifestation of diabetes are noteworthy. Approximately 30% of patients with diabetes mellitus develop a skin disorder that may be a "tip-

TABLE 95
Skin Lesions of Diabetes

Lesion	Feature
Diabetic dermopathy	"Shin spots"; flat, dull red papules on extensor surfaces of legs, heal spontaneously leaving a thin atrophic scar
Necrobiosis lipoidica diabeticorum (NLD)	Rare, but specific: oval plaque; shiny, irregular borders; yellow center, often ulcerates
Diabetic bullae	Blisters on plantar surface of feet
Granuloma annulare	Multiple, small ringlike lesions constituted by multiple papules
Skin infections	Fungal and bacterial infections (especially staphylococcal)
Acanthosis nigricans	Especially associated with insulin resistance, hirsutism, and amenorrhea
Gangrene	Skin changes associated with diabetic gangrene
Eruptive xanthoma	Crops of yellowish papules resulting from hypertriglyceridemia secondary to poor control

off" to the underlying disease or may complicate it. The skin lesions of diabetes are outlined in Table 95 with a brief description of the characteristics of each lesion.

From the foregoing, it is evident that the multisystem involvement and protean expressions of diabetes have appropriately earned the disease the aphorism once reserved for syphilis: "If one learns diabetes, one knows all of medicine."

47

Diagnostic Studies in Diabetes Mellitus

47.1. Introduction

The diagnostic studies in diabetes mellitus fall under three major categories: tests performed for diagnostic purposes, tests aimed at evaluating adequacy of glycemic control, and studies for evaluating the complications of the disease.

47.2. Studies Performed for Diagnosis of Diabetes

This category focuses on the screening as well as the definitive tests to establish the diagnosis of diabetes mellitus (or impaired glucose tolerance). The diagnostic studies that merit focus are the standard oral glucose tolerance test, the fasting blood glucose, and the 2-hr postprandial glucose. Of these, the most informative and perhaps the most sensitive is the standard oral glucose tolerance test, which is discussed first.

47.2.1. The Standard Oral Glucose Tolerance Test

The standard oral glucose tolerance test (OGTT), when performed properly, is an excellent method of evaluating glucose disposal following an oral glycemic challenge. The proper method of performing an oral GTT, the interpretation of the results, the criteria for diagnosis of diabetes versus impaired glucose tolerance, and the multiple nondiabetic causes of an abnormal glucose tolerance deserve emphasis.

The most important parameter that should be focused on during the performance of a standard OGTT is preparation of the patient. It is mandatory that for at least 3 days prior to the test, the patient be on a standard diet consisting of 3000 calories with 80 g of protein, and 300 g of carbohydrate.

399

This high-carbohydrate preparatory diet is crucial for proper interpretation of the OGTT, since hypocaloric diets tend to impair the ability of the normal subject to metabolize glucose. In nondiabetic subjects, the single most important variable that affects the rate of disappearance of postprandial hyperglycemia is the daily carbohydrate intake. A starved, anorectic patient is not at peak performance in terms of metabolizing glucose, a phenomenon that is being tested by the oral glucose load; the obvious reason is that the mechanism for metabolizing glucose is dormant in patients who are on low-carbohydrate diets, and the metabolic system cannot be expected to handle the sudden administration of a glucose load. Therefore, the OGTT curve of a patient on a low-carbohydrate diet will mimic the diabetic curve.

The procedure is done after an overnight fast by drawing blood for glucose determinations at specific time intervals following an oral load of glucose. The glucose load can either be a uniform 100 g or can be calculated as 1.75 g of glucose per kilogram body weight. (Glucola® solution is usually palatable and serves the purpose.) Blood specimens are drawn before and every half hour for at least 3 hr after ingesting the Glucola. Urine is tested for glucose, especially when renal glycosuria is suspected.

The criteria for interpretation of the results of the OGTT are different depending on the system used. Although there are several systems used by various authorities, the two most quoted and followed parameters are those established by Fajans and Conn 30 years ago and the more recent ones of the National Diabetes Data Group (NDDG). Table 96 outlines the criteria set forth by Fajans and Conn, which are simple to remember.

These cut-off points are based on plasma glucose levels, which are usually 15– 20 mg/dl higher than the whole-blood glucose. The measurement of true glucose by the Somogyi–Nelson method is preferred over other methods. It should be noted that the fasting level is not a crucial criterion for diabetes, since many patients with mild disease may demonstrate normal fasting level. However, a fasting plasma glucose in excess of 140 mg/dl is virtually diagnostic of diabetes.

The criteria for abnormality by the National Diabetes Data Group are slightly different from the criteria of Fajans and Conn. The NDDG is a consortium of specialists from United States and Europe created for the purpose of establishing simple and standard criteria that can be used worldwide. The

TABLE 96
Fajans' and Conn's Criteria for Normal OGTT

Time	Plasma glucose (mg/dl)
Fasting	<140
1 hr or peak value	<185
1½ hr	<160
2 hr	<140

TABLE 97
Criteria of NDDG for Abnormal GTT

Time	Diabetes (mg/dl)	Impaired glucose tolerance (mg/dl)
Fasting	>140	>140
1½ hr	>200	>200
2 hr	>200	140–199

plasma glucose standards established by the NDDG are higher than the previously used criteria; this has the advantage of including only patients with definitive diagnosis under the label of diabetes. Also, another category, "impaired glucose tolerance," has emerged based on NDDG criteria (Table 97).

According to the NDDG, the criteria for an abnormal oral GTT are the demonstration of a 2-hr plasma glucose value equal to or higher than 200 mg/dl and at least one value before 2 hr equal to or higher than 200 mg/dl. The criteria for "impaired glucose tolerance" are based on demonstration of a 2-hr plasma glucose level between 140 and 199 mg/dl and at least one value before 2 hr equal to or higher than 200 mg/dl.

The criteria for gestational diabetes by the NDDG are the same as the conventional criteria—the demonstration of two or more fasting glucose levels

TABLE 98
Nondiabetic Conditions That Affect Glucose Tolerance

Condition	Comment
Malnutrition, starvation	Undernutrition is associated with blunted insulin secretion
Chronic illness, physical inactivity	Glucose utilization is sluggish under these situations
Stress	Counterinsulin hormones at play impair glucose tolerance
Liver disease	Abnormal liver function impairs glucose tolerance
Hypokalemia	Impairs insulin release
Endocrinopathies	Acromegaly, Cushing's, primary aldosteronism, pheochromocytoma, and hyperthyroidism are associated with varying degrees of glucose intolerance
Renal failure	"Pseudohyperglycemia" because of non-glucose-reducing substances
Drugs	Glucocorticoids, diuretics, estorgens, nicotinic acid, diazoxide, etc.

exceeding 105 mg/dl and exceeding 190 mg/dl of plasma glucose at 1 hr, 165 mg/dl at 2 hr, and 145 mg/dl at 3 hr following 100 g of oral glucose.

In interpreting the oral GTT, attention should be paid to the several variables that can affect this test. The successful application of the oral GTT depends on proper performance of the test as well on awareness of the multitude of nondiabetic causes that affect one's ability to metabolize a glucose load. The crucial question that must be asked while studying the results of an oral GTT is whether any nondiabetic cause underlies the abnormality in glucose tolerance. Generally, when the patient is apparently healthy and ambulatory, the absence of other diseases that affect glucose tolerance can be assumed. However, the same cannot be said of the hospitalized patient, who may harbor one or more underlying disorders that can affect glucose tolerance. Table 98 outlines the disorders that should be considered while interpreting the results of an oral glucose tolerance test.

47.2.2. The Fasting Blood Glucose and the 2-Hour Postprandial Blood Glucose

Following an overnight fast (at least 10 hr) a blood glucose level above 130 mg/dl or a plasma glucose level above 150 mg/dl in an apparently healthy patient is diagnostic of diabetes. However, a normal fasting blood glucose does not exclude the disease. Normality in basal conditions and abnormality when challenged with glucose is the biochemical hallmark of early diabetes. The screening value of the postprandial blood glucose level depends on the

TABLE 99
Indications for Standard Oral GTT

Clinical
   Recurrent skin infections
   Abnormal obstetric history
     Repeated abortions, stillbirth
     Toxemia of pregnancy
     Delivery of "large" (>10 lb) babies
   "Reactive hypoglycemic" symptoms after meal
   Obesity with family history of diabetes
   Strong family history
   Premature cataracts
   Unexplained proteinuria or neuropathy
   Premature coronary or peripheral
     atherosclerosis
Biochemical
   Abnormal screening tests, e.g.,
     abnormal 2-hr postprandial
   Random glycosuria
   Random hyperglycemia
   Hyperlipidemia
   Unexplained hyperuricemia

type and amount of carbohydrate in the meal consumed and the interval since the meal. The preferred timing is 2 hr after a meal; the preferred glucose loads in descending order of preference are 100 g of glucose, 7 oz of Glucola (75 g) orally, or a meal consisting of large glass of fruit juice with added sugar, several sweet rolls, and coffee with extra sugar. The demonstration of a 2-hr postprandial blood glucose in excess of 120 mg/dl or a plasma glucose in excess of 140 mg/dl is abnormal. Because of the significant false positives and negatives with such screening, an abnormal postprandial value should be followed up with a standard oral glucose tolerance study. Table 99 outlines the indications for the standard oral GTT.

47.3. Diagnostic Studies Evaluating Glycemic Control

Since the bulk of animal experimental studies indicate that good glycemic control can delay (and may even prevent) the chronic complications of diabetes, assessment of "good glycemic control" is an integral part of diabetes care. Regardless of which therapeutic modality is used—dietary, sulfonylurea therapy, or insulin—attainment of normoglycemia throughout or through the most part of the day is the therapeutic goal. Several studies of patients on insulin pumps or intensified insulin regimens have indicated that idealization of goals is a means to an achievable end. The "motivation factor" is the single determinant and driving force that underlies many a good control. Measurement of fasting blood glucose, determination of postprandial glucose, careful urine testing for glycosuria, and measurement of glycosylated hemoglobin (hemoglobin A_{1c}) are all used to varying degrees in assessment of glycemic control.

47.3.1. Fasting Blood Glucose and Postprandial Blood Glucose

The fasting blood glucose (FBS) determination, although valuable, has been unduly and mistakenly perceived as an indicator of adequacy of the glycemic control. Although a clearly elevated FBS indicates lack of good control, a normal FBS can be misleading and conducive to promulgating a false sense of security. The difference between normal subjects and diabetics lies in the fact that the magnitude of fluctuations in the blood glucose levels in diabetics is far greater than in normals. The mean amplitude of glycemic excursions is several times greater in the diabetic than in normal subjects. This phenomenon underscores the fact that single fasting or single random blood glucose determinations cannot be used as indicators of control throughout the day, much less throughout the week or month between patient visits.

Measurement of postprandial glucose levels, when abnormal, indicates the severity of postprandial glycemic excursions. However, a single normal postprandial glucose level in the blood cannot and does not reflect the adequacy of glycemic control throughout the day. It should be pointed out that when the FBS and postprandial blood glucose levels are high, the glycemic control obviously leaves a lot more to be desired. The "ideal" FBS aimed for is below 100–110 mg/dl, and the postprandial blood glucose level below 130 mg/dl. When these goals are met, the next step is to delineate if these numbers are indicative of true control maintained throughout most of each day for a protracted period of time. This can be achieved by measurement of glycosylated hemoglobin level.

47.3.2. Glycosylated Hemoglobin

The glycosylated hemoglobins (A_{1a}, A_{1b}, and A_{1c}) are minor components of hemoglobin A, constituting approximately 6% of HbA in normals. Glycohemoglobins are so termed because of their inherent property of condensing with glucose. The rate of glycohemoglobin formation is a function of blood glucose levels. The portion of hemoglobin that condenses with glucose is the amino portion, the condensation reaction occurring in two stages; the first stage is the formation of the labile aldimine forms, and the second is the formation of the stable ketoamine by the so called Amadori rearrangement, which is irreversible. The glycosylated hemoglobin reflects the "time-averaged" integrated blood glucose values in the preceding 60 days. The obvious advantage is that it provides much more integrated information than a single blood sample. The interpretation of glycosylated hemoglobin should take into consideration the following facts:

1. There are several techniques in vogue for measuring HbA_{1c} (column chromatography, calorimetry, and even a radioimmunoassay). The development of a "rapid assay," while shortening the turnover time, is attended with cross reactivity from other "fast" hemoglobins such as HbA_{1a}, HbA_{1b}, and Hb-pre-A_{1c}.
2. The HbA_{1c} level reflects the quality of glycemic control in the preceding 60–90 days, the period of euglycemic maintenance required for the normalization of the previously elevated HbA_{1c} levels.
3. Hemolysis or a large volume of of immature cells will decrease the HbA_{1c} level.
4. Abnormal hemoglobinopathies affect the level of HbA_{1c}.
5. Acute hyperglycemic episodes (DKA) may lead to a disproportionate increase in glycosylated hemoglobin level if the method does not separate the unstable aldimine bases. When properly separated, the hemoglobin A_{1c} is not significantly affected by acute hyperglycemia.
6. In a patient who is clearly "out of glycemic control," measurement of HbA_{1c} is not indicated.

47.3.3. Urine Testing

Semiquantitative urine glucose monitoring and fractional quantitative urine analysis are also simple methods used to assess daily patterns of glycemic excursions. The correlation between urine glucose and blood glucose is not always concordant for two reasons: first, the renal threshold for glucose is often lowered in diabetics, precluding any meaningful correlation with blood glucose level; second, even with double-voided urine specimens, the varying amounts of residual urine in the bladder partially reflect the blood glucose several hours prior to collection.

Fractional quantitative analysis by collecting volumes of urine over a specific period of time and measuring the percentage of glucose in grams is superior to semiquantitative (or qualitative) urine analysis. These determinations, usually performed in aliquots of urine collected from meal to meal, correlate better with the mean blood glucose levels as obtained by continuous monitoring. The limiting factor is the renal threshold, especially when elevated as a result of the development of diabetic nephropathy. This procedure, although superior to qualitative urine testing, is cumbersome, expensive, and inferior to blood glucose monitoring by the patient.

47.3.4. Self Glucose Monitoring

The most effective method of monitoring control is by self (home) glucose monitoring by the patient. The advent of special reagent strips that permit color comparison following application of a drop of capillary blood obtained by finger prick permits excellent and accurate monitoring of blood glucose at various times of the day. Comparison can be done visually or by the use of a portable reflectance meter. Home blood glucose monitoring correlates extremely well with continuous glucose monitoring profiles. Brittle diabetics with extremely wide fluctuations cannot be monitored (and appropriately treated) by any modality other than self glucose monitoring. Patients are taught to determine blood glucose on their own seven times a day to establish the pattern of glycemic excursions. The therapeutic adjustments are made on the basis of the self-monitored results until a normoglycemic pattern is established, after which the frequency of monitoring can be reduced on an individual basis. The emergence of home glucose monitoring as a modality of adjusting therapy (insulin and diet) has literally placed the care of diabetes at the patient's fingertips. The combination of self blood glucose monitoring and glycosylated hemoglobin measurements has greatly enhanced the insulin delivery scheme in insulin-dependent diabetics.

47.4. Studies in the Evaluation of the Complications of the Disease

These studies, practically encompassing all areas of internal medicine, depend on the particular complication being suspected. Most of the diagnostic studies necessary for diagnosing target organ disease are discussed in individual sections dealing with complications of diabetes. These studies, done as part of a diagnostic workup or as follow-up parameters, are mostly related to micro- and macroangiopathic complications of the disease. Ocular (Section 49.2), renal (Section 49.3), neurological (Section 49.4), and vascular (Section 49.5) studies represent the bulk of diagnostic studies to detect the presence and severity of these complications.

Metabolic Decompensations in the Diabetic

48.1. Introduction

The three major metabolic decompensations in the diabetic are diabetic ketoacidosis (DKA), hyperglycemic hyperosmolar syndrome, and lactic acidosis (LA). Prompt identification and proper therapy are vital to prevent the complications from these metabolic derangements.

48.2. Diabetic Ketoacidosis

Diabetic ketoacidosis represents the most common reason for hospitalization in diabetics, accounting for 15% to 20% of all diabetic admissions. Diabetic ketoacidosis may be the first manifestations of diabetes; such a phenomenon constitutes 20–25% of all episodes of DKA.

48.2.1. Pathogenesis

The two hallmarks of DKA are increased ketone body production and metabolic acidosis. Therefore, the pathogenesis of DKA should be viewed in terms of these two phenomena. The critical event that sets the stage for DKA is augmented lipolysis. The hormonal milieu in DKA is highly favorable for augmented lipolysis, i.e., relative insulin deficiency and absolute increase in counterregulatory hormones. When the level of insulin, a predominantly antilipolytic hormone, is decreased, there is accentuated lipolysis. Several counterinsulin hormones such as glucagon or catecholamines contribute to lipolysis in a synergistic fashion, since the inhibitory effect of insulin is no longer present. In this regard, the role of glucagon and catecholamines should be placed in perspective; elevated levels of these lipolytic hormones in the absence of insulin deficiency does not result in DKA, underscoring the important role played by relative or absolute insulin deficiency in the pathogenesis of DKA.

As a consequence of lipolysis, the products of fat breakdown, particularly free fatty acids (FFA), accumulate and flood the liver. Hepatic ketogenesis (ketone body formation by the hepatic mitochondria) is regulated by several factors, the most important of which is the availability and amount of FFA flooding the liver. Equally important is activation of a mitochondrial enzyme called carnitine acyltransferase (CAT). The function of this enzyme is to effectively transfer the FFA that enters the liver cell into the hepatic mitochondria for oxidation into ketone bodies. The enzyme CAT presumably is under hormonal control, its activation occurring in response to insulin deficiency and/or glucagon excess. Another variable involved in the channeling of FFA into the mitochondria is the coenzyme malonyl-CoA. This cofactor normally directs the FFA into cytoplasmic pathways involving the combination of FFA, acetyl-CoA, and malonyl-CoA into hepatic triglyceride synthesis. Thus, it appears that the factors that decide whether the FFA will enter the mitochondrial system for oxidation to ketones or the cytoplasmic system for triglyceride formation depend on CAT and malonyl-CoA, respectively. A reciprocal relationship between CAT and malonyl-CoA has been established. Thus, when CAT levels increase in response to the hormonal milieu of DKA, there is a suppression of malonyl-CoA, augumenting the channeling of FFA into the mitochondrial pathway for ketogenesis. In summary, the augmentation of ketogenesis in DKA occurs for the following reasons: increased availability of the substrate (FFA), augmented activity of the mitochondrial enzyme system (CAT), and relative suppression of cytosol factors (malonyl-CoA) involved in hepatic triglyceride synthesis from FFA.

The next step following transfer of FFA into the mitochondria is β-oxidation of FFA into β-hydroxybutyric acid, which is progressively oxidized to acetoacetic acid and acetone. These three substances are collectively referred to as ketoacids. In addition to increased production of ketoacids, DKA is also associated with decreased peripheral utilization of ketoacids as a result of insulin deficiency.

β-Hydroxybutyric acid and acetoacetic acid are strong acids, dissociating at body pH into 1 mEq of hydrogen ion and 1 mEq of ketoacid ions. The result is exhaustion of the bicarbonate buffer, leading to metabolic acidosis and decreased bicarbonate. The relative production of β-hydroxybutyrate (B) and acetoacetate (A) is variable in patients with DKA, but in general the ratio of B/A is 3. The conversion of B into A may be reduced when the redox state of the cell is altered as in lactic acidosis. Under these circumstances, β-hydroxybutyric acid will be the only ketoacid produced in excess, and although this product is excreted in the urine, it cannot be detected by the routine testing measures for ketones or by the nitroprusside test.

The renal mechanisms for excreting the ketones and the blood glucose are usually excellent, accounting for the glycosuria and ketonuria and for the polyuria that is secondary to osmotic diuresis. Occasionally, the renal mechanism for clearance of plasma ketones can be so excellent that the patient

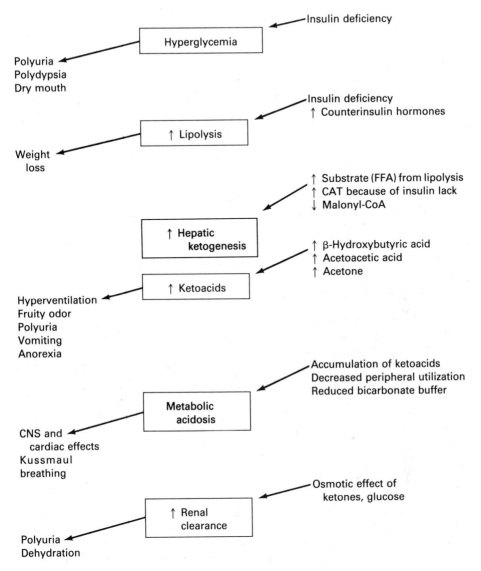

FIGURE 28. Pathogenesis of DKA.

may demonstrate strongly positive ketonuria as indicated by the nitroprusside test with absent or only a trace of ketonemia. Figure 28 outlines the key mechanisms of DKA.

48.2.2. Clinical Features

Several clinical features of DKA are outlined in Figure 28. Nonspecific symptoms such as malaise, dry mouth, weight loss, polyuria, and polydipsia predominate in the symptomatology of DKA. With progressive evolution of the process, shortness of breath, Kussmaul breathing, lethargy, and coma ensue.

Abdominal pain of a nonspecific nature is often encountered in DKA. This, coupled with vomiting (because of ketones) and guarding, may suggest a surgical problem. The picture may be complicated by enzyme elevations, particularly serum amylase, which are reversible on institution of insulin therapy. The reasons for nonspecific abdominal pain or the enzyme elevation have not been clearly elucidated.

Precipitating factors, particularly infections, should be carefully identified by physical examination.

48.2.3. Diagnostic Studies

The four abnormalities in DKA are hyperglycemia, ketonuria, ketonemia, and acid–base disturbance.

48.2.3.1. Hyperglycemia

The blood glucose is always elevated in DKA, with ranges between 350 and 750 mg/dl. The mean blood glucose concentrations in DKA average 500–600 mg/dl. Approximately 10–15% of patients with DKA may demonstrate blood glucose levels below 300 mg/dl ("euglycemic ketoacidosis"). These patients are no less severely ill than the patients with hyperglycemia, since the degree of metabolic acidosis of euglycemic ketoacidosis is as severe as or even worse than that in DKA. Three groups of diabetics are susceptible to euglycemic ketoacidosis: the alcoholic, the pregnant woman, and the child with insulin-dependent diabetes.

48.2.3.2. Ketonuria

The presence of ketones in the urine can be qualitatively detected by the nitroprusside reaction. The bedside methods of ketone testing detect only acetone, which is derived from acetoacetate. In general, the severity of ketonuria (graded from trace to 4+) correlates with the severity of ketosis. However, it should be underscored that when lactic acidosis complicates DKA, significant ketonemia can coexist with only a trace or even negative ketones in the urine. This is because when the redox state of the cell is altered by lactic acidosis, the predominant ketone produced is β-hydroxybutyric acid, which is not detected by the urine test. With the correction of lactic acidosis, the oxidative potential of cells is restored with effective oxidation of B into A resulting in ketonuria.

In DKA, when the plasma and urine ketones are monitored during therapy, β-hydroxybutyrate declines rapidly with therapy but is more readily oxidized to acetoacetate with replenishment of the acetoacetate pool. Hence, it is not surprising that acetone levels may remain unchanged (or even increase) with therapy and improvement in the DKA. Consequently, the observation of a progressively increasing plasma or urine acetone does not always imply a poor therapeutic response and may indicate a shift in B/A ratios.

48.2.3.3. Ketonemia

The serum acetone can be measured by using Acetest® tablets and can be tested in undiluted serum as well as in dilutions of 1 : 2, 1 : 4, 1 : 8, and so on. Diabetic ketoacidosis can exist with weak or negative ketones under three circumstances: when the renal clearance mechanism is so excellent that the plasma is rapidly cleared of ketones; when the DKA is complicated by lactic acidosis; and when the DKA is very early and mild.

Ketones in the diabetic do not always imply DKA; for instance, the diabetic may develop ketonemia and ketonuria with dieting (fasting), vomiting, or starvation, as can the nondiabetic. Measurement of blood glucose and blood gases is adequate to differentiate ketonemia of DKA from that of starvation.

48.2.3.4. Acid–Base Disturbances

Diabetic ketoacidosis is characterized by a reduction in the serum bicarbonate levels. This reduction is equal to the increase in β-hydroxybutyrate and acetoacetate. The anion gap $[Na - (Cl + HCO_3)]$ in DKA is increased, the increase being equal to the decrease in HCO_3 concentration. The serum chloride in DKA is normal since the renal tubular reabsorption of this ion is normal. This situation is sharply contrasted with the increased anion gap of lactic acidosis, where the increase in the anion gap cannot be accounted for by the decrease in the HCO_3 alone. Lactic acidosis is characterized by a decrease in the chloride concentration as well because of a loss of chloride in urine in exchange for lactate, which is absorbed by the renal tubule.

The blood gases in DKA are those of uncomplicated compensated metabolic acidosis. The PCO_2 is low because of the compensatory respiratory response. The respiratory response can be impaired with coexistent respiratory disease, electrolyte problems, and severe acidosis, which depresses the ventilatory drive and minute volume. Occasionally, the pH may be normal or only mildly acidemic or even alkalemic despite severe ketoacidosis. This is the classic situation when DKA is superimposed on a state of underlying metabolic alkalosis. In such a situation, the pH may be normal despite a drastic lowering of bicarbonate.

The PO_2 in DKA may be elevated as a result of the hyperventilation as well as factors that increase glucose metabolism. A decrease in PO_2 in DKA should indicate underlying respiratory pathology or ventilatory depression secondary to severe acidosis.

48.2.4. Treatment

The goals in the treatment of DKA are restoration of the fluid deficit and replenishment of intravascular volume, correction of hyperglycemia, prevention and correction of electrolyte imbalance, correction of acid–base imbalance, prevention of complications attendant with the DKA as well as with the therapy of DKA, and identification and treatment of precipitating factors.

Treatment of DKA represents an exercise in organization of data and monitoring. The patient with DKA is ideally managed in the medical ICU, where the system is geared for treatment based on monitoring. General measures such as continuing monitoring of vital signs or continuous EKG monitoring can be performed only in the setting of a MICU. Flow sheets should be maintained to provide information on the clinical status, fluid intake and output, electrolytes, chemistries, and blood gases. The question of aspirating the stomach contents of patients with DKA (to prevent aspiration as a result of gastroparesis) is somewhat controversial. The specific therapeutic measures are outlined below.

48.2.4.1. Restoration of Fluid Deficit

Replenishment of intravascular volume is the first priority in patients with DKA. These patients can be assumed to have at least 10% dehydration. Extreme care should be taken to monitor the urine output to determine fluid therapy. The initial choice of fluid is isotonic (normal, 0.9%) saline. It should be realized that the water losses in DKA far exceed the sodium losses; water loss can be of a significant magnitude (approximately 100 mg/kg body weight). Most patients with moderate to severe DKA require 2 to 3 liters of normal saline in the first 4 hr. Isotonic saline is relatively hypotonic in comparison to the hypertonic serum of patients with DKA and provides more water than solute.

48.2.4.2. Correction of Hyperglycemia

Correction of hyperglycemia with insulin in the treatment of DKA has undergone a drastic change since 1973, when several workers reported the therapeutic efficacy of "low" doses of insulin in management of DKA. The unphysiological nature of the conventional high-dose insulin therapy, practiced ever since the discovery of insulin, becomes apparent if one considers the half-life of insulin. When intravenously administered, the half-life of insulin is 3 to 7 min, and when given intramuscularly, the half-life is at best 2 hr. Administering unphysiologically large amounts of insulin is conducive to marked swings in the blood glucose levels, resulting in an erratic, unpredictable, and unstable progression towards the goal of gradually lowering the glucose level. It is believed that a smooth, orderly, and predictable lowering in blood glucose levels can be achieved by maintenance of plasma insulin concentrations at 50 to 60 μU/ml. This can be achieved by administering 0.1 U of regular insulin per kilogram body weight per hour. The route of administration does not matter (unless the patient is severely vasoconstricted), although the initial drop is greater with IV than IM administration. With the low dose, a gradual decline of blood glucose by 100 mg/dl per hr can be attained.

When the efficacies of low-dose and conventional high-dose insulin treatment for DKA are compared, the incidence of hypokalemia and hypoglycemia is extremely low (4%) in the low-dose in contrast to 29% in the high-dose group. The potential disadvantages of the low-dose therapy are nonresponsiveness in the resistant patient and delay in correction of acidosis. These factors are not particularly significant drawbacks if the patient is carefully monitored. The established safety and efficacy of the low-dose insulin therapy have rendered this form of insulin treatment the cornerstone of insulin delivery in treatment of DKA.

48.2.4.3. Prevention and Correction of Electrolyte Imbalance

The electrolyte imbalances can be viewed in terms of Na, K, phosphorus and magnesium.

The sodium losses in DKA are extensive, reaching as high as 7–10 mEq/kg body weight in severe cases. The serum sodium concentration in DKA, despite total body deficit, is normal in one-fourth of patients. In the rest, the serum Na may show a mild to moderate reduction. In interpreting a low serum Na in DKA, two factors should be remembered. First, hyperglycemia results in hyperosmolarity of the extracellular compartment, leading to a redistribution of water from the intracellular to the extracellular compartment with consequent "dilutional" hyponatremia. The calculation used is that for every 100-mg increase in blood glucose, the plasma sodium is expected to decline by 1.6 mEq/liter. Second, hypertriglyceridemia may also contribute to factitious hyponatremia by reducing the amount of Na measured in the aqueous phase.

Regardless of dilution or the hyperlipidemia, DKA is associated with significant urinary loss of Na, attributed to osmotic diuresis, insulin deficiency, or glucagon excess. The administration of normal saline and insulin is usually adequate to correct the hyponatremia.

Depletion of total body potassium is the most important electrolyte derangement seen in DKA. Yet, most patients admitted with DKA demonstrate normal or even mildly elevated levels of serum K^+. This paradox, in the light of a potassium deficit that occasionally borders on an average deficit of 3 to 5 mEq/kg body weight, arises from metabolic acidosis and volume contraction. Regardless of the initial K^+ level, the serum potassium will invariably decline with therapy for the following reasons:

1. Insulin derives K^+ intracellularly; the larger the dose of insulin, the greater is the drop.
2. Rehydration dilutes serum K^+.
3. Correction of acidosis enhances the intracellular entry of K^+.
4. Volume expansion leads to more Na^+ delivery to the distal renal tubule, which is already being exposed to high aldosterone concentrations, which cause kaliurisis.

The following general guidelines are applicable to potassium administration in DKA:

1. At the time of presentation, if the K is elevated (>6 mEq/liter), K supplements may be withheld for the first hour.
2. If the serum K is between 3.5 and 5.5 mEq/liter, potassium supplementation should be started with 10 to 30 mEq of KCl hourly, providing there is no renal failure.
3. When the serum K is below 3.5, vigorous supplementation should be started with 40 to even 60 mEq of KCL per hour.

Phosphorus depletion is an important phenomenon associated with DKA. The following observations are pertinent in terms of alterations of phosphorus metabolism in DKA.

1. The phosphate wasting of DKA is via phosphaturia.
2. Only a small percentage of patients are hypophosphatemic.
3. Insulin deficiency may contribute to decreased uptake of phosphorus by cells.
4. With therapy of DKA, a further decline in phosphorus levels may occur.
5. When the serum phosphorus declines below 0.5 mg/dl, the red cell 2,3-DPG (diphosphoglycerate) levels decline, resulting in a shift of the oxyhemoglobin dissociation curve to the left.

Based on the above, it appears reasonable to replenish phosphorus in DKA, yet the benefits to be derived from phosphorus replacement are mostly theoretical. Routine administration of phosphate to all patients with DKA is not recommended. Severe hypophosphatemia can be treated, but with care taken not to replace the entire deficit.

48.2.4.4. Correction of Acid–Base Imbalance

In uncomplicated DKA with pH above 7, bicarbonate therapy is not necessary. Correction of insulin deficiency with consequent prevention of lipolysis are adequate to diminish the ketonemia that is responsible for the acidosis. Bicarbonate therapy is indicated in the management of DKA if the pH is below 7, or, when the pH is between 7 and 7.2, the indications are (1) a comatose patient with DKA, (2) impending respiratory exhaustion from protracted hyperventilation, or (3) cardiac arrhythmia or a wide QRS or tall peaked T waves. When bicarbonate therapy is administered in DKA, the bicarbonate deficit is calculated by the following formula:

$$\text{Bicarbonate deficit} = (23 - \text{bicarbonate level}) \times 0.3 \times \text{wt in kg}$$

Half of the calculated deficit is administered intravenously, either as a bolus or 50 mEq every 10 min with pH monitoring or as an infusion. Nearly all patients with DKA respond readily to bicarbonate. Yet, bicarbonate administration should be restricted to the indications mentioned earlier because of the complications of such therapy. These include:

1. The development of sudden hypokalemia. For an increase of pH by 0.1, the serum K correspondingly falls by a factor of 0.6 mEq/liter because of a rising pH which drives the K intracellularly.
2. A paradoxical increase in the hydrogen ion concentration of CSF may occur with bicarbonate therapy, resulting in cerebral acidosis and dysequilibrium.
3. Correction of the acidosis may result in a shift of the oxyhemoglobin dissociation curve to the left, increasing tissue hypoxia.
4. Tetany may develop.

The above reasons preclude the indiscriminate use of bicarbonate therapy in DKA.

48.2.4.5. Prevention of Complications

The two major complications in the treatment of DKA are the development of hypokalemia and hypoglycemia. As indicated above, these are considerably reduced with the institution of the low-dose insulin therapy. Certain medical complications appear to predominate in DKA: myocardial infarction, cerebrovascular accidents, cerebral edema, and pancreatitis. Identification of these is often clouded by the urgency dictated by the metabolic emergency.

48.2.4.6. Recognition and Treatment of Precipitating Factors

Underlying precipitating factors can be found in only a minority of patients with diabetic ketoacidosis. When present, infections are the leading cause among underlying factors that trigger DKA. The source of infection can be obvious, as with urosepsis or respiratory tract infections, or can be occult, as with perinephric abscess, subphrenic abscess, or paracolic abscesses. In addition to infections, DKA can be precipitated by emotional stress, particularly in adolescents, and by physical trauma or anesthesia.

48.2.5. Prognosis

The mortality from DKA, although significantly reduced in comparison to the preinsulin era, still hovers around 5–8%. The cause of death from DKA is often related to nonmetabolic complications such as the development of acute myocardial infarction, pancreatitis, or cerebral edema. Cerebral edema complicating DKA is a rare event particularly occurring in children and young adults with DKA. The hallmark of this dreaded complication is that it develops after initiation of therapy. The usual presentation is characterized by obtundation in a previously conscious patient. The cerebral edema develops rapidly, with progressive stupor and coma, despite improvement in blood pH and glucose. Papilledema and a rise in temperature may be seen in some. The underlying mechanism for the development of this fatal complication is not completely understood. It is supposed that the accumulation of polyols (sorbitol) in the brain tissue results in water imbibing and resultant edema. The accumulation of these polyols is a reflection of the shift in glucose metabolism within the brain cells when insulin is lacking. Although the sorbitol hypothesis is plausible, it does not competely explain the evolution of this syndrome following therapy. It has been suggested, but not completely proven, that too rapid a correction of the hyperosmolarity with hypotonic solutions may result in fluxes of water into the brain, resulting in swelling of the brain. Other hypotheses, such as a breakdown in the blood–brain barrier or dysequilibrium caused by rapid correction of pH, have been suggested based on animal model studies. There appear to be no parameters that are predictive in identifying the group of patients at high risk for developing this lethal complication. Younger patients, especially those with initial hyponatremia, tend to be at a higher risk, although this complication can occur at any age and with any serum Na level.

The severity of the hyperosomolarity, acidosis, and hyperglycemia adversely affects the outcome, as do an older age and underlying medical problems.

48.3.   Hyperglycemic Hyperosmolar Syndrome

Hyperglycemic hyperosmolar syndrome (HHS), also known as hyperosmolar nonketotic coma (HNKC) or diabetic dehydration syndrome, is a serious metabolic derangement that can result in renal or CNS complications and even death. The criteria that characterize this syndrome are marked hyperglycemia, usually around 1000 mg/dl, minimal or absent ketonemia or ketonuria, absence of or minimal metabolic acidosis, and extreme hyperosmolarity with dehydration.

48.3.1.   Clinical Features

The clinical features of hyperosmolar nonketotic coma depend on the degree of hyperosmolarity. The syndrome usually evolves gradually, with several symptoms antedating the state of severe dehydration. Thus, quite similarly to DKA, polyuria, polydipsia, thirst, fatigue, and muscle weakness are experienced for a variable length of time before hospitalization.

The frequency of neurological symptoms, particularly coma, has earned the syndrome the term "hyperosmolar nonketotic coma." However, coma is less frequent in current practice, and a sizeable number of patients present with absolute lucidity. Several neurological findings may be evident and include transient hemiparesis, aphasia, hemianopsia, seizures, and positive Babinskis. The neurological signs are caused by extreme "dryness" of the brain tissue and are reversible on fluid replenishment. However, sometimes the development of a "stroke" may result from HNKC, rendering the patient permanently hemiplegic.

Gastrointestinal features occur in nearly half the patients with HNKC. Nausea, vomiting, abdominal discomfort, and ileus with or without gastric dilatation represent the major gastrointestinal abnormalities seen in HNKC. All of these are reversible on hydration.

The cardiovascular aspects of HNKC are those of severe dehydration and include hypotension, tachycardia, and sometimes a pericardial friction rub. When hyperosmolar nonketotic coma is complicated by hypothermia, bradycardia, hypotension, and atrial fibrillation may be seen. Hypothermia of varying degrees occurs in as many as one-third of patients with HNKC.

The renal effects of HNKC are secondary to extreme volume depletion (decrease in GFR and creatinine clearance with prerenal azotemia). When the decrease in GFR is protracted, acute renal failure may develop.

48.3.2. Pathogenesis

The profiles of the patient with the hyperglycemic hyperosmolar syndrome and DKA differ sharply. In contrast to DKA, which is predominantly a metabolic derangement seen in the insulin-dependent diabetic, HHS occurs in elderly individuals with mild non-insulin-dependent diabetes. In some instances, even a past history of diabetes may not be present. A history of medication use is obtained in 50% to 70% of patients with the hyperglycemic hyperosmolar syndrome. The drugs associated with the syndrome include diuretics (thiazides or furosemide), diazoxide, propranolol, cimetidine, glucocorticoids, and diphenylhydantoin (Table 100).

The differences between DKA and hyperosmolar nonketotic coma lie in the degree of hyperosmolarity (and dehydration), the ketosis, and the acidosis. Extreme hyperglycemia, profound hyperosmolarity, and severe dehydration characterize the hyperosmolar nonketotic state, yet with a paradoxical and conspicuous absence of significant ketosis or acidosis. The three phenomena that require explanation are the absence, or rather the relative absence, of ketosis; the severity of the hyperglycemia; and the profoundness of the dehydration. Each of these deserves brief mention.

The reasons for absence of ketosis in the hyperosmolar nonketotic state are ill understood, and several hypotheses have been advanced to explain this paradox. First, the amount of insulin in the circulation may be enough to prevent lipolysis but not adequate to prevent hyperglycemia. Second, the levels of counterinsulin (lipolytic) hormones in HNKC may not be as high as levels observed in DKA. In this regard, it should be noted that several studies have failed to show significant differences in glucagon levels between patients with DKA and HNKC. However, cortisol and growth hormone are usually lower in HNKC in comparison to DKA; whether this accounts for the lack of significant lipolysis and, consequently, ketosis remains unclear. Third, it is believed that extreme dehydration *per se* suppresses release of free fatty acids (FFA) from the adipose tissue. The serum levels of FFA in patients with HNKC are significantly and consistently lower than the FFA levels in DKA. Whatever the mechanism, the hormonal milieu in HNKC is that of an "insulinized liver

TABLE 100
Clinical Settings of HNKC

Patients
  Elderly
  Very young
  Institutionalized
  The thirst impaired
  Post-burns
  Mentally deficient
Drug history
  Glucocorticoids, thiazides, furosemide,
    propranolol, cimetidine,
    diphenylhydantoin, diazoxide
Post-procedures
  Postoperative
  Posthyperalimentation
  Post-peritoneal-dialysis
Associated diseases
  Acromegaly
  Hyperthyroidism
  CNS disease
  Hypothermia

with a diabetic periphery," meaning that hepatic ketogenesis is inhibited by ratios of glucagon/insulin in the portal vein that do not favor ketogenesis, while hyperglycemia continues to build up because of the lack of insulin.

The severity of the hyperglycemia is the second facet of the syndrome that deserves mention. Three factors contribute to the severe hyperglycemia, which usually exceeds 1000 mg/dl. First, the chronicity in the evolution of hyperosmolar nonketotic coma permits progressive accumulation of glucose in the blood. Second, a decrease in renal excretion of glucose, either from intrinsic renal disease or because of prerenal azotemia caused by extreme volume depletion, results in failure to excrete the glucose. Third, inadequate intake of fluids with a resultant shrinkage in the intravascular volume increases the tubular maximum for glucose reabsorption, leading to glucose retention. All these events contribute to life-threatening hyperosmolarity in HNKC.

The profoundness of dehydration in HNKC is also caused by a combination of factors. Persistent glucosuric osmotic diuresis leads to phenomenal losses of water and electrolytes through the urine. This loss is compounded by the inability to respond to thirst because of concomitant CNS symptoms such as confusion or stupor. The resultant dehydration is of a magnitude seldom seen with any other condition—the dry, hot skin can be lifted off the underlying tissue "like a tent," and the blood drawn from these patients is syrupy, resembling molasses.

The pictures of DKA and hyperosmolar nonketotic coma can overlap, resulting in the syndrome of HNKC being superimposed in an insulin-dependent young diabetic. When this happens, the differences in pathophysiology blur, as do the differences in management.

48.3.3. Diagnostic Studies

1. The blood glucose level in HNKC can range from 600 to 4800 mg/dl, averaging 1000–1200 mg/dl.
2. The serum Na usually exceeds 150 mEq/liter.
3. The serum osmolarity is usually in excess of 350 mOsm. The serum osmolarity can be calculated as 2(Na + K) + glucose/18 + BUN/2.8. The serum osmolarity can be accurately measured by the method of freezing osmometry.
4. The serum bicarbonate is usually normal or minimally decreased.
5. The urine and serum are negative for ketones or may show a trace.
6. The serum triglycerides are usually elevated, often with a "lipemic" serum.
7. The BUN and creatinine are invariably elevated because of the profound prerenal azotemia.
8. Polymorphonuclear leukocytosis is usually observed, at times to a marked degree.

48.3.4. Complications

The hyperosmolar nonketotic state can be complicated by three major events: acute tubular necrosis, vascular occlusions, and hypothermia. Acute tubular necrosis is more likely to occur in the patient with protracted severe volume depletion or with underlying chronic renal disease. Vascular occlusions involving the mesenteric or internal carotid arterial systems may complicate the course of the patient with HNKC. Some actually may develop a coagulopathy identical to disseminated intravascular coagulation (DIC). Hypothermia, as indicated earlier, may complicate the picture in as many as one-third of patients with HNKC. Normothermia or hypothermia are such common occurrences in HNKC that any rise in temperature should invoke a strong suspicion of infection.

48.3.5. Treatment

The cornerstones of therapy for HNKC are swift and aggressive fluid replacement with physiological (low) doses of insulin.

The volume of fluid losses in patients with HNKC averages 8 to 10 liters. Although there is a great deal of controversy as to the type of fluid selected for initial replacement, the majority of workers recommend brisk hydration with hypotonic (half-normal) saline. The advantages of using hypotonic saline are threefold: first, hypotonic saline represents the most effective method of providing additional free water; second, this type of fluid represents the most rapid means of lowering osmolarity without providing excess of sodium and chloride; third, it is the only fluid that can replace free water proportional to the electrolyte losses. The arguments against the use of hypotonic saline are also threefold. The most significant argument is the fear of too rapid a reduction in the osmolarity of extracellular fluid. Second, hypotonic saline is not as effective as isotonic saline in maintenance of extracellular fluid volume. The third argument is that isotonic saline in reality is hypotonic relative to the patient's hyperosmolarity and this, coupled with its ability to provide better defense for maintenance of blood volume, may be superior to half-normal saline.

Despite the above arguments, the following lines of reasoning are directed in choosing hypotonic saline as the initial fluid in the nonhypotensive patient with HNKC.

1. Although isotonic saline is relatively hypotonic in comparison to the patient's hyperosmolarity, the excessive sodium contained in this solution is conducive to the development of hypernatremia and hyperchloremia.
2. The level of consciousness in patients with HNKC closely correlates with hyperosmolarity of the serum, and, therefore, "reasonably rapid" reduction of this abnormality allows restoration of consciousness to normal. This goal is best attained with the use of hyptonic saline rather than isotonic saline, which also works well initially but loses effectiveness subsequently because of its high sodium content.
3. Although it is true that the glucose-lowering effect of insulin therapy is contemporaneously associated with a movement of fluid into the cells, thereby decreasing the extracellular fluid volume, the magnitude of this phenomenon in compromising blood volume is not large enough to give 0.9% saline.

If the patient is hypotensive, vigorous attempts to expand the intravascular volume with isotonic saline and/or colloid solutions such as albumin are indicated.

The rate of fluid infusion is variable, depending on the severity of the dehydration, degree of hyperosmolarity, age, and cardiac and renal status of the patient. In general 1000 to 2000 ml of fluid is administered in the first hour, 1000 ml in the second (and third) hour, followed by 500 ml per hour until the osmolarity and the hyperglycemia return to normal. Careful attention to detail is the key word in the management of HNKC. Monitoring the vital signs, urines output, central venous pressure, glucose, electrolytes, and serum osmolarity with the aid of an informative flow sheet is crucial for proper management.

With vigorous fluid replacement, three complications may be anticipated. These are the development of hypokalemia, hypophosphatemia, and late hypotension. These complications should be anticipated and treated with potassium, phosphorus solutions, and volume expansion as and when needed.

The administration of insulin for the treatment of HNKC is no different than that of DKA. Hourly administration of 5–7 U of regular insulin with careful monitoring of blood glucose to avoid hypoglycemia is the essence of insulin treatment in HNKC. The vast majority of patients who recover from the hyperosmolar nonketotic coma seldom require insulin after discharge, their diabetes being mild enough to be managed by diet alone or in combination with oral hypoglycemic agents.

48.3.6. Prognosis

The prognosis of HNKC depends on the severity of the hyperosmolarity, the duration of coma, the presence of underlying medical problems, and the complications that may evolve during the course of therapy. Despite aggressive therapy, the mortality of HNKC hovers around 20–40% when treatment is delayed. With early detection and treatment, the mortality of HNKC is still 10–15%, mostly because of the presence of underlying medical conditions.

48.4. Lactic Acidosis

Lactic acidosis represents an extreme example of metabolic acidosis, resulting from an increased production of lactate. For reasons that are ill understood, diabetics are more prone to develop lactic acidosis that nondiabetics. Although typically lactic acidosis occurs secondary to cardiovascular disease, infections, and poor tissue perfusion ("low-flow states"), it seems that diabetics are particularly susceptible to the development of lactic acidosis in the absence of these factors (idiopathic lactic acidosis).

48.4.1. Pathogenesis

Lactic acid is produced by almost all tissues, but the ones that are most actively involved in the production of lactic acid are the skeletal muscle, RBCs, and brain. Glycolysis, the process of energy derivation from glucose, requires oxygen and is mediated by several enzymes located in the extramitochondrial part of the cells. The key metabolites derived from glucose by oxidative glycolysis are glucose-6-phosphate, fructose-6-phosphate, glyceraldehyde-3-phosphate, phosphoglycerate, and pyruvate. Pyruvate is converted into CO_2 and water. When oxygen is not available, pyruvate is converted to lactate. Whenever there is tissue anoxia, the cellular mechanisms call for an increase in glycolysis (Pasteur effect). With continued tissue hypoxia, lactate continues to accumulate, resulting in hyperlactatemia and lactic acidosis.

Lactic acid in the blood quickly dissociates into hydrogen ion and the lactate ion. The hydrogen ion thus released combines with bicarbonate. With progressive accummulation, there is depletion of the bicarbonate buffer pool. The lactate ion is utilized by the tissues, particularly the liver and kidney, for gluconeogensis with regeneration of the bicarbonate ion that was consumed. Approximately 50% of the utilization of lactate is carried out by the liver and the kidney. The liver can utilize as much as 50% of the lactate released during exercise.

There are four important aspects in the diabetic that uniquely operate in predisposing to the development of lactic acidemia:

1. The enzyme pyruvate dehydrogenase, which normally regulates the conversion of pyruvate to acetyl-CoA, is reduced in diabetics. With ongoing glycolysis and reduced conversion to acetyl-CoA, the pyruvate generates more and more lactate.
2. The hepatic clearance of lactate by the liver may be impaired in diabetics. The exercise-induced hyperlactatemia is excessive in diabetics in comparison to normals. It has been speculated, but not proven, that the process of lactate reutilization by the liver may be insulin dependent.
3. The mild hyperlactatemia associated with DKA may be a reflection of low pH rather than insulin lack *per se*. When the extracellular pH approaches a range of 6.8 to 7, the liver ceases to extract lactate from the blood but instead begins to produce lactate. The combination of increased production and decreased reutilization is the reason for mild hyperlactatemia during severe DKA.
4. The incidence of lactic acidosis complicating DKA is relatively small. If a serum lactate level of 5 mM or above is used as a criterion for metabolically significant lactic acidosis, the incidence of lactic acidosis complicating DKA is less than 10%. Such a combination, however, does occur, particularly when DKA occurs in the background of hypotension, shock, severe cardiac failure, sepsis, alcohol, or therapy with the biguanide phenformin. The two hallmarks to suspect lactic acidosis in conjunction with DKA are the presence of a widened anion gap that exceeds the decrease in the bicarbonate and the presence of "weak" ketones (or no ketones) despite severe acidosis.

48.4.2. Clinical Features

The onset of lactic acidosis in the diabetic is usually acute, although occasionally the onset may be insidious. The symptoms are nonspecific and consist of malaise, anorexia, fatigue, nausea, and vomiting, bearing a close similarity to the prodromal symptoms of either DKA or HNKC. Gastrointestinal symptoms such as unexplained vomiting or abdominal pain in the diabetic may be a result of lactic acidosis. As the metabolic acidosis evolves, the invariable accompaniment is hyperpnea, which often is out of proportion to the degree of acidosis. Blunting of sensorium, lethargy, and coma may eventually develop.

48.4.3. Diagnostic Studies

1. The systemic pH is significantly depressed, often below 7.
2. The bicarbonate level is quite low. The anion gap is markedly widened. The reason for the increase in anion gap, which is greater than the decrease in bicarbonate, is probably the loss of chloride in the urine.

3. The serum chloride is usually low, since there is an increased reabsorption of lactate by the tubules in preference to chloride.
4. Blood lactate levels are usually in excess of 5 mM.

When DKA is complicated by lactic acidosis, the only ketoacid that is elevated is β-hydroxybutyrate. Because of a shift in the redox potential of the cell, there is an impairment in the conversion of β-hydroxybutyrate to acetoacetate and acetone. Since the nitroprusside test does not detect β-hydroxybutyrate, the classic combination of severe metabolic acidosis with minimal ketones in a diabetic should immediately suggest the coexistence of DKA with lactic acidosis. Measurement of plasma β-hydroxybutyrate and plasma lactate would readily reveal the dual nature of the problem.

48.4.4. Treatment

The successful treatment of lactic acidosis revolves around correction of the underlying problem that precipitated lactic acidosis and correction of metabolic acidosis by the administration of alkali. Unlike DKA, lactic acidosis requires extraordinary amounts of bicarbonate replacement because of the phenomenal depletion in the bicarbonate buffer. Persistent acidosis despite bicarbonate therapy can be frustrating. The adverse effects of persistent acidemia on myocardial irritability, ventricular function, and pulmonary vascular resistance are the major causes of death from lactic acidosis.

49

Chronic Complications of Diabetes

49.1. Introduction

In Chapter 48, the acute complications of diabetes are discussed. Improvement in diabetes care has certainly contributed to the decline in the mortality of DKA. However, the morbidity and mortality from the chronic complications of diabetes continue to prevail despite better care of the diabetic. The glimmering hope that tight metabolic control may contribute to decreasing and even preventing chronic microangiopathic complications is yet to be realized. These complications, involving the eyes, kidneys, and nervous system, are responsible for cutting down diabetics at the prime of their lives. With the discovery of insulin it was hoped that these complications could be prevented, but, unfortunately, the prolongation of life with insulin has also led to an increased chance for these complications to develop. If one objectively views the future prospects of the child with diabetes, the reality of the pain and sorrow facing the child come to focus with crushing force; thus, the chances of such a child becoming blind by age 50 or becoming uremic or impotent by age 40 and the chance of a decrease in the life span by 20% are high and real. Yet, the physicians caring for these youngsters should avoid permeating therapeutic nihilism, because the "cure" for diabetes may be within reach, and β-cell transplantation may be around the corner. Until that corner is reached, every attempt should be made to prevent these complications.

The major complications are diabetic retinopathy, diabetic nephropathy, diabetic neuropathy, large-vessel disease of diabetes, and chronic infections in the diabetic.

TABLE 101
Ocular Involvement of Diabetes

Retina	Diabetic retinopathy
	Nonproliferative (background)
	Preproliferative
	Proliferative
	Retinal detachment
Vitreous	Vitreous hemorrhage
Anterior chamber	Glaucoma
	Narrow-angle glaucoma
	Chronic open glaucoma
	Vascular glaucoma
Pupil	Internal ophthalmoplegia
	(myotonic pupil)
Iris	Rubeosis iridis
Cornea	Corneal striae, erosions, or ulcer
Optic nerve	Optic neuropathy
Extraocular muscle	External ophthalmoplegia resulting from
	cranial neuropathies

49.2. Diabetic Retinopathy

Diabetes can affect practically every part of the eye. Table 101 illustrates the protean manifestations of ocular involvement, any of which can contribute to visual deterioration.

Diabetes is related to visual loss in approximately 12–15% of the blind population of the United States. The diabetic faces a 25-fold risk of "legal" blindness and visual handicap in comparison to the nondiabetic. Between the ages of 45 and 74, 20% of all new cases of blindness are related to diabetes. The most frequent causes for visual deterioration in the diabetic are retinopathy, glaucoma, cataracts, and optic neuropathy.

49.2.1. Pathophysiology of Retinopathy

The pathogenesis of diabetic proliferative retinopathy is largely an unsettled issue, with several theories abounding. The increased capillary permeability is an established early phenomenon, not unlike the change in early diabetic nephropathy. Loss of capillary pericytes is thought to be an early event that may predispose to increased permeability. The stimulus for increased neovascularization is also unclear. Several factors such as glucose, growth hormone, and free fatty acids have all been proposed and discarded. The basis for retinal ischemia is also unsettled; abnormal platelet aggregation has been suggested as a factor predisposing to the microvascular occlusion. The lack of an experimental animal model for diabetic retinopathy (in contrast to nephropathy) has greatly impaired the understanding of its pathogenesis.

49.2.2. Clinical Features

Nearly all patients who have had diabetes for more than 20 years demonstrate some form of retinopathy. In general, the incidence of diabetic proliferative retinopathy correlates with the duration of diabetes and the degree of suboptimal control, the incidence increasing with duration of diabetes, more frequently in the diabetic with poor glycemic control. The incidence of diabetic retinopathy in the insulin-dependent diabetic with disease duration of 15 years is 60% to 65%. In this group, proliferative retinopathy develops in 18% to 20%, progressing to complete blindness.

The conventional classification of diabetic retinopathy into nonproliferative, preproliferative, and proliferative retinopathy is used in the following discussion.

Nonproliferative retinopathy, also known as background retinopathy, occurs more frequently in the non-insulin-dependent diabetic and consists of any of the following six changes:

1. Microaneurysms (red spots in the retina).
2. Changes in the retinal veins (dilation, beading, sausage formation, and loop formation).
3. Intraretinal hemorrhage (appearing as "dots and blots").
4. Hard exudates, which are fatty deposits (appearing as glistening yellow areas, often with ring formation).
5. Soft exudates (appearing as soft, fluffy white spots located in the nerve fiber layer of the retina and representing infarcts).
6. Macular edema representing accumulation of fluid in the retina in the macular region. Appearing as a "blister," this is the only nonproliferative lesion that can lead to acute visual loss because of its location.

All of the changes of nonproliferative diabetic retinopathy can be easily recognized by funduscopic examination. The only exception is macular edema, which can easily be missed. Careful examination of the fundus with an indirect opthalmoscope is needed to detect macular edema. The best instrument to detect even subtle grades of macular edema is the slit-lamp bimicroscope, which affords a high degree of magnification, resolution, and illumination.

Preproliferative retinopathy is regarded as a transitional phase in the evolution towards proliferative lesions. The two features of this phase are an increase in and striking clustering of background changes and a characteristic lesion referred to an intraretinal microvascular anomaly (IRMA). This lesion represents flattened but markedly dilated blood vessels within the retinal layers.

Proliferative retinopathy is characterized by proliferation and outgrowth of new blood vessels (neovascularization). The reason for proliferation of the endothelium of the retinal capillaries is unclear, but it is believed to be secondary to vasoproliferative substances released by the anoxic or hypoxic retinal tissues. These lesions start at the periphery of ischemic lesions and are particularly seen in the optic disk and the superior temporal quadrant of the retina. The two characteristics of the newly formed blood vessels are their friability, which makes them bleed easily, and the tendency to incite fibrous tissue proliferation around the vessels. Thus, the neovascularization, the tendency to bleed, and the fibroglial proliferation set the stage for some devastating sequelae. These devastating sequelae include retinal and vitreous hemorrhage, macular bleeding, and retinal detachment from contraction of the fibrous tissue. All three complications are severe and associated with sudden, often permanent, visual loss.

49.2.3. Diagnostic Studies

49.2.3.1. Direct Funduscopic Examination

A careful funduscopy is adequate for detecting microaneurysms, exudates, intraretinal hemorrhages, and changes in the veins. Proliferative retinopathy—the neovascularization and its complications (vitreous hemorrhage, retinal detachment, etc.)—can be identified by their characteristic funduscopic appearance. However, macular edema can easily be missed by routine funduscopy.

49.2.3.2. Indirect Funduscopy

This method provides an excellent means of detecting macular edema when the condition is suspected.

49.2.3.3. Fluorescein Angiography

This method detects early proliferative retinopathy long before fundal changes are evident by the opthalmoscope. Fluorescein angiography evaluates the permeability of the retinal vessels to contrast media. Following injection of a dye in the antecubital vein, the fundus is examined with blue light for dye leak. Normal retinal vasculature is impermeable to the dye, whereas early proliferative retinopathy is characterized by exudation of dye from the retinal vessels. Neovascular tissue is hyperpermeable and thus can be detected at an early stage. The sensitivity of the test is quite high, permitting not only detection but identification of all locations where neovascularization has begun. Photographs of the study are excellent aids for following the progression or regression of these changes.

49.2.4. Prognosis

The prognosis of background retinopathy is fair. Unless there are profuse lesions occurring in clusters, there in no reason to believe that these lesions progress to proliferative retinopathy. In contrast, the prognosis of proliferative retinopathy is poor. The detection of neovascularization, particularly in the region of the optic disk, is associated with a 40% chance of loss of vision unless the condition is treated early. Vitreous hemorrhage, once it has occurred, resolves slowly, often leaving behind residual visual impairment. Retinal detachment is a very serious sequel of proliferative retinopathy and leaves the patient permanently blind when it is complete.

49.2.5. Treatment

The treatment of advanced diabetic proliferative retinopathy is disappointing. Therefore, every attempt should be made to avoid the serious sequelae of chronic proliferation. In this regard, controlled trials (double blind) evaluating the role of photocoagulation indicate that it prevents progression and sequelae of neovascularization to a significant degree.

Photocoagulation is a procedure that uses high-intensity light (xenon arc or laser) to "burn" the points where neovascularization is noted. The beneficial effects of this form of therapy may be related to four mechanisms: first, the beam destroys the friable new vessels that are prone to bleed into the vitreous; second, the procedure possibly "seals" the leaks; third, the photocoagulation burn heals by scarring, resulting in chorioretinal adhesions that reduce the risk of detachment of retina; and, finally, photocoagulation destroys the ischemic retinal areas that presumably release vasoproliferative substances. Photocoagulation is not recommended in nonproliferative retinopathy except in the case of macular edema. The risk of visual loss from the burn is significant only when the macula is damaged by the beam.

Vitrectomy is another procedure being evaluated for its effectiveness in preventing retinal detachment. Vitrectomy is a microsurgical procedure performed with special instruments introduced through the ciliary body with the purpose of shredding the vitreous opacities and suctioning them off. During the entire procedure the intraocular pressure is maintained by a constant infusion of physiological solution. The beneficial effects of vitrectomy are related to removal of the opacities that block the path of the light beam and by severing and releasing the traction bands of fibrous tissue that tug at the retina. Generally, vitrectomy is not performed immediately after the vitreous hemorrhage because of its high rate of postoperative complications. The beneficial effects of "prophylactic" vitrecomy in patients with proliferative retinopathy but no vitreous hemorrhage have not been shown to be superior to photocoagulation.

Cataracts resulting from diabetes are quite amenable to cataract surgery.

The notion that tight metabolic control may reduce or even prevent proliferative retinopathy is gaining increasing acceptance as a motivating factor to advocate good glycemic control.

49.3. Diabetic Nephropathy

Diabetic nephropathy represents the most frequent chronic complication of diabetes that culminates in death. It also represents the most frequent reason for morbidity and disability in the diabetic.

49.3.1. Pathophysiology

The hallmark of diabetic nephropathy is microangiopathy, i.e., widespread small vessel disease. Histologically, this is identified by changes in the glomerular capillaries. The two characteristic changes in the glomerular capillaries are thickening of the glomerular capillary basement membrane and accumulation of PAS-positive (basement-membrane-like) material in the mesangium. These changes are caused by accumulation of glycoproteins in the mesangial region and the glomerular capillary basement membrane. The lesions can be focal, appearing as nodular lesions (Kimmelsteil–Wilson type) or diffuse with extensive involvement. Electron microscopic studies performed prospectively in children with diabetes indicate that the mesangial widening and the thickened glomerular basement membrane are direct consequences of abnormal glucose regulation, since these changes do not antedate diabetes but develop within $1\frac{1}{2}$ to $2\frac{1}{2}$ years after the onset of the disease.

The chemical nature of the abnormal basement membrane of the affected glomerular capillaries has generated considerable controversy. The glomerular and mesangial basement membrane glycoprotein of diabetics seems to contain an increased hydroxylysine content with a proportionate decrease in the lysine content. The significance of such a finding, however, has been disputed. An equally unresolved issue is the interpretation of studies that indicate a lack of the enzyme catalyzing the glycosylation of galactosylhydroxylysine in the renal cortex of animals rendered diabetic by alloxan; this enzyme reportedly can be modified with insulin treatment. The high association of hypertension and nephrosclerosis in the diabetic population further complicates matters.

There is a large body of animal experimental studies to support the concept that diabetic nephropathy occurs as a consequence of a derangement in metabolic factors. The problem extends beyond simple hyperglycemia as the sole mechanism of causation. Other factors, such as genetic predisposition, changes in microvascular hemodynamics, and tissue changes affecting prostaglandins or angiotensin, have all been variably implicated. A direct relationship to glycemic control and the development of diabetic microangiopathy is supported by the following lines of evidence:

1. Experimentally, when dogs are rendered diabetic, the frequency, severity, and progression of microangiopathy is greater in the group of animals whose glycemic control was poor.
2. Similarly, rats rendered diabetic by β-cell toxins or pancreatectomy develop lesions identical to human diabetic nephropathy. However, when insulin therapy is instituted early in the course of experimental diabetes, or if pancreatic β-cell transplantation is carried out, nephropathic changes either fail to develop or, if they do, are of a mild degree.
3. Several prospective and retrospective studies in diabetics have provided ample evidence to indicate a positive correlation between the degree of glycemic control and the presence, severity, and progression of diabetic nephropathy.

4. Finally, the vascular lesions of diabetes develop in normal healthy kidneys transplanted in diabetics; this implicates the host milieu involving glycemic or other factors. Within 2 years of transplantation, these transplanted kidneys demonstrate hyaline arteriolar changes in a significant number of patients. Within 4 years, almost all patients with transplanted kidneys demonstrate some histological change of diabetic microangiopathy.

Thus, the bulk of evidence favors the notion that poor metabolic control provides a deleterious metabolic milieu for the development of diabetic nephropathy. As to the reversibility of these lesions with "tight metabolic control," animal and human studies provide suggestive evidence that early changes can be reversed with excellent control. When "diabetic" kidneys of rats are transplanted into normal healthy rats, reversibility of lesions has been noted. Similarly, the early basement membrane changes in diabetic patients can be reversed by intensive insulin therapy or attainment of excellent glycemic control with second-generation sulfonylureas.

49.3.2. Clinical Features

The facets of renal disease in diabetes are outlined in Table 102 and reflect the consequences of proteinuria, renal failure, and a heightened proclivity to urinay tract infections.

In general, the longer the duration of diabetes, the greater are the chances of developing diabetic nephropathy. The apparent high incidence in insulin-dependent diabetics is a reflection of the onset of diabetes at an early age and prolongation of survival with insulin therapy. After 20 years of the disease, more than 60% of patients demonstrate significant proteinuria (>500 mg/day) and/or a decrease in the GFR. Usually, the renal involvement by diabetes evolves in a rather predictable fashion, going through three phases: asymptomatic mild proteinuria, significant proteinuria with or without the nephrotic syndrome, followed by the eventual development of slowly progressive glomerular and tubular failure. In patients with proteinuria in excess of 2.5 g, azotemia develops within 1 to 3 years. Each of these stages deserves brief mention.

TABLE 102
Renal Involvement in Diabetes

1. Asymptomatic mild proteinuria
2. Significant proteinuria
3. Nephrotic syndrome
4. Azotemia
5. Urinary tract infections
6. Acute papillary necrosis
7. Hydronephrosis secondary to bladder dysfunction
8. Associated changes of hypertension

49.3.2.1.   Asymptomatic Proteinuria

This stage is characterized by mild (<500 mg) proteinuria and occurs quite early in the course of diabetes. This stage may persist for years without any deterioration of renal function. At present, there are no histological or metabolic parameters that are helpful in identifying those patients at risk of progression into severe disease. The creatinine clearance and the GFR are often normal, even elevated. It is now evident that, paradoxically, the GFR is often increased in diabetics prior to the onset of significant proteinuria. In fact, several studies have demonstrated the persistence of elevated GFR for as long as a decade before significant proteinuria develops. The mechanism for such a phenomenon is unclear, but available evidence indicates a possible role for growth hormone and structural abnormalities of the glomerulus itself.

49.3.2.2.   Phase of Significant Proteinuria

Excretion of protein in the urine in excess of 500 mg per day marks the beginning of the end. The proteinuria is a result of increased permeability of the glomerular basement membrane, allowing the protein to leak. The GFR and creatinine clearance may be normal or decreased. Clinically, the nephrotic syndrome, characterized by edema, even anasarca, proteinuria in excess of 2.5 g, and hypoalbuminemia, develops in some patients. When the proteinuria exceeds 3 g daily, the ominous significance is that azotemia and renal failure will ensue within 1–3 years.

49.3.2.3.   The Phase of Renal Failure

Azotemia and a decline in renal function resulting in renal failure is the end stage of diabetic nephropathy. The development of renal failure is more prevalent when hypertension and atherosclerosis complicate diabetes; such is the case, unfortunately, in nearly 60% to 70% of instances.

The development of renal failure is heralded by symptoms such as nausea, vomiting, anorexia, weight loss, and a tendency to retain fluid. The patient often feels ill and is drained of all energy, motivation, and hope. The morale of patients with diabetic nephropathy is at an understandably low ebb. A characteristic feature is the ready development of hypoglycemic symptoms to doses of insulin that were well tolerated before. Azotemic diabetics are very sensitive to insulin, in part because of the longer circulating half-life of insulin in the presence of renal failure. The renal failure of diabetic nephropathy characteristically evolves slowly. However, rapid deterioration in renal function may develop in the presence of acute papillary necrosis, accelerated hypertension, and fulminant acute pyelonephritis.

In addition to nephropathy, the diabetic also faces the increased susceptibility to urinary infections, which take an independent toll. Asymptomatic bacteriuria, cystitis, and pyelonephritis are very common occurrences in the diabetic. Four observations are important as they pertain to the diabetic. First, the recurrent nature of these infections renders the organisms (usually gram negative) resistant to antibiotics commonly employed to treat such infections. Second, the urinary tract infections take longer to respond even when the organisms are treated with antibiotics to which they are sensitive. Third, a urinary tract infection deemed "simple and easy to treat" in the nondiabetic may evolve into a catastrophic illness in the diabetic, culminating in local complications (such as perinephric abscess or papillary necrosis) and systemic complications (such as septicemic shock) contributing to mortality. Metabolic control of the diabetic can be completely perturbed during urinary tract infections, contributing to poor healing. Finally, antibiotics used to treat the urinary tract infections can precipitate renal failure in the diabetic, a phenomenon only too familiar to recount.

One variety of urinary infection in the diabetic deserves special mention—acute papillary nacrosis. This disorder is characterized by the sudden development of high fever, chills, renal colic, hematuria, and in some cases rapidly progressive renal failure. The condition is readily diagnosed by the passage of actual bits of tissue in the urine when such a finding is evident; more often, the disorder is diagnosed retrospectively by intravenous pyelography, which demonstrates abnormal papillary pattern of the calyces. Other rare local complications include the development of perinephric abscess and renal carbuncle.

49.3.3. Diagnostic Studies

The four simple tests required in diabetics for evaluation of renal complications are urinalysis with examination of sediment, urine culture and sensitivity when bacteriuria or pyuria is seen on microscopic examination, quantitative evaluation of proteinuria, and measurement of blood urea nitrogen (BUN), creatinine, and creatinine clearance. The significance of the above features has already been discussed.

Caution should be exercised in recommending an intravenous pyelogram on a routine basis in diabetics because of the increased risk of contrast-medium-induced renal failure.

The indication for renal biopsy in diabetics mostly revolves around diagnostic purposes. The development of proteinuria or azotemia in a patient with longstanding diabetes signifies diabetic nephropathy and does not require a biopsy to establish the diagnosis. The indication for renal biopsy is when a coexistent disorder is suspected or when the need to establish diabetic nephropathy exists. One situation in which such a need exists is the development of glomerular or tubular abnormalities in presence of mild diabetes of short duration.

The three characteristics of the histological abnormalities in diabetic nephropathy are glomerular basement membrane thickening, mesangial widening with an increase in matrix, and immunofluorescent staining for albumin in the basement membrane of the glomerulus, tubule, and the Bowman's capsule. The intensity of the histological changes does not always correlate with the clinical severity.

49.3.4. Prognosis

In insulin-dependent diabetics with proteinuria greater than 2.5 g in 24 hr, azotemia develops within 1 to 3 years. The progression of renal disease can be assessed by serial determinations of serum creatinine, which bears a logarithmic relation to progression of renal failure.

49.4. Diabetic Neuropathy

The third important late complication of diabetes is neuropathy. This is perhaps the most common complication of diabetes, since its effects are far-reaching and involve several organ systems.

49.4.1. Classification

Customarily, diabetic neuropathy is classified into two major categories—somatic neuropathy and visceral neuropathy. The diversity of nerve involvement in diabetic neuropathy is such that practically any neurological disorder can be mimicked. Table 103 utilizes a simple clinical classification for the various neurological syndromes encountered in diabetic neuropathy.

TABLE 103
Diabetic Neuropathy

Somatic neuropathy
Peripheral neuropathy
Mononeuropathy
Cranial neuropathy
Diabetic amyotrophy
Diabetic neuropathic cachexia
Visceral neuropathy
Autonomic neuropathy
Orthostatic hypotension
Anhidrosis
Vasomotor instability
Genitourinary neuropathy
Bladder dysfunction (neurogenic bladder)
Retrograde ejaculation
Erectile dysfunction
Gastrointestinal neuropathy
Esophageal dysmotility
Gastroparesis diabeticorum
Diabetic diarrhea

49.4.2. Pathogenesis

The pathogenesis of diabetic neuropathy is the least understood of all the chronic complications of the disease. Although occasionally neuropathy may be the first manifestation of diabetes, in general it occurs in patients with longstanding disease. A correlation between degree of glycemic control and the degree of severity of neuropathy has not been convincingly established.

The two major theories in the pathogenesis of diabetic neuropathy are *vascular* and *metabolic*. The vascular theory is based on the observation that histologically, the vasa vasorum is involved in certain varieties of diabetic neuropathy, particularly the diabetic mononeuropathies. Histologically, the hallmark of diabetic neuropathy is segmental demyelination of the peripheral nerves. Although Schwann cell abnormalities appear striking, they probably represent a secondary phenomenon, the primary one being axonopathy. Axonal degeneration appears to be the earliest change observed in both the peripheral and the autonomic nerves of animals with experimentally induced diabetes. The distal parts of the neurons are the initial target of diabetic neuropathy. This observation has added credence to a vascular etiology, the distal parts of the neurons being more susceptible to avascularity.

The metabolic theory of diabetic neuropathy gained momentum when it was discovered that the *sorbitol* pathway for glucose metabolism exists in the nerves, particularly in the Schwann cells of the peripheral nerves. Experimentally, when diabetes is induced in animals, the resultant lack of insulin favors the accumulation of sorbitol in the Schwann cells, with a concomitant reduction in the nerve conduction velocity (NCV). The enzyme involved in conversion of glucose to sorbitol is aldose reductase; experimental use of drugs inhibiting aldose reductase has, at least in some studies, demonstrated a beneficial effect on the NCV.

Another observation in the peripheral nerve tissue of diabetics is a consistent decrease in the *myo*-inositol concentrations. This metabolite plays an important role in nerve conduction, since experimental reductions in *myo*-inositol are accompanied by sharp and reproducible decrements in NCV. Experimental studies in diabetic animals have provided some encouraging results in that rigid glycemic control has been shown to restore the *myo*-inositol content to normal.

49.4.3. Clinical Features

49.4.3.1. Somatic Neuropathy

49.4.3.1a. Peripheral Neuropathy. The most common manifestation of diabetic somatic neuropathy, here the presentation is characterized by sensory symptoms. These include parasthesias such as tingling and numbness, "glove and stocking" symmetrical anesthesia, cramps, and pain. The painful variety of diabetic polyneuropathy occurs predominantly at night. The pain can be of variable severity, ranging from a dull ache to excruciating lancinating or crushing pain. The nocturnal intensification is often relieved by "pacing floors." When sensory symptoms predominate, the patient may complain of "heaviness in the feet" and may describe a "feeling of walking on cotton wool."

The important neurological signs consist of decrease in the vibratory and thermal sense coupled with decreased stretch reflexes, especially in the ankle.

The motor involvement of diabetic polyneuropathy is characterized by weakness of hands and feet. Eventually, foot drop and muscle atrophy supervene. The muscle atrophy is striking in the interrossei muscles of the hands.

The importance of diabetic peripheral neuropathy lies in the fact that it predisposes to neuropathic ulcers; the poor perception of pain and temperature can result in the development of perforating ulcers at pressure points.

The loss of sensory, particularly proprioceptive, impulse conduction, coupled with intact motor component is unique for diabetes, tabes dorsalis, and rarely syringomyelia. One particular extension of this phenomenon relates to joints, which lose their protective mechanism of pain during weight bearing, leading to degenerative changes. Often triggered by repeated minor trauma, these degenerative changes result in the Charcot's joint. Eventually, there is disarticulation and dissolution of the joint. The most common cause of Charcot's joint today is diabetic neuropathy.

49.4.3.1b. Diabetic Mononeuropathy. Mononeuropathy is characterized by selective and asymmetric involvement of the sciatic, femoral, peroneal, and lateral femoral cutaneous nerves. Truncal mononeuropathies and cranial mononeuropathies can mimic other neurological syndromes, resulting in a needless and extensive workup to exclude tumors. The main symptom of mononeuropathy is pain along the distribution of the nerve, almost invariably unilateral. Dysesthesia along the distribution of the affected nerve is usually evident.

49.4.3.1c. Cranial Neuropathy. Cranial neuropathy represents a mononeuropathy of the cranial nerves. The most common cranial nerves involved are the third, fourth, and sixth nerves and rarely the seventh. Isolated cranial nerve palsies occur in 1% of diabetics. Although more common in older diabetics with longstanding disease, it can occasionally manifest in diabetic youngsters. Very rarely, cranial mononeuropathy can be the first manifestation in a person not known to be diabetic in the past. There are several unique characteristics of diabetic cranial neuropathy.

1. The onset is often acute and dramatic.
2. Localized (retroorbital or supraorbital) pain is very common.
3. Systemic symptoms are usually absent.
4. The cranial nerve palsies are unilateral, resulting in deviation of the globe with distressing diplopia.
5. Ptosis (from third nerve involvement) can be partial or complete.
6. The hallmark of cranial mononeuropathy involving the oculomotor nerves is "pupillary sparing." The pupils respond normally to light and accommodation.

7. The condition is self-limiting, often with complete restoration to normality within 12 weeks. A tendency to recur, especially on the contralateral side, has been noted.

49.4.3.1d. Diabetic Amyotrophy This rare entity is characterized by the development of progressive wasting and weakness of the muscles of the pelvic girdle and thigh. The quadriceps is particularly involved. The only sensory symptom is pain, with a characteristic preservation of all sensory modalities. The proximal myopathy should be differentiated from other causes of amyotrophy.

49.4.3.1e. Neuropathic Cachexia. This rare variety of diabetic neuropathy has several important characteristics:

1. The condition usually affects males in the fifth or sixth decade of life.
2. The predominant symptom is profound weight loss, at times approaching 60% of the normal weight ("cachexia").
3. Pain is a severe symptom, far out of proportion to the mild bilateral symmetrical neuropathy seen in these patients ("neuropathic").
4. The diabetes is mild, usually controllable without the need for insulin.
5. Depression and anorexia are integral parts of the syndrome, having nothing to do with the metabolic disturbance.
6. Paradoxically, despite the magnitude of this form of neuropathy, evidence of retinopathy or nephropathy is minimal.
7. The condition spontaneously resolves within a year or so after the onset.

Diabetic neuropathic cachexia is an important differential diagnosis of metastatic carcinoma and carcinomatous neuromyopathy.

49.4.3.2. Visceral Neuropathy

49.4.3.2a. Autonomic Neuropathy. One of the most distressing symptoms of diabetic autonomic neuropathy is dizziness secondary to orthostatic hypotension. In a normal subject, the assumption of the upright posture is attended by very minimal changes in the blood pressure. This is because several homeostatic mechanisms mediated by the autonomic system come to play in preventing a fall in the blood pressure when the subject stands. The four important mechanisms are:

1. Response of baroreceptors in the aortic arch and carotid sinus.
2. The response of arteriolar smooth muscle, innervated by the sympathetic system.
3. Response of catecholamines to posture.
4. Response of sympathetically mediated renin to upright posture.

The vasomotor and hormonal reflexes are responsible for preventing orthostatic hypotension in normals. Diabetic subjects with autonomous neuropathy characteristically lack these posture-related adaptive reflexes. As a consequence, the blood pressure drops, often to an alarmingly low level, on standing. Several general characteristics apply to the orthostatic hypotension experienced by diabetics.

1. In general, autonomic neuropathy correlates with the presence of somatic peripheral neuropathy. Abnormalities in NCV are present in the vast majority of patients with autonomic neuropathy.
2. Patients with orthostatic hypotension secondary to autonomic neuropathy fail to demonstrate an appropriate increase in the pulse rate when the blood pressure falls assuming the vertical position. This is because of a breakdown in the sympathetically mediated increase in cardiac output and vasoconstriction.
3. Static exercise such as hand-grip or Valsalva maneuver fail to evoke any blood pressure response in patients with autonomic neuropathy.
4. Biochemically, most patients with diabetic autonomic neuropathy fail to demonstrate an appropriate rise in plasma catecholamines or renin in response to upright posture.
5. Most patients with orthostatic hypotension secondary to diabetic autonomic neuropathy demonstrate other evidence of visceral neuropathy such as bladder dysfunction, diarrhea, or erectile dysfunction (impotence).

The main symptoms of orthostatic hypotension are dizziness, vertigo, or even syncope on standing. These can be mistaken for hypoglycemia, since they occur in the morning when the patient gets up from the horizontal position. When the compensatory mechanisms are severely impaired, momentary loss of consciousness and even seizures may occur as a result of marked reduction in cardiac output and reduction in the vasoconstrictor response of arteriolar smooth muscle. Not surprisingly, this may predispose to or trigger a cerebrovascular accident when cerebral atherosclerosis complicates the picture.

49.4.3.2b. Genitourinary Neuropathy.   The three facets of the genitourinary neuropathy of diabetes are the development of neurogenic bladder in both sexes and the occurrence of retrograde ejaculation of seminal fluid and erectile dysfunction in males.

The neurogenic bladder of diabetic neuropathy develops in patients with longstanding diabetes. The onset is insidious; the progression is gradual but relentless. The clinical picture is highlighted by urinary retention. The bladder develops a sluggish contractile response to even enormous amounts of urinary volumes. The early symptoms consist of infrequent voids, hesitation, poor urine stream, and incomplete evacuation, often with dribbling. Eventually, the sensation to micturate may be so impaired that severe urinary retention occurs, resulting in a distended bladder appearing as a lower abdominal mass. The inevitable complication of urinary stasis is infection.

The cystometric abnormalities of the neurogenic bladder are characteristic and consist of a long, low pressure curve with failure to sense filling until very large capacities are reached. The residual volume of urine from a catheterized bladder are invariably increased. Intravenous pyelography would reveal a large urinary bladder, often with changes of hydronephrosis.

Retrograde ejaculation is another complication seen in the diabetic male and is related to pelvic autonomic neuropathy. In the normal male, orgasm is immediately accompanied by two phenomena, emission and ejaculation. *Emission,* delivery of the seminal fluid to the posterior urethra by the contraction of smooth muscles, is part of male orgasm; *ejaculation* is a propulsion of the seminal fluid from the urethra externally by a forceful thrust from contraction of the bulbocavernosus muscle. During this forceful contraction, the internal vesical sphincter must remain closed. In the diabetic with bladder dysfunction, the internal vesical sphincter remains relaxed during contraction of the bulbocavernosus muscle, resulting in retrograde propulsion of seminal fluid from the urethra back into the bladder. The centrifuged urine following orgasm would reveal motile sperm when retrograde ejaculation exists. This phenomenon in an important cause of infertility in the diabetic male.

Impotence is experienced by at least 30–40% of patients who have had diabetes for more than 10 years and represents the single complication that is feared by the diabetic in the prime of life. The causes of erectile dysfunction in the diabetic are several:

1. Diabetic autonomic neuropathy involving the parasympathetic innervation to the penis (the nervi erigentes via S_2, S_3, S_4). Often, other facets of autonomic dysfunction such as orthostatic hypotension, bladder or bowel abnormalities, or anhidrosis are present.
2. Psychogenic impotence is not uncommon in a chronic disease such as diabetes. This is understandable, since depression is an extremely frequent accompaniment in the poorly controlled, frustrated diabetic falling prey to one complication or another. When psychogenic impotence occurs in the diabetic in the absence of organic causes, nocturnal penile tumescence studies are normal.
3. Vascular insufficiency is an overlooked cause of erectile dysfunction in the diabetic male. The diabetic patient is very prone to gradually develop atherosclerosis of the aortoiliac bifurcation (Leriche's syndrome). This results in a compomise in pudendal artery circulation, which supplies the corpora cavernosa of the penis.
4. Alcohol, drugs, and antihypertensive medications can complicate the organic erectile dysfuncion in the diabetic male.

49.4.3.2c. Gastrointestinal Neuropathy. Esophageal dysmotility, as demonstrated by abnormal manometry, is usually associated with somatic or autonomic neuropathy. The abnormalities consist of absence or reduced number of coordinated primary peristalitic waves or spastic contractions occurring in a random fashion. These abnormalities may occur in asymptomatic patients or may be associated with dysphagia or heartburn.

Gastric neuropathy secondary to autonomic dysfunction may result in a variety of symptoms such as abdominal discomfort, anorexia, nausea, vomiting, abdominal distension, and early satiety. Most patients with "gastroparesis diabeticorum" have evidence of peripheral or autonomic neuropathy. The hallmarks of gastroparesis diabeticorum are delayed gastric emptying and the presence of uncoordinated low-amplitude peristaltic waves replacing the normal strong 3-per-minute contractions. The basis for the delayed gastric emptying is probably vagal neuropathy.

Diabetic diarrhea is discussed in Section 46.3.

TABLE 104
Diagnostic Studies in Diabetic Neuropathy

Type of neuropathy	Diagnostic test	Results
Peripheral	Nerve conduction velocity (NCV) study; EMG study	Decreased conduction Decreased potentials
Autonomic Orthostatic hypotension	Pulse response to orthostasis or Valsalva	Impaired
	BP response to static exercise (hand grip)	Impaired
	Catecholamine response to posture	Impaired or absent
Neurogenic bladder	Measurement of residual urine volume	Increased (>350 ml)
	Cystometry	Increased bladder capacity
	IVP	Enlarged bladder, hydronephrosis, large residual urine in postvoiding film
Infertility	Examination of centrifuged urine following orgasm	Would reveal motile sperm as a result of retrograde ejaculation
Erectile dysfunction	Nocturnal penile tumescence (NPT) study	Normal when impotence is exclusively psychogenic
	Doppler study for penile flow	May be diminished when atherosclerosis complicates
	Aortogram	May demonstrate narrowing of aortoiliac junction (Leriche syndrome)
Esophageal neuropathy	Manometry	Poorly coordinated low-amplitude contractions or random contractions
Gastroparesis	Upper gastrointestinal series ("barium burger")	Sluggish, irregular peristalisis; delayed emptying of contrast medium; duodenal atony
	Gastric emptying study with isotope	Delay in gastric transit time
Small bowel neuropathy	Small bowel series	Increased intestinal transit time; small bowel segmentation
	Stool fat study	Steatorrhea
	Malabsorption workup	Varying degrees of malabsorption of vitamins and nutrients
	Antibiotic trial	Works when bacterial overgrowth underlies diarrhea
	Small bowel biopsy	To exclude other causes of malabsorption

49.4.4. Diagnostic Studies

The various diagnostic studies employed in the evaluation of the different facets of diabetic neuropathy are outlined in Table 104.

49.4.5. Treatment

The therapy of diabetic neuropathy is mostly unsatisfactory and frustrating. Further, spontaneous resolution of certain neuropathic syndromes makes it difficult to evaluate the efficacy of any therapeutic modality. The syndromes that demonstrate a proclivity for spontaneous resolution are diabetic neuropathic cachexia, amyotrophy, mononeuropathy, painful somatic neuropathy, and diabetic diarrhea.

The management of peripheral neuropathy, especially when painful, is particularly difficult. Attainment of "tight" glycemic control, the use of thiamine and B_6, a trial of diphenylhydantoin, experimentation with aldose-reductase inhibitors, and the liberal use of analgesics all may or may not be effective. Successful management of orthostatic hypotension is well nigh impossible. The use of 9-α-fluorohydrocortisone or pindolol (β-adrengeric agent) may be beneficial in some patients. The use of the U. S. Air Force antigravity suit may become necessary in some.

The diabetic male with impotence has several options. It is absolutely essential to exclude concomitant hormonal, vascular, and psychogenic etiologies of erectile dysfunction. This can be done by, respectively, measurement of testosterone, LH, FSH, and prolactin in plasma; Doppler studies for penile flow and, if indicated, arteriography; and nocturnal penile tumescence studies. When diabetic erectile dysfunction is localized to neuropathy, a penile prosthesis may be considered. There are basically two types of penile prostheses. In one type the surgeon places two small-caliber rigid silicone tubes, one in each corpora cavernosa. As a result, the patient has a permanent erection, which is a drawback of the procedure, but the penis can be held up against the pubis and lower abdomen by tight briefs. The procedure improves morale remarkably, and since the libido is normal, the patient is able to enjoy intercourse, limited by the inability to climax.

The second type of penile prosthesis involves an inflatable device. The advantage of this technique is that erection can be controlled. The components of the Brantley–Scot inflatable device include (1) two silicone cylinders placed in the corpora cavernosa, (2) a reservoir of fluid placed extraperitoneally beneath the lower abdominal muscles, and (3) a hydraulic pump placed in the scrotum. All these parts are connected by tubing. When the patient wants to have an erection, he squeezes the hydraulic pump in the scrotum, which moves the fluid from the reservoir into the silicone cylinders to inflate them. The inflated silicone cylinders give the patient an erection. After coitus he presses a certain spot in the pump that opens a valve and drives the fluid back from the silicone cylinders into the reservoir. This elegant device needs expertise and may cost up to $3000. The occurrence of mechanical malfunctions with the device has been a problem.

When infertility is a problem in the diabetic male and is caused by retrograde ejaculation of seminal fluid, artificial insemination of the spermatozoa retrieved from the urine can be successful.

The management of neurogenic bladder of diabetes can be quite a problem. Medical treatment with parasympathetic drugs and antibiotics are the usual modes of therapy in the early phases. When retention is a problem, catherterization or suprapubic cystotomy can be resorted to. Voiding every 3 to 4 hr aided by manual pressure (Crede method) coupled with parasympathetic drugs constitute nonsurgical management. The surgical management for the atonic diabetic bladder is by performing bladder neck resection by the transurethral route. The procedure weakens the vesical neck to a degree sufficient for the incompetent muscle to expel the contents completely. The procedure does not result in incontinence since the external sphincter of the bladder is not touched.

Gastroparesis diabetecorum and the symptoms caused by delayed gastric emptying respond well to metaclopramide, a dopamine antagonist. Similarly, the esophageal and colonic dysfunction resulting in dysphagia and constipation, respectively, respond fairly well to this drug. Diabetic diarrhea, on the other hand, is extremely unpredictable in terms of responding to medical therapy. A trial of broad-spectrum antibiotics is warranted, since bacterial overgrowth is a predominant association in this form of diarrhea.

The mainstay of therapy, it is obvious, in all forms of diabetic neuropathy is empathy from the physician's point of view coupled with hope that perhaps better glycemic control may hasten the attainment of spontaneous resolution.

49.5. Diabetic Macrovascular Disease

Whereas nephropathy, neuropathy, and reinopathy represent complications of diabetic *microangiopathy,* the disease also involves intermediate and large vessels. The three major targets are the coronary arteries, the peripheral vasculature, and the cerebral vasculature, all of which can be involved by atherosclerosis in diabetics.

49.5.1. Coronary Artery Disease

The prevalence of coronary artery disease (CAD) in diabetics is higher than that in the general population and represents the most common cause of death in maturity-onset diabetics.

The specific highlights of CAD occurring in diabetics are summarized below:

1. Although hyperlipidemia in diabetics may pose an added risk factor for the development of CAD, the independent influence of diabetes *per se* on the development of CAD has been well established.

2. The therapy for diabetes has no impact on the incidence of developing CAD in diabetes. It has not been established in any large-scale study that better glycemic control is conducive to lowering the incidence of CAD in diabetics.

3. Clinically "silent" infarctions occur more frequently in diabetics. Epigastric pain, vomiting, congestive failure, and loss of glycemic control may be the presenting features of myocardial infarction in diabetics.

4. The short-term and long-term mortality of myocardial infarction in diabetics is considerably higher than in nondiabetics who suffer myocardial infarctions.

5. A higher proportion of diabetics who suffer a myocardial infarction develop complications such as shock, life-threatening arrhythmias, congestive failure, and recurrence of infarction compared to nondiabetics.

6. The extent of atherosclerosis in diabetics is greater in comparison to the nondiabetic counterpart. Based on angiographic data, there is convincing evidence to support the notion that multiple vessel involvement is greater in diabetics than in nondiabetics with CAD.

7. Diabetics tend to demonstrate a higher prevalence of distal vessel disease than nondiabetic patients with CAD matched for age, blood pressure, and serum lipids.

8. At present, the indications for coronary revascularization in diabetics are the same as those in nondiabetics and are based on anatomic and hemodynamic parameters rather than the metabolic milieu.

49.5.2. Peripheral Vascular Disease

Approximately 45–65% of nontraumatic amputations occur in diabetics. Although neuropathy and infection contribute to this devastating incidence, the underlying abnormality that represents the major predisposing factor is peripheral vascular disease (PVD). The incidence of PVD in diabetics ranges from 10% to 50% depending on the intensity with which it is screened for.

Although atherosclerosis dominates as the histological hallmark of PVD encountered in diabetics and nondiabetics, the atherosclerotic lesions of diabetics differ in two respects: first, they occur at a much younger age in comparison to nondiabetics, and second, once they have occurred, the progression of atherosclerotic lesions in diabetics proceeds at a faster rate. To compound the problem, the atherosclerotic lesions of diabetics tend to occur in a generalized fashion, affecting multiple segments of multiple vessels, a phenomenon not unlike the vascular involvement in polyarteritis nodosa.

The pathogenesis of PVD in diabetes is not completely understood. In contrast to microangiopathy, where evidence for a correlation between hyperglycemia and angiopathy has been observed, no such correlation obtains for PVD. The vascular involvement of PVD in diabetes is characteristically a patchy involvement of the medium-sized and small muscular arteries below the knee. Although many patients with diabetic gangrene may demonstrate microangiopathy, no correlation has been established between these two types of vascular lesions. The risk factors in the development of PVD in the diabetic are primarily four: age of patient, duration of diabetes, hypertension, and hyperlipidemia. Diabetics over the age of 50 with longer duration (10–15 years) of disease, especially associated with hypertension, hypercholesterolemia, or hypertriglyceridemia, represent the groups with the highest risk of developing PVD.

The symptom of diabetic PVD is intermittent claudication, particularly in the calf. However pain in the buttocks or thighs can occur when high occlusions are present. Cold feet, nocturnal "rest pain," and loss of hair with atrophy of skin may also be indicative of underlying vascular disease in the diabetic. The single most important physical finding is decreased pulsations of dorsalis pedis. This, however, is a delayed occurrence.

Laboratory evaluation of peripheral vascular disease assumes importance when one considers that 30–35% of patients without symptoms may show evidence of arterial disease by noninvasive testing. Since a significant portion of diabetics with PVD are asymptomatic, routine periodic screening for PVD has been suggested. The noninvasive methods used for this purpose are the Doppler study, the pulse-volume recorder, measurement of temperature differences, and exercise testing with the treadmill. The relative merits and shortcomings of each, as well as a narrative description of these procedures, is beyond the scope of this work. Aortography is indicated only in patients with chronic, severe symptoms not relieved by conservative methods (such as discontinuation of smoking, vasodilators, etc.), and only when surgical intervention is being contemplated by the patient and physician.

Several techniques of vascular repair are currently available when surgery is deemed appropriate to correct poor outflow. These include endarterectomy, a procedure used for large vessels, and bypass operations that circumvent flow around the obstructed arterial lesion. One of the most commonly used bypass operations is the inverted saphenous femoropopliteal bypass graft. Although the success rate of restoring adequate vascular flow by this operation is 80–85% at the first year following surgery, recurrent blockage continues to remain a problem in the subsequent years. Catheter angioplasty is a technique by which an inflatable rigid balloon on a flexible catheter is inserted into the artery to split and disrupt the occluding plaques. This new procedure has not found wide application since the long-term effectiveness of the procedure has not been evaluated. Diabetic gangrene is treated with amputation.

49.5.3. Cerebrovascular Insufficiency

The third important vascular complication of diabetes involving the large vessels is the development of cerebrovascular insufficiency. The incidence of cerebrovascular disease is higher in the diabetic than in the nondiabetic. Residual paralytic strokes constitute a major reason for morbidity and disability in the diabetic.

There are three major factors that contribute to cerebovascular ischemia in diabetes:

1. Atherosclerosis of the internal carotid arterial system represents the major underlying lesion. Like its counterpart in the peripheral vasculature, the cerebral atherosclerosis in the diabetic occurs at an earlier age and tends to be rather diffuse.
2. Low cerebral flow induced by orthostatic hypotension and the consequences of autonomic neuropathy that result in abolition of cardiac reflexes needed to maintain blood supply to brain further complicate the picture. Transient ischemic attacks are much more common in the diabetic.
3. Hypoglycemia can precipitate a stroke in an already precariously compromised brain. Repeated mild hypoglycemic attacks can result in loss of higher function and, when severe or protracted, may result in hemiplegia.

There are no satisfactory methods for preventing the cerebrovascular atherosclerosis associated with diabetes. It is not known if attempts at good metabolic control impede or reverse the atherosclerosis of the cerebral blood vessels. Certainly, hypoglycemia should be avoided, since this can precipitate insufficiency in the "watershed" areas.

49.6. Infections in the Diabetic

Although several infectious diseases occur with equal frequency in diabetics as well as non-diabetics, certain infections are almost exclusively associated with the diabetic state. The diabetic state is characterized by an alteration in the host defense mechanisms that normally combat infection. Although inherently the defense mechanisms against infection is normal in diabetics, some mechanisms that are taken for granted in the normal healthy state are impaired in the diabetic by target-organ complications caused by disease. For instance, the impaired sense of touch (caused by sensory neuropathy) and circulatory problems (secondary to peripheral vasculopathy) contribute to a breakdown in the first line of defense against pathogens. Studies of humoral immunity in diabetes have only yielded inconsistent results; similarly, the relationship between hyperglycemia and impairment in cell-mediated immunity is also a controversial one. The one irrefutable piece of experimental evidence is that phagocytic function of the leukocytes is significantly impaired in diabetics. Using the classical "Rebuck skin window," several studies have convincingly demonstrated that chemotaxis, phagocytic engulfment, and the bactericidal properties of white blood cells are significantly impaired in diabetics. Reversibility of these defects with attainment of metabolic control has been proven in some but not all studies. Table 105 outlines the infections in diabetics based on the proclivity of these infections to complicate the diabetic state. The salient features of each are briefly presented.

TABLE 105
Infections in Diabetics

Category	Disease	Pathogen
Infections unique to the diabetic	Mucormycosis	*Rhizopus* or *Mucor* fungus
	Malignant otitis externa	*Pseudomonas aeruginosa*
	Emphysematous cholecystitis	*Clostridium perfringens; E. coli*
	Necrotizing cellulitis	*Staph. aureus;* gram-neg. rods; anerobes
Infections to which diabetics are more vulnerable	Pneumonia (necrotizing)	*Staph. aureus; K. pneumoniae*
	Urinary tract infections	*E. coli;* anerobes
	Skin infections (boil, carbuncle)	*Staph. aureus;* fungal infections
	Tuberculosis	*M. tuberculosis*

49.6.1. Mucormycosis

This devastating infection almost exclusively occurs in diabetics, particularly in ketoacidosis; the danger associated with mucormycosis resides in the ability of the fungus (mucor or rhizopus) to spread rapidly by contiguity. The path of spread of this "black mold fungus" originates in the upper end of the nasal cavity. Mucormycosis leaves a blazing trail as it spreads upward to the orbital tissues and then crosses over the cribriform plate of the ethmoid bone into the cranial cavity, where it involves the vascular system—cavernous sinus or internal jugular—eventually infecting the meninges and even the brain. The clinical features of mucormycosis closely parallel the "mucortrail"; thus, nasal discharge, often with a dark color, swelling of the upper eyelid, chemosis, and induration of the lids are features seen in the early course of the disease. With progression of the disease, vascular involvement sets in, highlighted by the striking, dramatic features of cavernous sinus thrombosis (proptosis, redness, paralysis of the extraocular muscles innervated by the oculomotor nerves as well as the ophthalmic division of the trigeminal nerve, etc.). In the final stages of the disease, meningitis with or without encephalitis may supervene.

The devastating effects of mucormycosis should be recognized early, since the therapeutic outcome depends on the early institution of antifungal therapy with amphotericin B.

49.6.2. Malignant Otitis Externa

This particular infection, usually caused by *Pseudomonas aeruginosa*, resembles mucormycosis in its invasive potential. The disease starts as pain in the ear with purulent discharge. The infection quickly spreads internally, laterally, and externally. The internal spread, the most serious sequel, is along the cleavage planes between the cartilage and bone of the petrous temporal bone. Thus, the bacterial infection may involve the inner ear, the temporal bone, the auditory nerve, and the vascular structures within. When the infection spreads laterally, it can involve the parotid glands, facial nerve, and the mastoids. Externally, the pinna can be involved, becoming red, swollen, and indurated.

Like mucormycosis, early recognition of malignant otitis externa is essential for a successful therapeutic outcome; culture of *Pseudomonas* from the greenish-yellow discharge or from the granulation tissue in the floor of the external auditory canal permits ready recognition. Therapy for this invasive condition is with carbenicillin and an aminoglycoside.

49.6.3. Emphysematous Cholecystitis

This rare inflammatory disease of the gallbladder is unique to diabetics and is characterized by invasive progression. The offending organisms are usually gram-negative bacteria (*E. coli*), clostridia, or anaerobes. The onset of the disease is no different from other forms of septic gallbladder disease (acute cholecystitis). However, in contrast to other forms of acute cholecystitis, patients with emphysematous cholecystitis appear more toxic with pronounced pain, tenderness, and guarding of the right upper quadrant. As the disease evolves, a necrotizing element is added to the process, resulting in cholangitis, empyema of the gallbladder, and perforation complicated by bile peritonitis. The condition can be suspected by the recognition of air in the gallbladder or biliary tree. Unless emergency removal of gallbladder is carried out, the condition usually results in death.

49.6.4. Necrotizing Cellulitis

A rare but serious and potentially lethal infection associated with diabetes is necrotizing cellulitis. This infection usually occurs as a result of infection with *Staph. aureus*, a gram-negative organisms, or gas-forming clostridia. An antecedent local infection (boil, infected injection site, etc.) may be the cause in some instances. The hallmark of necrotizing cellulitis is the alarmingly rapid rate at which it spreads, causing necrosis of entire areas of sheets of subcutaneous tissue and skin. Septicemia, fever, and metabolic acidosis quickly supervene, resulting in extreme morbidity and a very high mortality. Aggressive and early surgical debridement coupled with intense metabolic management and broad-spectrum antibiotic therapy may result in resolution of at least some cases.

49.6.5. Pneumonia in the Diabetic

The diabetic is particularly prone to the development of pneumonia from infection with *Staphylococcus aureus* and *Klebsiella pneumoniae*. The characteristics of these pneumonias in the diabetic are the necrotizing nature of the pneumonias, the longer duration taken for resolution, the tendency to develop bacteremia, the need to administer antibiotics for a protracted period (2 weeks), and the high incidence of postpneumonic complications such as bronchiectasis or residual interstitial disease.

49.6.6. Urinary Tract Infections in the Diabetic

The high prevalence of asymptomatic bacteriuria and the higher incidence of urinary tract infections in the diabetic are well-recognized facts. In addition, the following aspects of urinary infections in the diabetic bear emphasis.

1. Acute papillary necrosis is a rare sequel of acute pyelonephritis in the diabetic and is characterized by high fever, chills, severe tenderness in the costovertebral area, and the passage of "tissue" in the urine.
2. Upper tract infections are more common in the diabetic in contrast to nondiabetics. The development of renal abscess (cortical abscesses) or perinephric abscess is usually a result of staphylococcal infections. These infections may result from "ascending infection" or be a consequence of staphylococcal bacteremia. These abscesses may pose difficulties in detection and can become a chronic source of "smoldering sepsis."
3. Although gram-negative organisms (particulary *E. coli* and *Proteus*) predominate as the major pathogens responsible for urosepsis in the diabetic, two organisms deserve special emphasis: gas-forming organisms and *Candida albicans*. Gas-forming organisms (particularly clostridia) can cause a severe, rapidly progressive ascending urinary tract infection. This rare infection can be suspected when "air shadows" are seen in the kidney or bladder area. Regarding *Candida,* it should be recognized that colonization of the urinary tract by *Candida* is a not-infrequent occurrence in asymptomatic diabetics. The diagnosis of candidiasis of the urinary tract may be difficult and requires culture of a clean catch or catheter sample.
4. The urinary tract infections seen in diabetics show a tendency to result in septicemia, may require a longer course of antibiotics in comparison to the nondiabetic with a comparable infection, and tend to recur. The tendency for recurrence is particularly noted in diabetics with neurogenic bladder, where the increased residual volume and stasis favor bacterial proliferation.

50

The Treatment of Diabetes

50.1. Introduction

The therapy of diabetes is besieged by problems inherent to any chronic disease. An additional aspect that is unique in treatment of diabetes mellitus is the heterogeneous nature of this disorder. The variability in responses to the same form of therapy administered to apparently identical patients is, in part, attributable to the heterogeneity of diabetes. Another major problem in the long-term management of diabetes is the enormous amount of effort asked of the diabetic patient throughout his/her diabetic life. Understandably, the development of physician dependence complicates the perspectives of therapy. Clearly, well-educated diabetics under the "team care" of professionals in a specialized setting tend to do better, live more normal lives, require less frequent hospitalizations, and be more dependent on themselves than on their physicians. The role of the physician caring for the diabetic is an especially important one, always bordering on the thin line between doing too much and doing too little. The former attitude, especially in the child or youngster with diabetes, is conducive to fostering dependency, which in extreme cases can be manipulated for secondary gains. The latter attitude may be perceived by the patient as a license for laxity in dietary and other disciplines that should be rigorously practiced for good glycemic control.

The troika relationship among the patient, the physician, and the nonphysician health care professional has to be hormonious, synchronized, and practical in order to deliver the highest degree of care to the motivated patient who wishes to lead a life as close to normal. Constant reinforcement of therapeutic principles is essential to the process of learning to live with diabetes. The diabetes clinic or diabetes care center should be structured with the patient and diabetologist at its core; the support structures are several, the sheet anchor of which is the dietitian. The opthalmologist, podiatrist, nurse-practitioner, psychologist, and vascular surgeon constitute the periphery of the well-structured diabetes ambulatory care centers.

The first line of therapy for diabetes is dietary. The second and third lines of therapy are oral hypoglycemic agents and insulin, respectively. This is not to be construed as minimizing the importance of insulin, which is the "elixir of life" for insulin-dependent diabetics. The terms "first, second, and third lines of therapy" apply to the majority of ambulatory, nondecompensated, NIDDM patients, who constitute 80% of the diabetic population.

50.2. Dietary Principles in the Management of Diabetes

The nutritional management of the diabetic constitutes the sheet anchor of diabetic therapy. Yet, it is least understood by a significant faction of physicians. Although it is true that the nutritionist serves as the counselor, consultant, or specialist in this setting, there are some basic principles that every physician who treats diabetics must be aware of. This section outlines the major "core concepts" of dietary therapy for the diabetic. Although at the present time our knowledge about the metabolic consequences of various dietary regimens for diabetes must be regarded as incomplete, the conventional concepts are underscored in this section.

The goals of dietary therapy in diabetes include the following:

1. Meal planning should be based on cultural, social, ethnic, and life-style considerations and should be individually tailored to suit the patient's needs. There is no simple, single generic plan suitable for all diabetics.
2. The caloric intake should be adjusted to render the patient as close to the ideal (or "desirable") body weight. Thus, overweight patients should be placed on a diet with a caloric content aimed at weight reduction, and vice versa.
3. The planning of meals should take into consideration the activity of the patient and the timing of meal with the administration of insulin.
4. The protein content of the diet for growing children should be favorable to promote growth.
5. The fat content should be curtailed in the hope of preventing atherosclerosis.
6. The implementation of any diet plan should be facilitated by the use of exchange lists, which provide diversity.
7. The meal plan should be nutritious enough to provide the diabetic with vitamins and minerals.

The meal plan for the insulin-dependent diabetic (type I) revolves around one major objective, i.e., the assurance of precise timing of the meals in synchrony with the dose of insulin. The coordination of meals with insulin is vital for the prevention of wide swings in blood glucose excursions. The total caloric intake in these patients is aimed at maintaining ideal body weight. Most of the well-insulinized diabetics tolerate carbohydrate fairly well, provided the total caloric intake is kept constant, and are able to regulate glucose disposal similarly to normals. The caloric intake should be adequate to assure normal linear growth in the growing diabetic.

The dietary therapy for the non-insulin-dependent diabetic constitutes the mainstay of therapy, since obesity is an associated feature in most NIDDM patients. Steady weight reduction is the first line of therapy in the obese type II diabetic. The specific aspects of diet for the patient with NIDDM revolve around several issues such as total caloric intake, carbohydrate composition of diet, the role of fiber in the diet, the timing of meals, and the dietary considerations under special circumstances such as pregnancy and growth.

50.2.1. Total Caloric Intake

Conventionally, this is based on the "ideal body weight," which is calculated on the following basis: for females, 100 lb for the first 5 ft of height plus 5 lb for every additional inch of height; for males, 106 lb for the first 5 ft, and 6 lb for every additional inch. These apply for the person with medium build. Addition or subtraction of 10% is applied for the person with a large or small frame. Basal calories are calculated as ideal body weight (in pounds) × 10. Activity calories are added to the basal caloric requirement in the following manner: for sedentary activity, the number of calories added is IBW × 3; for moderate activity, the added calories are IBW × 5; and for strenuous activity, the number of calories added is IBW × 10. Further addition is indicated in the presence of growth, pregnancy, or lactation; further subtraction is necessary when weight loss is desired.

These calculations, crude as they may be, provide a starting point. It is well recognized that two individuals with identical body size doing an identical work load may widely differ in their food energy requirements. This method of calculating the caloric needs based on ideal body weight may be supplemented by an attempt on the part of the physician to determine the patient's customary food energy consumption over a protracted period of time, based on interviews and "food diaries."

50.2.2. Carbohydrate Content

In recent years, there has been considerable controversy over the content of carbohydrate in the diabetic diet. The traditional concept that diabetics should restrict carbohydrates has undergone modification in the past decade. This is mostly based on the observation that as long as the total caloric content is kept constant, liberalization of carbohydrate content of the diet does not adversely affect the glycemic control. Most dietitians recommend a carbohydrate content of 50–55% of the total caloric intake. Patients with hypertriglyceridemia may require less. The term "carbohydrate" is a generic one and encompasses several nutrients: monosaccharides (glucose, fructose), disaccharides (sucrose, as in table sugar), and polysaccharides (such as glycogen, starches, etc.). The ingestion of high concentrations of sucrose or glucose alone (not as part of a mixed meal) is associated with a rapid rise in blood glucose; however, when glucose or sucrose is consumed with a mixed meal, the glycemic rise is not as rapid. The concept that diabetics should be completely denied the pleasure of refined sugar is under attack. The recent observation that different carbohydrates possess widely variable "glycemic potential" has opened up an entire area of polemics. This glycemic potential is determined by the rate and degree of glucose absorption from the gut, which in turn is modified by several variables such as polysaccharide content and fiber content of the carbohydrate and whether the food is raw or cooked. For instance, carbohydrates consumed as potatoes or fresh vegetables cause lesser increments in blood glucose levels than an equivalent amount of oral glucose. Also, carbohydrates with a high fiber content favor less absorption of glucose.

50.2.3. Protein and Fat Content

There is unanimity of opinion regarding how much protein should be contained in the diabetic diet; for adults, 1 g of protein per kilogram body weight, and more for growing children. The fat content of the diabetic diet should not exceed 35% of total calories. Recently, the trend has been to liberalize the carbohydrate calories at the expense of fat calories, limiting these to approximately 25% of total caloric intake. This appears to make sense, given the atherogenic risk of diabetics as a group. Although some uncertainty looms over the diet-lipid–atheroma hypothesis, most lipidologists would favor restriction of fat in diet, limitation of cholesterol in the diet to 300 mg daily, and increasing the polyunsaturated fat in the meal plan.

50.2.4. Fiber in the Diet

Ingestion of a diet rich in fiber content has a salutary effect on glucose excursions, insulin requirements, and lipid levels of patients with NIDDM. The proposed mechanisms for these effects of fiber on glycemia are the induction of delay in gastric emptying (and perhaps intestinal transit time) and the formation of a "gel" that sequestrates glucose. Legumes (peas and beans) are rich in soluble fiber, but large amounts of soluble fiber need to be consumed to produce a significant impact on blood glucose or blood lipid levels. The current fervor in liberalization of fiber in the diet appears to be warranted based on short-term studies. The impact of a long-term high-fiber diet on the absorption of calcium, magnesium, and trace metal cations has not been clearly defined.

50.2.5. Timing of Meals

This is crucial in insulin-dependent diabetics. The total calories should be distributed as breakfast (20%), midmorning snack (10%), lunch (20%), afternoon snack (10%), dinner (30%), and bedtime snack (10%). The timing of meals with the administration of insulin is vital for effective glucose disposal as well as for prevention of hypoglycemia. Each patient should individualize the caloric distribution based on the activity and schedule of work.

50.2.6. Diet in Special Circumstances

The growing child or adolescent requires more protein calories than the adult. Standard charts that compare the age, weight, height, and protein requirement are available to the physician to calculate these needs.

Pregnancy in the diabetic is a situation in which caloric restriction is contraindicated. The protein needs during a normal pregnancy are increased in addition to the increased caloric needs. Most pregnant women require an added 300 kcal/day over the basal 2000 kcal of the nonpregnant weight-stable female.

The general goal of the "diabetic diet" is to provide a nutritious balanced diet low in fat, low in calories, low in simple sugar content, and high in fiber. The foodstuffs to cut down on (or eliminate altogether) are fatty meats, fried food, butter, margarine, cream, eggs, cheese, and peanut butter. Meat, when consumed, should be eaten after trimming. Skimmed milk and low-fat milk are lower in calories than regular milk. Polyunsaturated fats (vegetable oils like corn oil or sunflower oil) are superior for cooking purposes than oil from animal fat. Although restriction of simple sugars (refined sugars) is a conventional recommendation for "sugar diabetics," many experts believe that complete elimination of the pleasures of desserts or pies is punitive and should be individualized. High-fiber foods such as bran, whole wheat bread, lentils, pinto beans, etc. should be included in the diet. "Free foods," i.e., foods so low in calories that they can be consumed without restriction, such as celery, cabbage, green peppers, lettuce, and spinach, should be encouraged. These foods help the patient feel full and therefore may suppress appetite as well as provide a source of plant fiber, albeit in limited quantities.

The diverse "exchange lists" used by dietitians can provide tremendous versatility. The diabetic who is well educated in the dietary principles learns to formulate menus that are palatable and easy to prepare. It has been the experience of many that so-called "noncompliance" is often encountered when the dietary instructions are limited as a consequence of either limited help or physician ignorance or apathy.

50.3. Oral Hypoglycemic Agents

In the United States, the term "oral hypoglycemic agents" is synonymous with sulfonylureas. The accidental discovery during World War II that a certain sulfonamide (on trial for its efficacy in the treatment of typhoid fever) possessed a glucose-lowering effect spurred the synthesis of sulfonylureas. These drugs, popularly called "the antidiabetic pills," were liberally used in the late 1950s and 1960s; they represented the major form of therapy for the obese maturity-onset diabetic until the University Group Diabetes Program Study (UGDP) cast a giant shadow on oral hypoglycemic agents. This study incriminated oral agents, particularly tolbutamide, as causal factors in the "unusually" high incidence of cardiac deaths among sulfonylurea-treated patients. For several years thereafter, there was considerable reluctance to use oral hypoglycemic agents in any diabetic. The resurgence of oral agents (sulfonylureas) in the treatment of diabetes mellitus is a consequence of three phenomena. First, the statistical validity of the UGDP study has been questioned by several reputable authorities, casting a shadow on the conclusions of that study. Second, the burgeoning information regarding the role of insulin receptors in the causation of NIDDM and the effect of sulfonylureas in reversing some of these abnormalities have added a new dimension to the action of sulfonylurea. Third, the emergence of a second generation of sulfonylureas with more potency and fewer adverse effects has spurred an interest in evaluating the role of these drugs as a viable alternative. The pharmacology, actions, efficacy, side effects, indications, contraindications, and guidelines for therapy with these agents are discussed in this section.

50.3.1. Pharmacology of the Sulfonylureas

The basic molecule of sulfonylurea consists of a sulfonated benzene ring with elimination of NH_2 substitution and the opening of the heterocyclic nitrogen ring.

$$R_1 \longrightarrow - SO_2 - NH - CO - NH - R_2$$

The R_1 and R_2 rings, when substituted with various groups (CH_3^-, Cl^-, CH_3CO) or larger rings, yields the various sulfonylureas with variability in potency, half-life and metabolic degradation. The four first-generation sulfonylureas are tolbutamide, chlorpropamide, tolazamide, and acetohexamide. The two important second-generation sulfonylureas are represented by glipizide and glibenclamide. Table 106 illustrates the differences in these compounds. The second-generation sulfonylureas, as a group, tend to be more effective in terms of their pancreatic and extrapancreatic effects, are bound less to serum proteins, are less uricosuric, and tend to have negligible effects on ADH release or action. The sulfonylureas are readily and rapidly absorbed from the gastrointestinal tract and circulate in the plasma with a variable degree of binding to albumin. Most sulfonylureas are metabolized by hepatic carboxylation or reduction. Importantly, the metabolites of certain sulfonylureas can be quite active, sometimes even more than the parent compound. This is particularly true of acetohexamide and chlorpropamide. All of the sulfonylureas are excreted by the kidneys except glibenclamide, which is also excreted in bile. Since chlorpropamide and acetohexamide are characterized by circulating hepatic metabolites that are active, and since their excretion is largely dependent on intact renal function, these are particularly contraindicated in renal failure. Generally, there is poor correlation between plasma

TABLE 106
The Sulfonylureas

Name	Dosage (mg/day)	Duration of action (hr)	Site of degradation	Activity of metabolites	Comments
Tolbutamide	500–2000	6–12	Liver	Inactive	—
Chlorpropamide	100–500	24–60	Liver; renal excretion	Active	SIADH "Alcohol flushing"
Acetohexamide	250–1500	12–18	Liver; renal excretion	Active	Uricosuric; diuretic action
Tolazamide	100–1000	12–14	Liver	Inactive or weak	Diuretic; nonuricosuric
Glipizide	2.5–40	Up to 24	Liver	Inactive	Potent
Glibenclamide	1.25–20	Up to 24	Liver	Inactive as well as active	—
Glibornuride	12.5–100	Up to 24	Liver	—	—

level of the sulfonylurea and the administered dose. The reason for this may in part be that sulfonylurea disposal may be a genetically determined phenomenon.

50.3.2. Actions of Sulfonylureas

Table 107 outlines the pancreatic and extrapancreatic effects of the sulfonylureas.

The β-cytotrophic effect of the sulfonylureas is an acute one, since this

TABLE 107
Actions of Sulfonylureas

Pancreatic β-Cytotrophic	Improves "glucose sensing" of receptors on the β cell Increases rate of ion fluxes Enchances insulin secretion of β cell in response to rising blood glucose
Extrapancreatic Enhancement of insulin action on receptors	Enhancement of insulin-mediated glucose transport in muscle and adipocyte Potentiation of actions of insulin on the liver (decreased gluconeogenesis and glucose output from liver) Inhibition of lipolysis

particular effect wanes with chronic use. The exact mechanisms of β-cell stimulation are not completely understood, but several hypotheses have been put forth to explain such an effect. The sulfonylureas primarily interact with the β-cell membrane and stimulate the first phase of glucose-mediated insulin release. This involves the release of the preformed, stored pool of insulin within the β cell. The most accepted mechanism for this phenomenon is redistribution of intracellular calcium ion either directly by increasing calcium influx or secondary to potassium–sodium fluxes. Electron microscopic studies have demonstrated that the acute insulin-releasing effect of the sulfonylurea drugs is associated with degranulation of β cells. An alternate mechanism, via stimulation of adenylate cyclase or inhibition of phosphodiesterase, does not appear to be the mediator of sulfonylurea-induced insulin release.

It should be emphasized that the stimulatory effects of sulfonylurea drugs on insulin release diminish with time. Several investigators have demonstrated a striking decrease in the glucose-mediated insulin release, when compared with the initial response, in patients controlled well with chronic sulfonylurea drug therapy. Therefore, the glucose-lowering effects of sulfonylurea drugs used on a chronic basis can not be explained by the pancreatic (β-cytotrophic) effects of the drug. The reasons for such an attenuation in response are unclear, but animal evidence suggests that changes in the β cell (degranulation) with concomitant decreases in insulin content may account for such an effect.

The extrapancreatic effects of sulfonylureas revolve around the unique ability of these drugs to "up-regulate" the insulin receptors throughout the body. Indeed, the bulk of current evidence favors the notion that the major antidiabetic effect of the sulfonylurea drugs is mediated by this receptor enhancement. Thus, it is not surprising that the drug works best when insulin is present in the circulation and when receptor insensitivity underlies the mechanism of glucose intolerance. Both of these phenomena are seen in a high proportion of patients with non-insulin-dependent diabetes mellitus, a disorder that ideally lends itself to treatment with sulfonylureas. It should be recognized that the effect of sulfonylureas is not the same in all insulin-sensitive tissues. The potentiation of insulin action in terms of carbohydrate transport in the muscle and adipose tissue is the best documented and probably the most potent extrapancreatic effect of sulfonylureas. On the liver, these drugs cause an enhancement of insulin action. A large body of animal data supports the tenet that these drugs potentiate insulin action on the liver, decreasing gluconeogenesis and decreasing hepatic glucose output.

The exact locus at which the action of sulfonylureas on the receptors is expressed is not clear, and it could be either enhancement of receptor binding of insulin or enhancement of the postreceptor actions of insulin. It is believed that the β-cytotrophic effect of sulfonylureas (enhancement of the glucose-mediated insulin response) is mediated by the binding of the drug to the plasma membranes of the β cell, whereas the potentiation of insulin-mediated glucose transport at the periphery is mediated at the postreceptor level.

50.3.3. Efficacy of the Sulfonylurea Drugs

Despite nearly 30 years of existence, the efficacy and role of sulfonylureas in treatment of diabetes has remained controversial. The reasons for this uncertain status and disparate opinions include the heterogeneity of NIDDM, the heterogeneity in patient response to sulfonylureas, the relatively few comprehensive studies, spread over a long duration, the lack of enough placebo-controlled studies and poor judgment in selection of proper patients for therapy. The consensus of opinion is that proper selection of patients for sulfonylurea treatment is the single most important parameter to predict success. The ideal patients for sulfonylurea therapy consist of NIDDM patients with disease onset after age 40, with disease duration less than 5 years at time of initiating therapy, diabetics with excess or normal weight, and diabetics with prior history of insulinization at a dose less than 20 U. In carefully selected patients, a good response to the drug will occur in 70–75% in the first few years of therapy.

The therapeutic usefulness of the first- and second-generation sulfonylureas has been the subject of several clinical studies. Four types of studies have attested to the therapeutic efficacy of this class of drugs.

1. Clinical studies of patients on long-term sulfonylurea therapy. The incidence of "primary" and "secondary" failure to sulfonylureas has been evaluated by several investigators. The term primary failure indicates no response to the drug at all, whereas the term secondary failure implies loss of response to the drug following a variable period of initial responsiveness. In large-scale studies boasting of patient participation as large as 3000 to 5000 patients, the primary failure to first-generation sulfonylureas ranged between 10% and 30%. The lowest incidence of primary failure (<5%) is noted when rigid criteria are applied for patient selection. The rate of secondary failure, again variable, ranges between 10% and as high as 40%. The highest incidence of secondary failure occurs in the first and second years of therapy. Nearly 40% of patients who manifested a successful initial response to sulfonylurea drugs can be expected to maintain the responsiveness at the end of 5 or 6 years. In those who develop secondary failure to sulfonylureas, a high proportion of patients demonstrate complications of diabetes or serious dietary noncompliance. Long-term studies with the second-generation sulfonylureas are not available, but judging from their enhanced potency, the result should be the same as or better than those with the first-generation sulfonylureas.

2. Studies evaluating the role of sulfonylurea in enhancing receptor sensitivity to insulin. Several methods are currently available to evaluate the receptor sensitivity to insulin. These range from measurement of insulin binding to monocytes to elegant studies using "glucose-clamp" techniques to evaluate the effects of injected insulin on various parameters. Numerous studies have demonstrated that the decreased

insulin binding to monocytes can be doubled and in some instances even normalized by the use of chlorpropamide in patients with NIDDM. Since some patients may show normal insulin binding but an impaired postreceptor mediation of insulin action, the glucose-lowering effect of insulin administered to patients with NIDDM can be studied by the use of glucose clamp techniques. These studies also demonstrate that sulfonylureas potentiate the peripheral action of insulin.

3. Receptor studies evaluating the independent roles of diet and sulfonylureas. Several investigators have demonstrated that the second-generation sulfonylureas increase the absolute number of insulin receptors on the monocytes of patients with NIDDM. In comparisons between diet alone and diet combined with sulfonylurea, the latter group demonstrated a striking restoration in insulin responsiveness.

4. The influence of short-term and long-term use of sulfonylureas on the glycosylated hemoglobin (hemoglobin A_{1c}) has also been evaluated by several workers; the results indicated a positive correlation between responsiveness to the drug and normalization of glycosylated hemoglobin levels in comparison to the pretreatment levels.

Thus, the bulk of evidence favoring a salutary response to sulfonylurea drugs on glycemic control of NIDDM patients can no longer be ignored. In properly selected patients, the drug has a 70–80% chance of succeeding, and half to two-thirds of these patients continue to respond satisfactorily up to as long as 5 years following therapy. The causes of primary and secondary failure are unknown. The degree of responsiveness to these drugs 5 years after therapy is unpredictable.

50.3.4. Side Effects

The incidence of side effects to sulfonylureas is low (between 3% and 6% overall). Table 108 illustrates the potential side effects of these drugs. Hy-

TABLE 108
Adverse Effects of Sulfonylureas

Category	Side effects
Gastrointestinal	Nausea, vomiting; heartburn; abnormal liver function; jaundice
Hematological	Agranulocytosis; red cell aplasia (aplastic anemia)
Skin	Rash; pruritus
Vasomotor	Disulfiramlike effect and flushing with alcohol (esp. chlorpropamide)
Endocrine	Thyromegaly; subclinical hypothyroidism; SIADH-like syndrome

poglycemia with sulfonylureas is most likely to occur with overdose, with concomitant renal or hepatic failure, and with drug interaction.

Several drugs affect the metabolism of sulfonylurea by multifactorial mechanisms. The half-life of sulfonylurea drugs can be shortened by enzyme induction in the liver. This is the mechanism by which rifampin and alcohol diminish the effect of sulfonylureas. The effects of sulfonylureas can be antagonized by thiazides, furosemide, propranolol, steroids, and diphenylhydantoin. In contrast, several drugs can potentiate the action of sulfonylureas and lead to profound hypoglycemia; the most important mechanism by which the hypoglycemic action of sulfonylureas is potentiated is by displacement of sulfonylureas from their binding sites in the plasma proteins (salicylates, sulfonamides, phenylbutazone, and clofibrate belong in this category). Another mechanism by which the action of sulfonylureas can be prolonged, is by prolonging the half-life of the drug. This is brought about by drugs such as dicumarol, phenylbutazone, chloramphenicol, and MAO inhibitors, which compete for the same enzymes that inactivate the sulfonylureas. Finally, the urinary excretion of sulfonylureas can be impaired by probenecid, pheylbutazone, and salicylates. Thus, it is extremely important to obtain a history of other medications taken with sulfonylureas, particularly sulfonamides, salicylates, and phenylbutazone.

50.3.5. Indications

The ideal patient for sulfonylurea therapy is the obese or normal-weight patient with NIDDM, 40 years or older, with disease duration less than 5 years. In such a patient, therapy with sulfonylurea is the second line of treatment. The first line of therapy is a 6- to 8-week course of intense dietary therapy and exercise. When these modalities fail, sulfonylurea therapy is a logical second step. Approximately 80% of patients with NIDDM will respond well to a continued regimen of dietary therapy combined with sulfonylureas. The continuing need for the drug is best determined by demonstrating that discontinuation of the drug renders the patient hyperglycemic (in the absence of weight gain) and that reinstitution normalizes the blood glucose. This maneuver would obviate the question of diet *per se* providing the benefit. The ideal goals of therapy are aimed at a fasting glucose below 100 mg/dl, a 2-hr postprandial glucose below 140 mg, and a normal glycosylated hemoglobin. The period of lasting responsiveness to the sulfonylureas varies from patient to patient (1–8 years).

The therapeutic use of the sulfonylureas must be underscored by recognizing that they are no substitute for a properly devised dietary program, they should be promptly abandoned when hyperglycemia persists, they are absolutely contraindicated in pregnancy and in insulin-dependent DM, they are relatively contraindicated in patients with renal and hepatic disease, and the safety of the sulfonylureas in patients with cardiovascular disease is still controversial.

Therapy with sulfonylureas should be abandoned under the following circumstances: when it is proven that diet alone is working, as evidenced by persistence of good glycemic control after the oral agent has been temporarily discontinued, when the blood glucose control is not satisfactory, during the presence of stress (infection, surgery, etc.), during the supervention of pregnancy, and when "secondary failure" develops or when the diabetes evolves into "insulin-requiring" diabetes mellitus.

Considering the metabolic derangements of NIDDM, the sulfonylureas appear to correct the three major abnormalities encountered in most patients with this disorder: these drugs improve insulin sensitivity by enhancing either the number of receptors or the postreceptor activity; these drugs improve the "glucose-mediated insulin response" of the β cell; and these drugs decrease the hepatic output of glucose.

Thus, the sulfonylureas are a sensible alternative to insulin in patients with NIDDM after an unsuccessful trial of diet therapy. Insulin therapy in the obese diabetic whose receptor affinity is suboptimal appears doubly unwarranted because of the well-known effect of insulin in terms of further "down-regulating" insulin receptors. As a consequence, more and more insulin will be required to achieve the same effect. The accompanying weight gain, a reflection of the lipogenic effect of insulin, further compounds the problem. Insulin therapy for the obese NIDDM patient becomes a tenable choice only after failure to sulfonylureas has been demonstrated.

50.4. Insulin Therapy

The discovery of insulin 1923 ranks as one of the most significant discoveries of this century and represents to many insulin-dependent diabetics the proverbial "new lease on life." This discovery is single-handedly responsible for decreasing the rate of acute death from diabetic ketoacidosis and for improving the day-to-day quality of life for insulin-dependent diabetics. Although the impact of insulin on therapy of diabetes has been significant, the notion that the incidence of microangiopathy in diabetes continues to remain high despite insulin therapy had minimized this impact in the past. However, the recent emergence of highly sophisticated insulin delivery systems for good glycemic control may change this outlook and may favorably influence the development of late complications. Work done in several laboratories has supported the tenet that various aspects of microangiopathy (abnormal nerve conduction velocity, basement membrane thickening, etc.) can be delayed or prevented and, in some instances, even reversed with "tight" metabolic control. In insulin-dependent diabetics, who are most often young, this glimmer of hope has added a tremendous note of optimism for dealing with the disease.

The four cornerstones that have served to integrate good therapeutic principles for such patients are:

1. The development of self-monitoring systems for glucose determination.

2. The emergence of HbA$_{1c}$ determinations to assess control.
3. The availability of highly purified insulins such as purified pork and human insulins.
4. The availability of insulin infusion systems (insulin pumps) that can synchronize insulin needs with insulin delivery.

This section outlines the indications for insulin therapy, the conventional types of insulin preparations, the factors that affect the action of insulin, the programs for insulin administration with practical pointers, the complications of insulin therapy, and, finally, the role of human insulin in the treatment of diabetes mellitus.

50.4.1. Indications for Insulin

The indications for insulin use are straightforward. The indications for "acute" use of insulin are diabetic ketoacidosis, hyperosmolar coma, and hyperglycemia complicated by infection, trauma, or surgery. All these situations require the use of regular insulin preparations that act rapidly.

The chronic use of insulin is restricted to the chronic deficiency states and includes several types of diabetics.

1. Characteristically, the insulin-dependent diabetic (type I) is the ideal candidate for insulin, since such a patient will lapse into DKA without it.
2. The symptomatic diabetic (type I and II) with polyuria, polydipsia, and weight loss coupled with severe (>400 mg) hyperglycemia.
3. The type II obese diabetic who continues to remain hyperglycemic despite a trial of diet and oral hypoglycemic agent. In this group, although insulin is not the ideal choice, it becomes the only one after the first two modalities have failed.
4. The pregnant diabetic not controlled by diet, needs to be on insulin throughout the pregnancy. This is so in light of the fact that attainment of good glycemic control, particularly during the early part of pregnancy, is associated with a decrease in the incidence of congenital malformations in the fetus. Also, good control throughout pregnancy reduces the risk of fetal death, premature labor, and other complications.

50.4.2. Insulin Preparations

Several types of insulin are marketed in the United States by different companies. In general, preparations of insulin used can be viewed in a three-dimensional fashion—its effect in terms of time (short, intermediate, or long acting), its source, and its purity. Each of these dimensions of the particular type of insulin preparation has considerable clinical impact.

The terms "short-acting," "intermediate," and "long-acting" insulins are derived on the basis of the time taken for the injected hormone to act, the

TABLE 109
Types of Insulin Based on Action

Type	Onset (hr)	Peak (hr)	Duration (hr)	Preparation of insulin
Rapid acting	½–1	3–6	6–8	Regular
				Semilente
Intermediate acting	3	8–12	18–20	NPH
				Lente
Slow acting	4	16–18	30–36	Protamine zinc
				Ultralente

peak time of its effect, and the duration for which the effects linger in the circulation. Thus, the short-acting preparations have an onset of action within an hour, reaching a peak in 3 to 6 hr, and may last up to 8 hr. The intermediate-acting insulins have an onset of action by 3 hr, with a peak attained in 8 to 12 hr, the effects lasting as long as 20 hr. The long-acting preparations take 4 hr to begin working and reach a maximal effect by 16–18 hr, the effects lingering up to 36 hr. The prototypes of "short"-acting insulins are the regular crystalline insulin and the semilente insulin; the examples of intermediate insulins, the most frequently employed variety of preparation used for chronic treatment, are NPH insulin and lente insulin; and examples of long-acting insulins, used seldom, are protamine zinc insulin (PZI) and ultralente insulin. It must be added that the time durations quoted above are subjected to tremendous intersubject and even intrasubject variations. Therefore, compartmentalizing the duration of action of any insulin preparation as "short," "intermediate," or "long" is, at best, an estimate subject to error.

TABLE 110
Classification of Insulin Based on Species

Species	Types of insulin available		
	Rapid acting	Intermediate	Long acting
Purified beef	Regular	NPH	PZI
		Lente	Ultralente (ultratard)
Purified beef and pork	—	Lente (lentard)	—
Purified pork	Regular (crystalline)	NPH	PZI
	Actrapid	Lente (monotard)	
Improved insulins USP beef–pork	Regular	NPH	PZI
	Semilente	Lente	Ultralente
Human (rDNA)	Regular	NPH	—

The source of insulin can be beef, pork, or "human." The amino acid sequence of bovine insulin differs from human insulin at three loci (A8, A10, B30). Porcine insulin, on the contrary, differs from human insulin only at one amino acid residue (B 30). Human insulin possesses an amino acid sequence homologous to native insulin secreted by the β cells. The synthesis of human insulin involves production by recombinant DNA technology. The purified pork insulin is practically identical to human insulin with the obvious drawback that it is dependent on the availability of the porcine source.

The purity of insulin is a reflection of the amount of proinsulin present in the insulin preparation. All insulins labelled "purified" contain less than 10 parts per million of proinsulin, often 0–5 ppm; all other insulins contain 20 to 35 ppm of proinsulin. When cost is not a factor, clearly all patients requiring insulin should be on only the purified preparations. Beef, pork, and beef–pork combinations of insulin are all available in the purified form. Tables 109 and 110 outline the various insulin preparations available in the United States.

50.4.3. Factors That Affect the Action of Insulin

Several factors affect the bioavailability and action of the insulin injected into the body. The site of injection to some extent influences absorption. For instance, peak concentrations of insulin are attained more quickly following abdominal injection of insulin as opposed to injections in the anterior thigh or in the buttocks. Exercise of the limb where insulin was injected may enhance absorption, as may warmth and massage of the injection area. Indeed, better absorption and quicker onset of action can be seen with deeper injection. Rarely, inactivation of the subcutaneously injected insulin can occur because of increased insulinase concentrations in the subcutaneous tissue, leading to "on-the-site degradation" of the injected insulin. A more common reason for impaired absorption of the injected insulin is when the injection is given at sites of insulin lipoatrophy.

The action of the absorbed insulin can also be modified by several factors. Intrasubject variation in the day-to-day absorption of the same dose of administered insulin can be significant. The reason for this variability is unclear. The two factors that exert a significant impact on the action of injected insulin are the presence of high titers of insulin antibodies and the degree of responsiveness of insulin receptors. Insulin antibodies bind and hold on to exogenous insulin for variable lengths of time, resulting in a delay in the onset and duration of insulin. In fact, one variety of insulin response, termed "delayed response," in which the onset of intermediate insulin is delayed but protracted, is thought to occur as a consequence of this "holding-on" effect of insulin antibodies. This phenomenon is unusual when purified pork or human insulins are used.

In addition to humoral antibodies, the responsiveness of insulin receptors also has a considerable impact on the action of exogenously administered insulin. Obesity is the major predisposing factor that down-regulates insulin receptors. Hyperinsulinemia, whether attained by endogenous secretion or exogenous administration, is also an important determinant that further down-regulates receptors. Rarely, antireceptor antibodies in the circulation may prevent insulin binding with the receptors. On the other hand, exercise and weight reduction enhance the responsiveness of the insulin receptors, accounting for the hypersensitivity to insulin seen in athletes.

In addition to the above factors, the development of renal failure is associated with a prolongation of the half-life of insulin, rendering the patient susceptible to hypoglycemia.

50.4.4. Programs for Insulin Administration

Unlike other replacement therapies in endocrinology, insulin treatment of the diabetic is characterized by extreme heterogeneity in the response to insulin among different patients; even in the same patient, there may be significant variations on a day-to-day basis. Although it is true that insulin therapy cannot be mastered from any textbook, there are some general principles regarding insulin therapy that need to be outlined.

Realistically, the true insulin-dependent diabetic, without any insulin reserve, cannot be expected to be rendered normoglycemic throughout the day with a single dose of intermediate insulin in the morning. This is because physiologically, the normal β cell secretes insulin in synchronicity with each meal. One dose of NPH or lente insulin given in the morning can hardly be expected to mimic the pulses of insulin peaks needed to metabolize each meal. The ideal method to mimic the meal-associated pulses of insulin is to administer regular insulin before each meal. This method obviously has practical limitations.

The type of diabetic who can be maintained euglycemic throughout the day with a single dose of NPH probably has some endogenous insulin on board.

The starting dose of NPH or lente is approximately 0.2 to 0.5 U/kg administered before breakfast. Since the NPH or lente will not provide coverage to metabolize the load of breakfast or lunch, it is advisable to combine regular insulin with NPH; usually the dose of regular insulin in the morning is approximately one- to two-thirds of the NPH dose.

Adjustments in the morning dose of NPH are made on the basis of the blood glucose level obtained presupper; the adjustments in the morning dose of regular insulin are made on the basis of prelunch blood glucose levels.

Adjustments in the morning dose of NPH can also be made, albeit indirectly, on the basis of the fasting blood glucose. For every 20 mg/dl of FBS exceeding 140 mg/dl, the prebreakfast NPH or lente dose can be increased by 1 U.

When the morning dose of NPH (or lente) exceeds 50 U, the dose should be "split." This can be done by reducing the morning dose of NPH by 20% and giving that 20% dose before supper.

When persistent fasting hyperglycemia is present despite an increase in

TABLE 111
Insulin Dosage Administration Patterns, Problems, and Suggested Modifications

Present Rx	FBG	Prelunch BG	Presupper BG	Bedtime BG	Modification
a.m. NPH	↑	↑	↑	↑	↑ a.m. NPH
a.m. NPH	N	↑	N	N	Add regular insulin in a.m.
a.m. NPH					↑ NPH; "Split"
a.m. Reg	↑	N	↑	↑	dose if a.m. dose exceeds 50 U
a.m. NPH	↑	N	N	↑	Add p.m. Reg
a.m. Reg					
a.m. NPH	↑	N	N	N	Add p.m. NPH
a.m. Reg					
a.m. NPH	N	N	N	N	Lower dose

the presupper NPH dose, the Somogyi effect should be suspected, i.e., post-hypoglycemic hyperglycemia from rebound. This can be excluded by checking the patient's blood glucose between midnight and 6 a.m. for hypoglycemia.

Adjustments in the dosage and schedule of insulin should be made gradually, one change at a time. Table 111 illustrates the various types of problems that may arise in patients treated with insulin. The changes or modifications suggested are made on the assumption that dietary considerations are reliably and strictly enforced. An additional problem not outlined in Table 111 is persistent postbreakfast hyperglycemia despite good glycemic control throughout the day. This is caused by the normal surge of cortisol in the early morning ("dawn phenomenon"). This problem can be handled by administering the dose of a.m. regular insulin 1–2 hr before breakfast.

In a patient previously well controlled with insulin, the development of "loss of control" should be evaluated with a multifactorial and systematic perspective. Thus, careful attention to dietary history, evaluation for stress factors (particularly infection), the search for a history of alcohol or drugs in the background, and a careful physical examination with focus on weight changes or coexistent endocrinopathies are essential facets in the differential diagnostic considerations. The possibility of Somogyi effect and antibody-mediated humoral resistance should also be carefully excluded.

Finally, in patients with wide glycemic excursions that preclude making therapeutic decisions based on single blood glucose or urine glucose determinations, the patient should be taught self blood glucose monitoring. Algorithms based on patterns derived by observing the self-glucose values immensely aid in controlling the glycemic excursions.

50.4.5. Complications of Insulin Therapy

The main complications of insulin therapy are outlined in Table 112. Each of these deserves brief mention.

TABLE 112
Complications of Insulin Therapy

1. Hypoglycemia
2. Somogyi phenomenon
3. Insulin allergy
4. Insulin resistance
5. Insulin lipoatrophy
6. Insulin edema

50.4.5.1. Insulin Hypoglycemia

Insulin-induced hypoglycemia occurs from inadvertent overinsuliniza-tion. Every diabetic receiving insulin should be familiarized with the symptoms of hypoglycemia. The sympathomedullary symptoms as well as the neurogly-copenic symptoms of hypoglycemia can be easily corrected by the oral or intravenous administration of glucose. In some insulin-dependent diabetics, the counterregulatory mechanisms to combat hypoglycemia can be severely impaired. The reason for this is not clear. The hypoglycemia in such a setting can be protracted and severe, resulting in altered consciousness without the warning signals of hypoglycemia such as nervousness, tremors, etc. Every diabetic receiving insulin should carry an emergency kit containing glucose (candy) and a vial of glucagon; this is a potent glycogenolytic hormone that rapidly mobilizes glucose from the liver, making it available for the tissues.

50.4.5.2. The Somogyi Phenomenon

The Somogyi phenomenon refers to the development of posthypogly-cemic hyperglycemia. Although the frequency of the Somogyi phenomenon complicating glycemic control is not exactly clear, it is particularly common in young insulin-dependent diabetics. The classic situation that sets the stage for Somogyi phenomenon is when the morning dose of NPH (or lente) is gradually increased based on the persistence of fasting hyperglycemia. As a result of overinsulinization, hypoglycemia occurs in the late night or early morning hours. There is some correlation between the size of the dose of intermediate insulin and its half-life. The symptoms of hypoglycemia are often missed since the patient is usually asleep. The hypoglycemia results in the release of several counterinsulin hormones, such as glucagon, epinephrine, growth hormone, and cortisol, in an attempt to raise the blood glucose. This results in rebound hyperglycemia. Since these hormones are also lipolytic, the resultant increase in the free fatty acids mobilized from the fatty tissue leads to ketosis. Therefore, the patient wakes up with hyperglycemia and ketonuria. This phenomenon creates a vicious cycle in which progressively increasing doses of insulin (mistakenly given in the assumption of insulin deficiency) result in further perpetuation of the problem. The Somogyi phenomenon should be kept in mind in the differential diagnosis of apparent "insulin resistance" and apparent "brittle" diabetes.

The features that should raise the suspicion of Somogyi phenomenon are:

1. Symptoms of nocturnal hypoglycemia.
2. Marked ketonuria in the prebreakfast sample.
3. Persistent hyperglycemia in the morning.
4. Weight gain, reflecting overinsulinization, is often present. However, when the Somogyi phenomenon is chronic, weight loss may be seen because of the lipolytic effects of the counterinsulin hormones.
5. When a child with insulin-dependent diabetes receives more than 1 to 1.5 U of insulin per kg body weight, Somogyi phenomenon should be suspected.
6. Wide swings in urine glucose and ketones throughout the day should also invoke the suspicion of Somogyi phenomenon.

Once this is suspected, the blood glucose levels during late night or early morning should be obtained to document hypoglycemia. This should be relatively easy and practical in the patient well versed with home glucose monitoring. The therapeutic approach for the documented Somogyi effect is gradual decrease in the dose of the intermediate insulin.

50.4.5.3. Insulin Allergy

Local allergy to insulin is manifested by pruritus and the subsequent development of erythematous indurated lesions at the injection sites. This reaction is mediated by IgE antibodies. The incidence of local allergy to insulin has considerably declined since the introduction of purified pork insulins, supporting the notion that these local reactions may be secondary to impurities or, rarely, to protamine or zinc. Local reactions to insulin generally tend to improve with the continued use of insulin.

Generalized insulin allergy, on the other hand, can be of variable severity, ranging from a generalized urticarial rash to angioneurotic edema, bronchospasm, and death from circulatory collapse. The generalized insulin reactions represent the interaction between insulin and IgE antibodies bound to the mast cells in various tissues. Generalized insulin allergy is, thankfully, rare and is probably a reaction to the insulin molecule *per se*. If the patient with systemic insulin allergy can be managed by dietary means or by oral hypoglycemic agents, avoidance of insulin is preferred. If this is not feasible, then desensitization to insulin should be undertaken in the ICU setting. Intradermal testing is performed using purified pork and purified beef insulin, 1/1000 and 1/500 U, respectively; unless the results indicate greater reactivity to pork than to beef, desensitization is initiated using the materials in the insulin allergy desensitization kit. The success rate of desensitization is 90–95%. The ability of the desensitization procedure to eliminate insulin allergy is probably based on depletion of the mediators of immediate hypersensitivity.

50.4.5.4. Insulin Resistance

Although all patients receiving beef or pork insulin will develop antibodies to these insulins, the problem becomes clinically significant in a minority of patients in whom such antibodies neutralize the effects of insulin. This form of "insulin resistance" is also termed "humoral resistance," since it is mediated by humoral antibodies belonging to the IgG class. As anticipated, humoral (or antibody-mediated) resistance is most pronounced with beef insulin, since this differs from human insulin in the sequence of three amino acids. Humoral antibodies occur less significantly when the purified forms of insulin are used. The tendency to generate antibodies is greater with NPH and lente insulin in comparison to regular insulins. Finally, the intermittent use of insulin is associated with a higher incidence of humorally mediated immunologic resistance.

The term "insulin resistance" used to be applied to situations in which the insulin requirements exceed 200 U in the absence of stress, infection, Somogyi phenomenon etc. In reality, insulin resistance occurs with much lower doses and should be suspected when more than 1 U of insulin per kg body weight is being required. It is hoped that with the use of purified pork or human insulin, the problem of antibody-mediated insulin resistance would decline significantly.

The measurement of insulin antibody titers does not correlate with the severity of the resistance. This is because it is the ability of these antibodies to neutralize the insulin that determines clinical resistance, not the mere titers. A possible etiologic link between insulin antibody titers and microangiopathic complications of diabetes was once suggested but has been currently discarded.

The treatment of insulin resistance secondary to antibodies is approached by switching to purer forms of insulin such as purified pork insulin or human insulin. The use of sulfated or dealanated insulins and glucocorticoid therapy is rarely resorted to today.

50.4.5.5. Insulin Lipodystrophy

There are two forms of lipodystrophy associated with the use of insulin: insulin lipoatrophy characterized by loss of subcutaneous tissue at the sites of injection and insulin hypertrophy, which consists of a spongy swelling at the site of injection. It is believed that insulin lipoatrophy is a result of "impurities" in the insulin preparation. The incidence of both forms of lipodystrophy is considerably lower in patients treated with purified and "single-peak" insulins. (The single-peak insulins are derived by careful chromatographic separation, which elutes only insulin.)

Insulin lipoatrophy is characterized by "dimples," which represent localized areas of loss in the subcutaneous fat. The loss of fat can occur at sites other than the injection sites. The condition is slowly progressive and can result in considerable disfigurement. Insulin lipoatrophy is almost always preventable by rotating the sites of injection and by using purified forms of insulin. Once it has occurred, the treatment consists of injecting purified forms of insulin (purified pork or human) into the affected area. The success rate of this form of therapy is high (>80%).

Insulin hypertrophy, less common than lipoatrophy, can occur in conjunction with lipoatrophy. The condition, which starts as a spongy swelling, eventually transforms into a fibrous, avascular area, often with anesthesia in the overlying skin. The importance of insulin hypertrophy lies in the fact that insulin injected into these sites is inadequately absorbed. The therapeutic response of insulin hypertrophy to the use of purified insulins is much lower in comparison with insulin lipoatrophy.

50.4.5.6. Insulin Edema

Insulin edema is a rare, self-limiting complication of insulin therapy. When seen, insulin edema almost invariably is associated with the use of insulin in patients with very poor glycemic control. The edema, usually localized to the legs, occurs within 1 week after initiating or adjusting therapy and dissipates within a week or two. The mechanism is unclear and bears a resemblance to the edema of refeeding associated with malnutrition.

From the foregoing, it is apparent that several complications that are associated with the use of insulin therapy can be expected to decline significantly with the use of more and more purified forms of insulin, the ultimate representation of which is human insulin. Human insulin is produced by recombinant technology, either by linking the separately produced A and B chains or by single fermentation to synthesize proinsulin, which is subsequently cleaved to form insulin. Human insulin is chemically, physiologically, and immunologically equivalent to native insulin and is free of several pancreatic peptides such as proinsulin, somatostatin, pancreatic polypeptide (PP), and vasoactive intestinal polypeptide (VIP).

When human insulin is compared to purified pork insulin in terms of potency, both insulins are identical. Although human NPH insulin is absorbed faster than pork NPH and has a slightly shorter duration of action, these changes in absorption and duration of effects are not particularly advantageous. Although human insulin is less immunogenic than pork, the clinical impact of this difference is arguable. The superiority of human insulin probably lies in its risk-free potential in the development of allergy and lipodystrophy.

In the absence of insulin allergy or lipodystrophy, there is no valid reason to switch patients on purified pork insulin to human insulin (which is considerably more expensive). When short-term insulin treatment is contemplated, human insulin with its negligible immunogenic potential is an ideal choice. Human insulin is also the ideal alternative in diabetics with lipodystrophy and allergy. It has been suggested, but not proven, that human insulin is superior to pork insulin in the gestational diabetic. Finally, the tenet that all newly diagnosed diabetics who need insulin should be placed on human insulin because of its immunogenic advantages is theoretically sound if cost were not a consideration. The immunologic advantages and superiority of human insulin should be tempered by scattered reports of the development of insulin allergy to synthetic human insulin in patients who have shown allergy to animal insulins. The real advantage of human insulin production by recombinant DNA technology is that it provides an inexhaustible resource of a highly purified product. The excitement generated by human insulin synthesis is that it represents the first successful product of recombinant DNA technology, marking the first step in this area of biotechnological revolution.

No section on insulin therapy would be complete without mentioning the newer methods of insulin delivery. The "insulin pump" currently used is an open-loop system devised for the delivery of insulin by continuous subcutaneous insulin infusion. After several modifications, the development of a small, technically advanced, and practically usable pump is currently a reality. Regardless of the company manufacturing the pump and the "options" available in the hardware, the principle of continuous subcutaneous insulin infusion is the same: the patient receives a basal small amount of insulin on an hourly basis, augmented by timed boluses in synchronicity with meals. Thus, the insulin delivery mimics the physiological secretion of insulin by the β cell. The programming of the pump is done by the patient and physician based on the blood glucose levels obtained by self blood glucose monitoring. Pump therapy is not to be considered an alternative to dietary and other ancillary modes of therapy. Rather, pump therapy should be viewed as an alternative to provide a most physiological means of insulin delivery to the "brittle" diabetic.

Selected Readings

Anderson, J. W., and Ward, K.: Long term effects of high carbohydrate high fiber diets on glucose and lipid metabolism. A preliminary report on patients with diabetes, *Diabetes Care* **1**:77, 1978.

Arieff, A. I., and Carroll, H. J.: Nonketotic hyperosmolar coma with hyperglycemia—clinical features, pathophysiology, renal function, acid base balance, plasma–CSF equilibria and the effects of therapy in 37 cases, *Medicine* **51**:73, 1972.

Bloodworth, J. M. B., and Engerman, R. L.: Diabetic microangiopathy in the experimentally diabetic dog and its prevention by careful control with insulin, *Diabetes* **22**:290, 1973.

Bottazzo, G. F., Florin-Christensen, A., and Doniach, D.: Islet cell antibodies in diabetes mellitus with autoimmune polyendocrine deficiencies, *Lancet* **2**:1279, 1974.

Burde, P. M.: Diabetic ophthalmoplegia, *Am. Ophthalmol. J.* **27**:48, 1977.

Carroll, P., and Matz, R.: Protocol for treating diabetic ketoacidosis and hyperosmolar nonketotic coma, *Diabetes Care* **6**:579, 1983.

Craighead, J. E.: The role of viruses in the pathogenesis of pancreatic disease and diabetes mellitus, *Prog. Med. Virol.* **19**:161, 1975.

DeFronzo, R. A., and Ferrannini, E.: The pathogenesis of noninsulin dependent diabetes. An update, *Medicine* **61**:125, 1982.

The Diabetic Retinopathy Study Research Group: The third report from the diabetic retinopathy study, *Arch. Ophthalmol.* **97**:654, 1979.

Ellenberg, M.: Impotence—what it is—four major misconceptions about impotence and diabetes, *Diabetes Forecast* **31**:36, 1978.

Ensinck, J. W., and Bierman, E. L.: Dietary management of diabetes mellitus, *Annu. Rev. Med.* **30:**155, 1979.

Faerman, I., and Glocer, L., Fox, D., *et al.:* Impotence and diabetes: Histological studies of the autonomic fibers of the corpora cavernosa in impotent diabetic males, *Diabetes* **23:**971, 1974.

Felig, P., and Bergman, M.: Intensive ambulatory treatment of insulin dependent diabetes, *Ann. Intern. Med.* **97:**225, 1982.

Felig, P., and Bergman, M.: Insulin pump treatment of diabetes, *J.A.M.A.* **250:**1045, 1983.

Foster, D. W., and McGarry, J. D.: The metabolic derangements and treatment of diabetic ketoacidosis, *N. Engl. J. Med.* **309:**159, 1983.

Fraser, D. M., Campbell, I. W., Edwing, D. J., *et al.:* Mononeuropathy in diabetes mellitus, *Diabetes* **28:**96, 1979.

Galloway, J. A., and Bressler, R.: Insulin treatment in diabetes, *Med. Clin. North Am.* **62:**663, 1978.

Gerich, J. E., Martin, M. M., and Recant, L.: Clinical and metabolic characteristics of hyperosmolar nonketotic coma, *Diabetes* **20:**228, 1971.

Home, P. D., and Alberti, K. G. M. M.: The new insulins. Their characteristics and clinical indications, *Drugs* **24:**401, 1982.

Jackson, R. L., Hess, R. L., and England, J. D.: Hemoglobin A_{1c} values in children with overt diabetes maintained in varying degrees of control, *Diabetes Care* **2:**391, 1979.

Job, D., Eschwege, E., Guyot-Argenton, C., *et al.:* Effect of multiple daily insulin injections on the course of diabetic retinopathy, *Diabetes* **25:**463, 1976.

Jovanovic, L., and Peterson, C.: The clinical utility of glycosylated hemoglobin, *Am. J. Med.* **70:**331, 1981.

Kahn, H. A., and Hiller, R.: Blindness caused by diabetic retinopathy, *Am. J. Ophthalmol.* **78:**58, 1974.

Kitabchi, A. E., Ayyagari, V., and Guerra, S. M. O.: The efficacy of low dose versus conventional therapy of insulin for treatment of diabetic ketoacidosis, *Ann. Intern. Med.* **84:**633, 1976.

Kreisberg, R. A.: Diabetic ketoacidosis: New concepts, and trends in pathogenesis and treatment, *Ann. Intern. Med.* **88:**681, 1978.

Kussman, M. J., Goldstein, H., and Gleason, R. E.: The clinical course of diabetic nephropathy, *J.A.M.A.* **236:**1861, 1976.

Lambert, A. E.: The regulation of insulin secretion, *Rev. Physiol. Biochem. Pharmacol.* **75:**98, 1976.

Lebowitz, H. E., and Feinglos, M. N.: Sulfonylurea drugs: Mechanism of antidiabetic action and therapeutic usefulness, *Diabetes Care* **1:**189, 1978.

Liang, J. C., and Goldberg, M. F.: Treatment of diabetic retinopathy, *Diabetes* **29:**841, 1980.

Mauer, S. M., Steffes, M. E., and Brown, D. M.: The kidney in diabetes, *Am. J. Med.* **70:**603, 1981.

McCurdy, D. K.: Hyperosmolar hyperglycemic nonketotic diabetic coma, *Med. Clin. North Am.* **54:**683, 1970.

McGarry, J. D., and Foster, D. W.: Ketogenesis and its regulation, *Am. J. Med.* **61:**9, 1976.

Mecklenburg, R. S., Benson, J. W., Becker, N. M., *et al.:* Clinical use of the insulin infusion pump in 100 patients with type I diabetes, *N. Engl. J. Med.* **307:**513, 1982.

Najarian, J.S., Sutherland, D. E. R., and Simmons, R. L.: Ten year experience with renal transplantation in juvenile onset diabetes, *Ann. Surg.* **190:**487, 1979.

Nerup, J., Platz, P., Anderson, O. O., *et al.:* HL-A antigens and diabetes mellitus, *Lancet* **2:**864, 1974.

Nuttal, F. Q.: Diet and the diabetic patient, *Diabetes Care* **6:**197, 1983.

Okiye, S. E., Engen, D. E., Sterioff, S. S., *et al.:* Primary and secondary renal transplantation in diabetic patients, *J.A.M.A.* **249:**492, 1983.

Oliva, P. B.: Lactic acidosis, *Am. J. Med.* **48:**209, 1970.

Osterby, R., and Gundersen, H. J.: Glomerular size and structure in diabetes mellitus—early abnormalities, *Diabetologia* **11:**225, 1975.

Porte, D., Jr., and Bagdade, J. D.: Human insulin secretion: An integrated approach, *Annu. Rev. Med.* **21:**219, 1970.

Reaven, G. M.: Therapeutic approaches to reducing insulin resistance in patients with noninsulin dependent diabetes mellitus, *Am. J. Med.* **74:**109, 1983.

Rubenstein, A. H., and Steiner, D. F.: Proinsulin, *Annu. Rev. Med.* **22:**1, 1971.

Schmidt, M. I., Georgopoulous, A. H., Rendell, M. *et al.:* The dawn phenomenon, an early morning glucose rise: Implications for diabetic intraday glucose variation, *Diabetes Care* **4:**579, 1981.

Somogyi, M.: Exacerbation of diabetes by excess insulin action, *Am. J. Med.* **26:**169, 1959.

Sotile, W. M.: The penile prosthesis and diabetic impotence—some caveats, *Diabetes Care* **2:**26, 1979.

Steiner, D. F.: Insulin today, *Diabetes* **26:**322, 1977.

Tattersall, R. B., and Fajans, S. S.: A difference between the inheritance of classical juvenile-onset and maturity-onset diabetes of young people, *Diabetes* **24:**44, 1975.

Varner, M. W.: Efficacy of home glucose monitoring in diabetic pregnancy, *Am. J. Med.* **75:**592, 1983.

West, K. M.: Diet therapy of diabetes: an analysis of failure, *Ann. Intern. Med.* **79:**425, 1973.

Zimmett, P. Z., Taft, P., Ennis, G. C., *et al.:* Acid production in diabetic ketoacidosis—a more rational approach to alkali replacement, *Br. Med. J.* **3:**610, 1970.

IX

Miscellany

51

Islet Cell Tumors

51.1. Introduction

Islet cell tumors can originate from different cell types of the islets of Langerhans. Depending on the cell type from which they originate, islet cell tumors can hypersecrete insulin, gastrin, glucagon, or vasoactive intestinal polypeptide. In this chapter, the physiological control of glucose homeostasis is discussed first as a prelude to understanding the manifold presentations of the β-cell tumor, insulinoma. This is followed by an overview of the physiological control of gastrin secretion as a background for understanding the Zollinger–Ellison syndromes. Finally, the features of the rare Verner–Morrison syndrome and glucagonoma are presented.

51.2. Glucose Homeostasis

An overview of the regulatory mechanisms that control glucose homeostasis is essential for understanding the mechanisms of hypoglycemia. The sources of glucose are exogenous (from the dietary sugars) and endogenous (from the liver, which synthesizes and releases glucose). In the postabsorptive state, when endogenous mechanisms are the prime source for glucose production and release, several organ systems compete for the plasma glucose; i.e., the central nervous system utilizes 60% of the glucose in the postabsorptive state, 20% is utilized by the bone marrow, the formed elements of blood, the kidney, and the peripheral nerves, and the remaining 20% of utilized by the adipose tissue and muscle. During a fast there are several adjustments made that shift the metabolic gears in an extremely coordinated fashion. The goal is to maintain the blood glucose with no more than a 10–15% variation from normal.

The metabolic adjustments made during the fasting state are the following:

1. Change in the metabolic fuel used. In order to preserve whatever glucose is left, adipose tissue, muscle, and liver completely stop utilizing it and rapidly switch to utilizing fatty acids as the source of their energy requirements. The brain initially continues to use glucose as fuel, as do the other glycolyzing tissues—red cells, kidney, and the bone marrow. With extreme prolongation of the fast, even the brain adapts to using ketones as an energy source.

2. Glycogenolysis. This mechanism is the first to be activated. The liver is rich in glycogen stores, and the glycogenolytic enzymes are activated to produce glucose from the breakdown of glycogen. Endogenous glucose release is possible only from the liver, and approximately 75% of the glucose released from the liver during fasting comes from glycogen breakdown. This process of glycogenolysis obviously depends on the amount of glycogen stores in the liver, the integrity of the enzymes, and the mediation of a number of hormones, most importantly glucagon and to a lesser extent catecholamines, glucocorticoids, and growth hormone. All these hormones are glycogenolytic.

3. Gluconeogenesis. If the subject continues to fast, within 48 hr the glycogen stores get depleted. The liver must now look for some other method to keep supplying glucose. When the glycogenolytic reserve is strained, the liver switches to actually producing glucose via a vital process called gluconeogenesis. This process, although initially accounting for no more than 25% of hepatic glucose output, becomes the sole mechanism when the glycogen stores become depleted. The later can happen with prolonged fast, in a malnourished cachectic state, or when glucagon is not available. Gluconeogenesis is an extremely involved process requiring three basis factors. First, the substrate to make glucose must be available. The major precursors of gluconeogenesis are lactate, the amino acid alanine, and, to a lesser extent, pyruvate and glycerol. When the substrate is not available, as in hypoalaninemia seen with chronic malnutrition, prolonged fasting, or in renal failure, gluconeogenesis becomes impaired. Second, the enzymes needed for gluconeogenesis must be available. There are several enzymes involved, but two are particularly important, pyruvate carboxylase (PC) and phosphoenolpyruvate carboxykinase (PEPCK). These are the enzymes involved in the initial steps of incorporating lactate and alanine into pyruvate, oxaloacetate, and phosphoenolpyruvate. When there is liver disease severe enough to impair availability of these enzymes, gluconeogenesis becomes impaired (e.g., fulminant hepatitis). More importantly, these enzymes need adequate NAD (disphosphopyridine nucleotide) to function efficiently. For instance, when ethanol is metabolized to acetaldehyde and acetate, tremendous amounts of NAD are used, which in turn is converted to NADH (reduced diphosphopyridine nucleotide). The resultant lack of available NAD is the reason for impaired gluconeogenesis in ethanol-induced hypoglycemia. Third, the liver must be able to release glucose into the

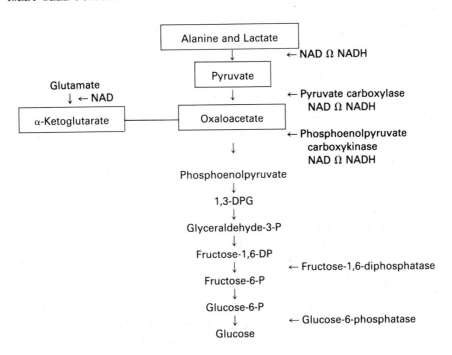

FIGURE 29. Pathway for gluconeogenesis.

circulation. This action can be modified by various hormones. Glucagon facilitates glucose output from the liver, and insulin suppresses it. Therefore, hyperinsulinemia in the fasted state has an adverse effect on hepatic glucose release. The various steps involved in gluconeogenesis are outlined in Figure 29. Despite its complexity, the gluconeogenic process is an extremely viable one, the major deterrent being lack of NAD.

4. Ketone utilization. If the person continues to fast (longer than 1 week), even the amazing ability of the liver becomes strained, and the rate of glucose production begins to decline. It is now that the brain begins to use ketones (which are provided by the breakdown of fat). The kidney now joins forces with the liver and assumes production of glucose by gluconeogenesis.

5. Hormonal adjustments. The role of insulin and glucagon in the fasted state are reciprocal; i.e., with fasting, insulin is promptly suppressed (the net effect being decreased utilization of glucose by tissues and increased glucose output by the liver), and glucagon levels are elevated (with the net effect being increased glycogenolysis, release of hepatic glucose, and lipolysis to provide fatty acids as energy source for the liver).

To summarize, the five adjustments required for glucose homeostasis during fasting are:

1. Shift in glucose utilization by various tissues.
2. Increased heptic glycogenolysis.
3. Increased hepatic gluconeogenesis.
4. Ketone utilization.
5. Hormonal adjustments (↓ insulin, ↑ glucagon).

Because of the elegant balance of hormonal interplay, starvation *per se* does not cause hypoglycemia in normal subjects. With starvation, there is a prompt decrease in insulin levels with a concomitant increase in glucagon levels. In the first 24 hr of starvation, accelerated glycogenolysis results in increased hepatic output of glucose, which prevents hypoglycemia. After the liver glycogen stores are depleted, gluconeogenesis serves as the major mode of glucose homeostasis.

Hypoglycemia, defined as a drop in blood glucose levels below 40%, can occur from either impaired hepatic glucose production or increased glucose utilization. The several causes of hypoglycemia are listed in Tables 113 and 114, with the respective mechanisms outlined. The features of some common varieties of fasting hypoglycemia deserve emphasis.

Alcohol-induced hypoglycemia is an extremely common etiology of fasting hypoglycemia. The mechanism of ethanol-induced hypoglycemia is impaired gluconeogenesis. Alcohol affects three aspects of gluconeogenesis:

1. When alcohol is metabolized, it "steals" the NAD needed for gluconeogenesis. Individuals who are nutritionally compromised already have depleted glycogen stores. When such individuals imbibe ethanol, especially when not eating, the only resource to maintain euglycemia is gluconeogenesis. By utilizing NAD and therefore increasing the ratio of NADH/NAD, alcohol precludes proper conversion of precursors into lactate. This results in stymieing of gluconeogensis.

TABLE 113
Etiology and Mechanisms of Fasting Hypoglycemia:
Impaired Glucose Production

1. Alcoholic hypoglycemia	Impaired gluconeogenesis because of lack of NAD, which is utilized for alcohol metabolism
2. Hypopituitarism, Addison's disease	Impaired gluconeogenesis because of cortisol lack
3. Myxedema	Impairment in enzymes needed for glycogenolysis and gluconeogenesis
4. Liver disease	Fulminant or severe disease impairing hepatic function
5. Renal disease	Lack of availability of amino acid precursors for gluconeogenous
6. Glycogen storage disease	Impaired glycogenolysis because of lack of glycogenolytic enzymes

TABLE 114
Etiology and Mechanisms of Fasting Hypoglycemia:
Increased Glucose Utilization

1. Insulinoma	Autonomous production of insulin by tumor of the β cell
2. Insulin or sulfonylurea overdose	Increased utilization of glucose by tissues
3. Nonislet tumors Hepatoma Retroperitoneal mesenchymal tumor	Glucose sequestration by tumor or production of insulinlike growth factor II
4. Immunologic	Autoantibodies to endogenous insulin that bind and release insulin
5. Septicemia	Unclear

2. Alcohol diminishes efflux of alanine from the skeletal muscle, thereby diminishing the supply of available substrate.
3. In addition, alcohol diminishes the uptake of alanine, lactate, and glycerol by the hepatocytes.

It must be realized that one does not have to consume extreme quantities of alcohol to become hypoglycemic. In a malnourished, cachectic individual who is not eating and whose liver glycogen is depleted, even moderate amounts of alcohol can precipitate dangerously low levels of blood glucose. The clinical presentation is not much different from other etiologies of hypoglycemia. Two important facets of ethanol hypoglycemia should be remembered. First, there is a paucity of symptoms of sympathomedullary discharge, and second, severe hypothermia is seen more often than in other etiologies of hypoglycemia. The CNS manifestations can be protean and include coma, convulsions, conjugate deviation of eyes, extensor rigidity, trismus, and positive Babinski reflexes.

There are two important aspects to be remembered with regard to therapy. First, even though these patients usually respond well to intravenous glucose, the mortality rate of alcoholic hypoglycemia is 11% in adults and 25% in children. Second, coma may recur if the glucose infusions are discontinued prematurely. Therefore, these patients should have continuous 5% or even 10% dextrose intravenously until adequate oral carbohydrates can be tolerated.

Fasting hypoglycemia secondary to liver disease is seen only when hepatic function is markedly compromised. The mechanism of hypoglycemia is related to generator failure and inadequate gluconeogenesis. In general, destruction of more than 75% to 80% of liver mass is required to produce significant hypoglycemia. Thus, even with widespread liver disease such as cirrhosis, metastatic liver disease, or sarcoidosis, hypoglycemia is seldom seen. The classical settings in which hypoglycemia occurs from liver failure are hepatitis of pregnancy, toxic hepatitis (from halothane, tetracycline, carbon tetrachloride, or phosphorus burns), and severe fatty liver with malignant malnutrition. In all these settings, the output of glucose from the liver is markedly diminished, and gluconeogenesis is severely compromised because of poor uptake by functionally impaired hepatocytes.

The hypoglycemia of renal failure is multifactorial. The most important reason is poor availability of substrate for gluconeogenesis. For instance, alanine turnover can be markedly diminished in chronic renal failure, resulting in diminished alanine delivery to the liver. This can be compounded by poor nutrition and low-protein diets prescribed for renal failure. Diminished degradation of insulin may also play a contributory role.

The fasting hypoglycemia of hypoadrenalism reflects the important role of glucocorticoids in hepatic glucose production and release and is seen only with severe hypoadrenalism caused by either hypopituitarism or Addison's disease. Hypoglycemia is particularly seen with panhypopituitarism, in which the loss of ACTH and growth hormone have a synergistic effect in causing hypoglycemia.

The hypoglycemia seen in association with nonpancreatic tumors is rare. The hypoglycemia in some of these settings results from ectopic secretion of insulin or insulinlike substances. Four, in particular, have been described: primary hepatocellular carcinoma, retroperitoneal tumors, bronchogenic carcinoma, and adrenocortical carcinoma.

Primary hepatocellular carcinoma (HCC) is the malignancy most frequently reported to be associated with hypoglycemia. The high incidence of this phenomenon reported from the Far East has not been found in the United States.

The mechanisms are probably multiple and include (1) excessive secretion of insulin, (2) impaired gluconeogenesis because of hypoalaninemia, (3) depleted glycogen content secondary to the disease process in the liver as well as the nutritional status of the patient, and (4) occasionally, increased glucose utilization by the tumor.

The hypoglycemia seen with retroperitoneal tumors of mesenchymal origin is a well-recognized entity. These tumors are usually fibrosarcoma, leiomyosarcoma, or rhabdomyosarcoma. They are large and often palpable. These tumors are highly malignant and render the patient rapidly cachectic. It is believed that these tumors utilize large quantities of glucose. The presence of nonsuppressible insulinlike activity has been demonstrated in these patients by a sensitive radioreceptor assay. Thus, these tumors, although not really secreting insulin, seem to secrete some substance with insulinlike activity. It is currently believed that this substance represents insulinlike growth factor II, a peptide with properties similar to the peptides of the somatomedin family. These tumors also possess high rates of anerobic glycolysis.

Adrenal carcinoma is also known to secrete insulin or insulinlike substances. Adrenal carcinoma is a very malignant tumor and can present with abdominal pain, weight loss, and hepatic metastases. The majority of adrenal carcinomas are of the nonsecretory variety; i.e., they do not cause virilization of Cushing's syndrome. The condition should be kept in mind when metastatic disease presents in the absence of an overt primary. Most carcinomas of the adrenal gland can be visualized by CT scanning.

The occurrence of hypoglycemia in bronchogenic carcinoma is a relatively rare phenomenon and can be seen with both squamous and anaplastic bronchogenic carcinomas.

The hypoglycemia of islet cell tumor is discussed in the following section.

51.3. Insulinoma

Insulinoma is a tumor arising from the pancreatic β islet cell that normally secretes insulin.

51.3.1. Etiology

Islet cell tumors are rare. The peak incidence of these tumors is in the fourth or fifth decade of life. In 80% of cases, a single adenoma is responsible. In the remaining 20%, the etiology is multiple adenomas, hyperplasia, or carcinoma of the islet cells. In addition, carcinoid tumors of the islet cells also constitute a small percentage. The term nesidioblastosis is used to denote autonomous hypersecretion secondary to β-cell hyperplasia. A small percentage of insulin-secreting islet cell tumors are associated with multiple endocrine adenomatosis I. The incidence of malignancy in β-cell tumors ranges from 10% to 25%.

51.3.2. Clinical Features

The clinical presentations of an insulinoma can be extremely variable, ranging from a dramatic acute presentation with severe hypoglycemia to highly subtle presentations that elude the diagnosis.

51.3.2.1. Acute Presentation

Acute hypoglycemia developing when the patient fasts or following exercise characterizes the major presentation of β-cell tumors. In 80–85% of patients with insulinoma, abnormal behavior is noted during an "attack." The abnormal behavior may consist of confusion or temporary amnesia coupled with any of the following: sweating, palpitations, blurred vision, diplopia, or weakness. Grand mal seizures are seen in 10–15% of patients with β-cell tumors. The symptoms of acute neuroglycopenia occur most often in the morning and late afternoon. A careful history may reveal the temporal association between the symptoms and fasting or exercise. The latter is an important clue in differentiating organic hyperinsulinism from "functional hypoglycemia." Exercise precipitates or aggravates the hypoglycemia of insulinoma, whereas it often improves the symptoms in functional hypoglycemia.

51.3.2.2. Chronic Neuroglycopenia

Many patients with insulinoma have vague symptoms occurring only intermittently, making the diagnosis extremely difficult. These are the patients with chronic neuroglycopenia and an array of intermittent symptoms that include nervousness, listlessness, depression, altered behavior, mood changes, sweating, fatigue, weakness, and chronic ill health. These are the patients who are often labeled as hypochondriacs or hysterical or have been evaluated for epilepsy, thyrotoxicosis, or neuropsychiatric disorders. In the absence of a documented episode of hypoglycemia, the diagnosis can be readily missed and, even if suspected, can be quite difficult to establish.

Insulinoma is a disorder in which the diagnosis can be suspected only by the history. The physical examination of these patients is characterized by a paucity of physical findings. Enlargement of the liver in a patient with β-cell tumor signifies metastases to the liver. Patients with insulinoma tend to be overweight, since they learn to consume more sugar to ward off their "attacks."

51.3.3. Diagnostic Studies

Establishing the diagnosis of insulinoma can be extremely easy or frustratingly difficult, depending on whether or not the patient was properly evaluated during a spontaneous episode of hypoglycemia. When the patient presents with spontaneous hypoglycemia, a properly performed hormonal evaluation can establish or exclude the diagnosis of β-cell tumor in 95% of instances.

51.3.3.1. Studies During an Acute Episode

The most crucial test in a hypoglycemic patient is the measurement of immunoreactive insulin (and C-peptide). The principle is based on the fact that in normal people (with nonautonomous production of insulin by the β cells), hypoglycemia is a powerful suppressor of insulin secretion. In contrast, patients with autonomous secretion of insulin, i.e., those with β-cell hyperfunction, continue to secrete insulin despite hypoglycemia. Therefore, the demonstration of inappropriately elevated circulating insulin levels in a hypoglycemic patient would be strong evidence to implicate hyperinsulinism as the etiology of hypoglycemia. The hallmark of insulinoma is the persistence of elevated insulin levels in the presence of hypoglycemia. The physiological response to a decline in the blood glucose level to below 30 mg/dl is an immediate decline in the immunoreactive insulin level to below 6 μU/ml. Most workers agree that a plasma level of insulin in excess of 6 μU/ml in a hypoglycemic patient with a blood glucose level below 30 mg/dl is strong pre-

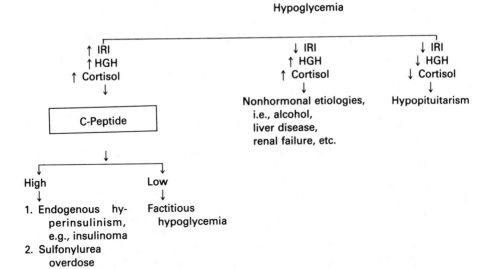

FIGURE 30.   Endocrine approach to hypoglycemia.

sumptive evidence for an islet cell tumor secreting insulin. Of all the parameters used to document hormonal evidence for an insulinoma, this seems to be the strongest one.

The measurement of C-peptide would provide the definitive proof that the hyperinsulinism is of endogenous origin. C-Peptide and insulin are released in equimolar proportions from their single-chain precursor, proinsulin. Therefore, when hyperinsulinemia results from a β-cell tumor secreting insulin, one would expect a simultaneous increase in C-peptide as well. The importance of C-peptide measurement lies in its ability to differentiate endogenous hyperinsulinism (β-cell tumor) from exogenous hyperinsulinism (factitious hypoglycemia from surreptitious administration of exogenous insulin). This stems from the fact that measurement of immunoreactive insulin is technically difficult when exogenous insulin is administered, whereas measurement of C-peptide remains unaffected. Since the plasma level of C-peptide is an accurate reflection of β-cell function, one would expect undetectable or low C-peptide levels in factitious hypoglycemia because the hypoglycemia induced by exogenous insulin administration promptly turns off β-cell function. In contrast, patients with truly endogenous hyperinsulinism caused by an islet cell tumor demonstrate elevated C-peptide levels.

There are two areas of exception that deserve comment. First, hypoglycemia induced by acute sulfonylurea overdose may be associated with elevated C-peptide levels (even though it is a form of factitious hypoglycemia) because of the stimulatory effect of sulfonylureas on β-cell function; second, in patients with the rare syndrome of hypoglycemia caused by autoantibody production to endogenous insulin, the results of immunoreactive insulin and C-peptide may be difficult to interpret. In general, however, measurement of immunoreactive insulin and C-peptide is the most valuable information in the evaluation of the hypoglycemic patient.

Since hypoglycemia is a potent stimulus for release of ACTH (and cortisol) and HGH, these hormones would be expected to be elevated when hypoglycemia is caused by an islet cell tumor secreting insulin (see algorithm for hypoglycemia, Figure 30).

51.3.3.2. Manipulative Studies in the Evaluation of β-Cell Tumor

51.3.3.2a. Prolonged Fast. This test is based on the principle that in normal subjects the physiological adjustment to prolonged fasting is a suppression of endogenous insulin levels. The aim of the test is to unmask the abnormal insulin–glucose relationship by fasting. A mere overnight fast may not be helpful, because the insulin–glucose ratio is normal in approximately 80% of patients with an insulinoma, and more protracted fasting is essential to unmask the abnormal insulin–glucose relationship. The insulin levels should be viewed in terms of the glucose level, as a ratio. The normal fasting IRI/glucose ratio is below 0.3. It must be realized that an elevated fasting level of insulin *per se* is not diagnostic unless the blood glucose is low. Many obese subjects have fasting hyperinsulinemia, but with normal or elevated fasting blood glucose level. It is therefore important to emphasize that hyperinsulinism is meaningful only when the blood glucose levels are low. An amended IRI/G ratio has been utilized for better discrimination of normals from patients with an islet cell tumor; this ratio is derived by the formula: plasma IRI × 100/(plasma glucose − 30). The rationale for subtracting 30 mg is based on the observation that in normal subjects when the blood glucose falls below 30 mg/dl there is prompt suppression of endogenous insulin levels. According to this formula, patients with a fasted amended ratio in excess of 50 should be suspected of harboring an insulin-secreting tumor. However, it should be noted that the interpretation of the amended ratio depends on the method of immunoassay for insulin. (The amended ratio employs an IRI method using activated charcoal, whereas most laboratories today employ the double-antibody radioimmunoassay.)

Regardless of the formula used, the purpose of the prolonged fast is to demonstrate insulin levels inappropriate to the degree of hypoglycemia by subjecting the patient to a supervised prolonged fast. The endpoint is the development of hypoglycemia below 40 mg/dl. When this is evident, it serves as an excellent parameter to evaluate the simultaneous circulating insulin level. The endpoint may be reached in 12, 24, or 48 hr. In 75–80% of patients with an insulinoma, Whipple's triad (symptoms of hypoglycemia, a blood glucose below 40 mg/dl, and relief of symptoms with glucose administration) can be demonstrated within 24 hr. In some patients the fast may have to be extended. The inherent problems of the prolonged fast include patient acceptance and compliance, the need for determining blood glucose levels every 2 hr, sampling for insulin levels if the blood glucose is below 40 mg/dl, and the need for personnel to supervise the patient.

51.3.3.2b. Tolbutamide Test. The tolbutamide test is based on the fact that islet cell tumors hyperrespond to the administration of intravenous tolbutamide. The pathognomonic triple parameters seen in patients with an insulinoma are a rapid drop in the blood glucose levels to below 40 mg/dl within 30 min, a persistent hypoglycemia for a protracted period of time, and concurrent hyperinsulinism. Better discrimination between normals and patients with islet cell tumors can be attained by viewing the insulin and glucose levels 150 min after tolbutamide, using the formula: glucose − (IRI × 0.5). Patients with insulinoma have scores below 43, whereas normal individuals have values greater than 43. The tolbutamide test is not frequently resorted to since it can be dangerous and since other, safer maneuvers are available; for instance, measurement of C-peptide levels before and after induction of hypoglycemia with exogenous insulin is a much safer method of attempting to demonstrate inappropriate hyperinsulinism in the presence of hypoglycemia than using intravenous tolbutamide.

51.3.3.2c. Glucagon Stimulation Test. The administration of glucagon results in a marked increase in the plasma insulin levels of patients with insulinoma. However, the application of this test as a provocative maneuver to diagnose insulin-secreting tumors has not found wide use because of the high incidence of false positives and negatives.

51.3.3.2d. Hypoglycemia Induction. The induction of hypoglycemia by the use of regular insulin with the concomitant measurement of C-peptide is another method for evaluating β-cell suppressibility. The characteristic of endogenous hyperinsulinism is the demonstration of an elevated C-peptide despite hypoglycemia.

51.3.3.3. Studies for Localization

Following the establishment of endogenous hyperinsulinism by hormonal methods, the next step is localization. Ultrasonography and computerized tomography assist in this process, albeit with a low yield. Visceral angiography identifies the islet cell tumors(s) with a 65% to 80% accuracy.

51.3.4. Prognosis

The prognosis of islet cell tumor is dictated by two factors. First, recurrent hypoglycemia, especially if severe, can result in neurological damage; second, the incidence of malignancy in insulinomas ranges from 10% to 25%.

51.3.5. Treatment

The treatment for benign islet cell tumor is surgical extirpation. The best surgical results are obtained when the tumor is single and located in the tail or the distal portion of the body. The results are less impressive when insulin hypersecretion is secondary to multiple tumors, hyperplasia, carcinoma, or carcinoids.

Drug therapy to block insulin release from the tumor can be employed by the use of diphenylhydantoin or diazoxide. The results, however, are highly variable and seldom complete or protracted.

Palliative treatment for inoperable malignant insulinoma can be provided by the use of streptozotocin, a broad-spectrum antibiotic obtained from *Streptomyces archromogenes*. Chemically this chemotherapeutic agent resembles the nitrosourea family of drugs. This drug, when given on a weekly schedule in a dose of 0.6 to 1 g/m^2 body surface area, causes biochemical improvement in 60–65% of patients with malignant insulinomas. Further, measurable disease response may be encountered in as many as 50% of patients on therapy. In those who thus respond to therapy, a doubling in the median survival with a significant increase in the 1-year survival rate has been seen. The side effects of the drug are severe nausea and vomiting in the acute phase. The main chronic side effect is renal toxicity, with azotemia developing in approximately 50% of patients receiving the drug. The next side effect is myelosuppression, which occurs in 20% of patients with prolonged use. In addition, mild hepatic enzyme elevation occurs in 60–67% of patients.

As would be expected, abnormal glucose tolerance, or even overt diabetes, would occur in a high proportion of patients taking the drug for a prolonged period because of destruction of the islet cells. A consistent observation in patients treated with streptozotocin is amelioration of the hypoglycemia. This represents a substantial benefit with the use of this drug.

51.4. Gastrin

Gastrin is a hormone that is normally secreted by the G-cells of the antrum. Even though the main source of gastrin is the antral mucosa of the stomach, gastrin has also been extracted from the duodenum. Pancreatic extracts also contain a very small amount of gastrin. Gastrin circulates in several forms, and the amount measured depends on the ability of the immunoassay to "see" the particular fragment that circulates in the plasma. There are four immunologically heterogeneous fragments of gastrin that have been characterized: minigastrin (G-14 gastrin), little gastrin (G-17), big gastrin (G-34 gastrin), and big-big gastrin (amino acid sequence uncertain). The gastrin extracted from the duodenol mucosa is G-17 gastrin. The predominant fragment of fasting gastrin in patients with Zollinger–Ellison syndrome is G-34 gastrin.

The release of gastrin by the antral G-cells of the stomach is mediated by a variety of factors, food, distension of the stomach, alkaline pH, and hypercalcemia representing the major ones.

1. Intake of food, particularly protein, is the single most important provocative factor for the release of gastrin from the stomach. Because gastrin is a potent stimulator of the acid-secreting parietal cells of the

stomach, the digestive process is aided by food-mediated gastrin release.

2. Distension of the stomach and vagal stimulation also stimulate gastrin release; however, these stimuli have more pronounced effects in animals than in humans.

3. An alkaline pH also serves as a potent releaser of gastrin. This is mostly the mechanism of hypergastrinemia associated with the retained antrum following a Billroth II, where the antral tissue retained in the duodenal stump is chronically stimulated by the alkaline pH of duodenal contents.

4. Acute or chronic hypercalcemia also stimulates gastrin release, and this may be relevant to the hypergastrinemia seen in patients with hyperparathyroidism.

Of the factors that suppress gastrin release, the two most important ones are an acid pH in the stomach and secretin, a gut hormone secreted by the duodenum.

1. The potent inhibitory effect of acidity on gastrin secretion is evidenced by the fact that when the pH of the stomach is lowered, the effects of provocative stimuli that release gastrin are blunted in normal subjects. Thus, even the demonstration of "normal" gastrin levels in a patient with marked hyperacidity can be viewed as inappropriate.

2. Secretin, the other factor that suppresses gastrin release, is important in differentiating normal G-cell function from pathological autonomic hyperfunction. In normals, the intravenous administration of secretin is association with a prompt and impressive decline in circulating gastrin levels, in contrast to patients with gastrinoma who not only fail to do so but actually increase the gastrin level paradoxically.

Less important factors that inhibit gastrin production are the hypothalamic peptides somatostatin and thyrotropin-releasing hormone (TRH). The triple controls of food, gastric acidity, and secretin work in a concerted fashion to facilitate digestion. When food reaches the stomach, there is a prompt release of gastrin by the antral G-cells. As a consequence, there is stimulation of the parietal cells to secrete acid. As the acidity of the stomach contents increases (pH declines), the gastrin release is inhibited, resulting in a gradual decline of gastrin levels *pari passu* with decreasing acid production by the parietal cells. As the food reaches the duodenum, secretin is released, which further inhibits gastrin production and restores the G-cells to the preprandial state.

The actions of gastrin extend throughout the gastrointestinal tract:

1. The prime action of gastrin on the stomach is its ability to stimulate acid. Gastrin stimulates gastric hypersecretion by increasing the secretion of hydrogen ions from the gastric parietal cells. The potency of G-17 gastrin is five times greater than that of G-34 in terms of

TABLE 115
Hypergastrinemia

Hypergastrinemia with hyperacidity
  Zollinger–Ellison syndrome (gastrinoma)
  Antral G-cell hyperplasia
  Retained excluded antrum syndrome
  After massive small bowel resection (transient)
Hypergastrinemia with hypoacidity
  Gastric ulcer
  Posttruncal vagotomy
Hypergastrinemia with achlorhydria
  Gastritis
  Pernicious anemia
Miscellaneous
  Chronic renal failure
  Chronic hypercalcemic states
  Chronic gastric outlet obstruction

    stimulating the gastric parietal cells and is 2.5 times greater than that of G-14 gastrin. There is experimental evidence to indicate that in animals exogenous gastrin stimulates gastric mucosal growth by increasing *de novo* synthesis of DNA and RNA.

2. Physiologically, gastrin decreases the rate of gastric emptying. Paradoxically, quite the reverse is seen in patients with Zollinger–Ellison syndrome.

3. Physiologically, gastrin stimulates contraction of the lower esophageal sphincter.

4. Gastrin stimulates the motility of the small intestines and, in supraphysiological amounts, will increase secretion of water and ions into the lumen.

5. Gastrin is a strong stimulant of the pancreatic enzyme secretion and a weak stimulant of gallbladder contraction.

Fasting hypergastrinemia should be interpreted in terms of gastric hyperacidity. Table 115 outlines the conditions characterized by hypergastrinemia in the presence of hyperacidity, hypoacidity, and achlorhydria.

51.5. Zollinger–Ellison Syndrome

    In 1955, Zollinger and Ellison described two patients with recurrent peptic ulceration, marked gastric hyperacidity, and a non-β islet cell tumor of the pancreas. Since the original description of the syndrome, several developments have altered the approach to the diagnosis and management of this entity. These include the immunoassay for gastrin and a variety of manipulations to evaluate gastrin dynamics; the development of sophisticated localizing techniques such as percutaneous transhepatic portal pancreatic venous catheterization; the discovery of the H_2 receptor antagonist cimetidine; the emergence of high-resolution computerized tomography of the pancreas; and the pharmacological discovery of a new group of "second-generation" H_2 receptor antagonists such as ranitidine.

51.5.1. Etiology

Currently, ZES occurs in four forms:

1. The sporadic form, caused by a non-β-cell tumor of the pancreas (gastrinoma of the pancreas, ZES II).
2. Hyperplasia of the antral G-cells (ZES I).
3. Gastrinoma occurring in nonpancreatic tissue, usually the duodenum.
4. Gastrinoma associated with the multiple endocrine adenomatosis syndrome (MEA I).

Each of the above entities can result in a clinical presentation characterized by the triad of peptic ulceration, marked hyperacidity, and hypergastrinemia.

The most common etiology of ZES is the gastrinoma of the pancreas (ZES II). The islet cell type from which the gastrinoma originates is a matter of controversy. The gastrinoma arises either from the rare islet D_1 cell (the type IV islet cell) or the endocrine ductular cells of the pancreas. However, there are cells in the pancreas with characteristics identical to those of the antral G-cells. Therefore, the ectopic versus eutopic origin of gastrinoma is an open question. Tumors of the pancreas are found in fewer than 50% of patients with hormonal data suggestive of a ZES-II-type syndrome. This underscores the difficulty in recognizing the tumor preoperatively or even intraoperatively. To compound the problem it may be difficult microscopically to differentiate normal tissue from hyperplastic or even tumorous tissue. The fact that ZES is being diagnosed at an earlier stage may have an impact on the incidence of finding tumors of the pancreas.

The syndrome of antral G-cell hyperplasia, also referred to as ZES I or pseudo-ZES, is characterized by the following five features:

1. Peptic ulceration with moderate to severe fasting hypergastrinemia.
2. Marked elevation of gastrin following a protein meal.
3. No pancreatic lesion.
4. Increased numbers of the antral G-cells.
5. A decline in serum gastrin following reaction of the antrum.

The importance of recognizing this rare syndrome lies in the fact that therapy for this entity is exceedingly simple (antrectomy), in contrast to the treatment of ZES II. The diagnosis of antral G-cell hyperplasia can be made on the basis of gastrin dynamic data (response to a secretin test and protein meal). The existence of this entity has been debated in the literature because the patients described as having the syndrome had undergone vagotomy, a procedure known to cause hypergastrinemia and increased population of the antral G-cells. Nevertheless, the consensus of opinion is that antral G-cell hyperplasia does exist, albeit rarely, and should be considered in any patient with hypergastrinemia and peptic ulceration.

Gastrinoma occurring in nonpancreatic tissue (especially the duodenum) is also a rare entity but an important one, since surgical excision of the lesion is usually associated with a "cure" for the hypergastrinemic state; it therefore carries a good prognosis.

The association between ZES and multiple endocrine adenomatosis (Wermer's syndrome, MEA I) is a well-established one. Evidence of parathyroid or pituitary hyperfunction if encountered in 20–40% of the patients with ZES. The most common association is hyperparathyroidism followed by pituitary adenomas secreting prolactin, growth hormone, or ACTH. The spectrum of pituitary involvement also includes chromophobe adenomas without clinical or hormonal evidence of hypersecretion of pituitary hormones.

51.5.2. Clinical Features

The two features of Zollinger–Ellison syndrome are peptic ulcer disease and diarrhea.

The presentation of the peptic ulcer disease of ZES can be quite variable. The ulcer disease can be aggressive, with a virulent course associated with complications, but the ulcer disease can also be unremarkable, presenting exactly like the usual patient with duodenal ulcer. This unremarkable "routine" presentation often is responsible for the delay in the diagnosis of ZES. Zollinger–Ellison syndrome should be suspected whenever the ulceration is multiple or when ulceration occurs at unusual sites such as the distal duodenum or jejunum. However, 38–68% of the patients with ZES have a solitary duodenal ulcer no different in size, location, or behavior than the average "routine" duodenal ulcer.

Diarrhea is a much more important discriminatory factor than ulcer disease or abdominal pain. Diarrhea alone may be present as the initial symptom in as many as 20% of patients during the early part of the illness. The reasons for diarrhea are threefold:

1. The most important reason for diarrhea is the increased volume of acid entering the gut. This high acid content irritates the small bowel mucosa with a resultant impairment of the absorptive processes. The above reasoning is supported by the fact that continuous aspiration of the gastric contents relieves the diarrhea. Further, small-bowel biopsies in ZES reveal abnormalities in the mucosa with blunting of the villi and varying degrees of edema, hemorrhage, and superficial erosions.

2. The high acid milieu in the duodenum resulting from the high gastric acid output denatures pancreatic lipase and precipitates the bile acids. As a consequence, the dietary triglycerides are not adequately broken down to mono- and diglycerides, and the bile acids are unable to

suspend the dietary fat in a micellar solution, a process needed for fat digestion. The end result is steatorrhea.

3. Gastrin in supraphysiological doses can increase the motility of the intestines.

51.5.3. Diagnostic Studies

The diagnostic studies involved in evaluation of Zollinger–Ellison syndrome can be categorized into those involving fasting gastrin level, those involving gastrin dynamics, gastric acid secretory studies, and radiological and localizational studies.

51.5.3.1. Fasting Gastrin Level

The fasting gastrin level is always elevated in patients with all forms of ZES and serves as the marker for the syndrome. The following clinical settings should raise the suspicion of ZES, thus mandating screening with fasting gastrin levels:

1. Peptic ulcer disease in a patient with a family history of peptic ulceration, renal calculous disease, or hyperparathyroidism.
2. Peptic ulceration associated with diarrhea of hypercalcemia.
3. Peptic ulceration of the distal duodenum or jejunum or multiple ulcerations.
4. Aggressive ulcer disease with severe abdominal pain or with complications such as bleeding or perforation.
5. Intractable ulceration resistant to conventional antacid therapy.
6. Recurrent ulceration following surgery.
7. Unexplained chronic diarrhea.
8. Radiological or endoscopic evidence of hypertrophy of rugal folds.

51.5.3.2. Gastrin Dynamic Studies

In patients with Zollinger–Ellison syndrome caused by a gastrinoma, the intravenous administration of secretin (in a dose of 2 U/kg) causes a prompt, marked, and paradoxical increase in the gastrin levels. Blood is assayed for gastrin before and 2, 5, 10, 20, and 30 min following the I.V. bolus of secretin.

There are several criteria used for characterizing the response of a gastrinoma:

1. An absolute increase of 200 pg over the basal gastrin level is considered diagnostic of ZES of pancreatic origin.
2. A peak level of 500 pg/ml of gastrin following secretin permits a 100% separation between the gastrinoma patients and those with duodenal ulcer disease.
3. An increase of gastrin by at least 100 pg/ml above the basal level postsecretin is highly suggestive of gastrinoma.

In contrast to patients with gastrinoma, the patients wih duodenal ulcer and those with retained excluded antrum generally demonstrate a decrease in serum gastrin level following the intravenous administration of secretin. Patients with ulceration secondary to antral G-cell hyperplasia generally demonstrate a decrease, no change, or occasionally a very small rise in gastrin following secretin administration. Thus, the secretin test has enormous diagnostic value in delineating the various etiologies of hypergastrinemic states with peptic ulceration. If the criterion of an absolute increment of 200 pg/ml over the basal value post-secretin is employed, the rate of false-positive responses is negligible. Occasional false-negative responses may be encountered in patients with gastrinoma.

The protein meal test is primarily used to make the diagnosis of antral G-cell hyperplasia (ZES I). In such patients, following a meal containing one slice of bread, 200 ml of milk, 50 g cheese, and one boiled egg, there is a dramatic increase in the gastrin level. This contrasts sharply with patients harboring a gastrinoma (autonomous secretion of gastrin by a pancreatic islet cell tumor), in whom there is no response or, at best, the response is no more than 50% greater than the basal preprandial level. This test would not be of help in the patient in whom the differential diagnosis is between ZES and retained excluded antrum. In both of these conditions only a minimal postprandial increase in the serum gastrin level would be expected.

51.5.3.3. Gastric Acid Secretory Studies

Gastric acid secretory studies, i.e., the determination of basal and stimulated acid output, are simple and time-honored tests in the evaluation of a patient with peptic ulcer disease and hypergastrinemia, especially when the gastrin levels are only marginally elevated. Several general comments apply to gastric acid secretory studies in the diagnosis of ZES.

1. A basal acid output that exceeds 15 mEq/hr is highly diagnostic of ZES. However, as many as 10% of the patients with simple duodenal ulcer may show basal acid outputs as high as 15 mEq/hr. In 4–12% of the patients with ZES, the basal output of gastric acid can be below 15 mEq/hr.

2. A ratio of basal acid output (BAO) to maximal acid output (MAO) greater than 0.6 is strongly suggestive of ZES. However, there is overlap between patients with duodenal ulcer and ZES, a small but significant number of patients with ZES having ratios of BAO/MAO less than 0.6.

3. The gastric secretory studies are difficult to interpret when prior gastric surgery and or vagotomy have been performed. A basal acid output greater than 5 mEq/hr in a patient who has had prior gastric surgery is strongly suggestive of ZES. However, hypersecretion is to be expected in patients with retained excluded antrum, sometimes to the extent seen in ZES.

51.5.3.4. Radiological Studies

The upper gastrointestinal series reveals ulcer disease, which can be quite diagnostic. The presence of jejunal ulcers, multiple ulcerations, or ulcers at atypical locations as well as the presence of rugal fold thickening are highly suggestive of Zollinger–Ellison syndrome.

51.5.3.5. Localizational Studies

The emergence of high-resolution computerized tomography has improved localization, but still only 20% to 40% of gastrinomas are visualized by this method. Visceral angiography continues to remain the mainstay in localizing pancreatic gastrinoma. The availability of percutaneous transhepatic portal pancreatic venous catheterization is limited to few centers in the United States.

51.5.4. Differential Diagnosis

When the presentation is characterized by recurrent ulceration following surgery, the major differential diagnosis of ZES is the syndrome of retained excluded antrum. The gastrin levels are elevated in both. The gastrin response to secretin is different and assists in the differential diagnosis; the serum gastrin of patients with retained excluded antrum demonstrates physiological suppression to secretin, whereas it paradoxically increases after secretin in patients with gastrinoma.

When diarrhea is the major manifestation, ZES has to be differentiated from other conditions characterized by "secretory diarrhea," such as VIPoma, villous adenoma, and medullary carcinoma of the thyroid.

51.5.5. Treatment

The therapy for ZES is controversial and constantly evolving. The standard therapy in the past was total gastrectomy, but in the last decade, the options of therapy have broadened. The two major factors that have been responsible are the increasing awareness of the long-term morbidity of radical gastric surgery and the emergence of effective drugs that lower gastric acidity. It is too soon to say whether medical therapy will render total gastrectomy a superfluous procedure, since this question cannot be answered without long-term observations on the natural history of ZES with chronic cimetidine therapy.

In a patient with peptic ulcer, documented ZES, and a positive localization of a tumor in the pancreatic body, the choice of therapy would be a combination of cimetidine with removal of the pancreatic tumor. Preoperative cimetidine is indicated to improve symptoms and to start reduction of gastric hyperacidity. During surgery, the tumor identified by angiography should be located by palpation. The pancreas should be carefully palpated for the presence of additional tumors. In addition, the paraaortic nodes and the liver should be carefully palpated and biopsied if indicated, since 30–63% of patients have metastatic disease at operation. If, at surgery, there is no evidence of metastatic disease, and the tumor appears to be solitary, enucleation of the tumor should be performed if technically possible. If the tumor is in the tail and enucleation is not feasible, a distal pancreatectomy is recommended. It should be noted that when a solitary gastrinoma is found in the head, a pancreatic doudenectomy is not recommended by most surgeons since the surgical mortality and morbidity of this procedure are considerably greater than the possible consequences of an unoperated solitary gastrinoma.

The long-term use of cimetidine alone in controlling the symptoms of gastrinoma as well as other forms of ZES has been the subject of several reviews. The initial experience with this drug in the United States is that more than 80% of patients can be controlled with cimetidine alone. Similarly encouraging results have been reported from Scandinavia. It is important to realize that even though the enthusiasm for cimetidine therapy appears to be justified, the following facts regarding cimetidine should not be overlooked:

1. It has to be given for life. The patient should be extremely compliant, since therapy involves q.i.d. dosage and the nuisance of frequent intragastric pH monitoring.
2. It should be remembered that the initial dosage of the drug that caused remarkable amelioration may, with time, have to be increased, often to a dose greater than 10 g daily. Such massive dosages are naturally associated with side effects. These include gynecomastia, impotence, oligospermia, and occasionally hepatic damage, mental confusion, and bizarre behavior in the elderly. The antiandrogenic activity of cimetidine is the most disconcerting, but the newer H_2 receptor antagonists appear to be free of this antiandrogenic effect.
3. Resistance to the continual use of the drug is a possible occurrence.
4. Fatal complications, i.e., GI hemorrhage, may develop in patients who interrupt therapy and in those who develop resistance.
5. The studies that have established cimetidine therapy as an excellent form of medical therapy have observed these patients for a mean period of only 2–4 years. It would require strict double-blind randomized studies with extensive follow-up before cimetidine therapy becomes established as *the* alternative to surgery.

Notwithstanding the above limitations, the indications for cimetidine therapy are:

1. As adjunctive therapy for relief of all symptoms caused by gastrin excess.
2. As the cornerstone therapy in inoperable ZES.
3. In patients with localized pancreatic gastrinoma, the drug should be used pre- and postoperatively.

Total gastrectomy as a choice is a last-resort option and one that is made with reluctance because of the extremely high potential of rendering the patient a gastric cripple. The nutritional problems following total gastrectomy are frustrating and often insurmountable.

A total gastrectomy seems appropriate under the following situations:

1. A patient with ZES in whom no lesions are found in the pancreatic bed or the duodenal wall *and* who has failed to respond to cimetidine therapy.
2. A patient in whom a pancreatic lesion has been found and resected but, following surgery, there is recurrence of ulcer disease *and* cimetidine therapy has failed.
3. Patients with malignant ZES but in whom the general condition is good, since regression of the metastases can occur following total gastrectomy.
4. The patient who has been on cimetidine but develops resistance to the drug or is not compliant in taking the drug every 6 hr and in whom no pancreatic tumor can be localized.

51.6. Verner–Morrison Syndrome

In 1958, Verner and Morrison described a patient with refractory watery diarrhea and marked hypokalemia caused by a non-β islet cell tumor of the pancreas. Since then, this condition has come to be known by a variety of names and acronyms: WDHA syndrome (watery diarrhea, hypokalemia, achlorhydria), WDHH syndrome (watery diarrhea, hypokalemia, hypochlorhydria), and VIPoma (vasoactive intestinal polypeptide-secreting tumor). None of these terms completely or accurately describe this entity. For example, hypochlorhydria or achlorhydria is not a prerequisite for making the diagnosis of the syndrome; vasoactive intestinal polypeptide, the humoral marker for the syndrome, may be unelevated in some patients with this syndrome. Further, a tumor in the pancreatic bed may not be found despite a careful search during exploratory laparotomy, underscoring the fact that at least in some cases, diffuse hyperplasia may be the underlying lesion.

51.6.1. Etiology

The etiology of the Verner–Morrison syndrome can be viewed in terms of the anatomic lesions that underlie the syndrome as well as the humoral principle(s) involved in the expression of the syndrome.

Verner–Morrison syndrome is most often caused by a non-β cell *tumor* of the islets of Langerhans. However, it should be emphasized that tumors are not always found, and the disorder can be a consequence of *diffuse hyperplasia*. Rarely, a *carcinoma* of the islet cells can also be the etiology of the Verner–Morrison syndrome. Further, Verner–Morrison syndrome has been described with nonpancreatic neoplasms. The reported tumors that have been associated with this syndrome are retroperitoneal ganglioneuroma, pheo-chromocytoma, bronchogenic carcinoma, and ganglioneuroblastoma. Al-though rare, these extrapancreatic lesions are important to recognize in order to avoid needless pancreatic surgery.

In terms of the humoral etiology, there has been considerable controversy in the literature as to the nature of the humoral mediator involved in this syndrome. It is now generally accepted that the diarrheagenic hormone of the Verner–Morrison syndrome is vasoactive intestinal polypeptide (VIP). The other contenders for the role—secretin, serotonin, prostaglandins, and glucagon—have been discarded since 1975, when patients with Verner–Morrison syndrome demonstrated consistent and significant elevations of assay-able VIP in the plasma. The reasons for conflicting reports in the literature are twofold: first, the variances in methodology for measurement of VIP have posed difficulties; second, isolated reports of the demonstration of other pep-tides in patients with the syndrome have clouded the true identity of the diarrhea-genic peptide involved. There are four lines of evidence to attribute a causal role for VIP in the Verner–Morrison syndrome:

1. When a sensitive and standard assay for VIP is used, the consistency with which this peptide is shown to be elevated in the plasma of patients with this syndrome is convincing.
2. Following successful extirpation of the tumor, the symptoms alleviate *pari passu* with a decline in the VIP levels to normal. Indeed, failure to achieve symptomatic relief is attended by a persistent elevation of serum VIP levels, rendering the assay a valuable parameter for defin-ing "cure."
3. The tumor extracts from patients with Verner–Morrison syndrome are rich in VIP, often several hundredfold greater than normal pan-creatic tissue extracts.
4. The most important evidence that links VIP to Verner–Morrison syn-drome is a comparison of the experimental effects of VIP infusion to the clinical features of the syndrome. The spectrum of actions of this peptide is consistent with the clinical effects seen when it is hyperse-creted: VIP has profound effects on the stomach, intestines, colon, bile flow, and pancreatic secretion.

The action of VIP on the stomach is potent inhibition of gastric secretion. Following intravenous administration of VIP, there is a marked inhibition in the gastric acid secretory response to histamine or pentagastrin.

The action of VIP on the small intestine is one of potent stimulation. The intravenous infusion of VIP is attended by a remarkably prompt (within 5 min) stimulatory response of intestinal secretion. The VIP-mediated stim-ulation of intestinal secretion is cyclic AMP dependent.

Vasoactive intestinal polypeptide also stimulates pancreatic bicarbonate and water secretion. This action, however, is less potent than the action of secretin on pancreatic exocrine secretion. The effect of VIP on the gallbladder

TABLE 116
Comparison of Experimental and Clinical Effects of VIP

Organ	Experimental effect of VIP	Clinical counterpart in V–M syndrome
Stomach	Gastric secretion inhibition	Achlorhydria; hypochlorhydria
Intestines	Stimulates intestinal secretion	Secretory diarrhea
Pancreatic exocrine function	Stimulates bicarbonate and water secretion	Profound bicarbonate loss; metabolic acidosis
Gallbladder	Relaxation of gallbladder	Dilated gallbladder
Liver	Glycogenolysis	Hyperglycemia
β Cell	↑ Insulin release	Hypoglycemia
Mineral metabolism	Hypercalcemia in dogs	Hypercalcemia

is to relax this organ, and this effect has been documented in experiments using isolated guinea pig gallbladders.

There are three metabolic effects of VIP that have been experimentally documented, i.e., glycogenolytic effect, insulinotrophic effect, and hypercalcemic effect. Vasoactive intestinal polypeptide has been shown to promote glycogenolysis. The intravenous administration of VIP to dogs is associated with an increase in the blood glucose levels. This effect has been compared with that of glucagon, and *in vitro* studies have demonstrated that although VIP is glycogenolytic, it is less potent than glucagon. Vasoactive intestinal polypeptide also stimulates insulin release by a direct mechanism, independent of the blood glucose levels.

Administration of VIP to dogs is associated with a slight increase in the serum calcium level; the mechanism(s) for the hypercalcemic effect are unclear.

The experimental effects of VIP and the clinical counterparts of these effects in the Verner–Morrison syndrome are outlined in Table 116, clearly supporting the causal role of VIP in this syndrome.

In spite of convincing evidence to implicate VIP, rarely, the levels may be normal in patients with Verner–Morrison syndrome. The demonstration of elevated serotonin or prostaglandins in serum or tumor extracts of such patients is a well-recognized phenomenon.

51.6.2. Clinical Features

Verner–Morrison syndrome is a very rare disease, typically occurring in middle-aged females, although it has been described in patients as young as 17 and as old as 74. There are two types of presentations of Verner–Morrison syndrome: the intermittent, in which the patient obtains relief from the diarrhea for periods of variable duration, and the chronic form, characterized by continuous watery diarrhea that relentlessly progresses to death from electrolyte imbalance. This form is not punctuated by quiescence. The symptomatology of Verner–Morrison syndrome can be viewed in terms of the diarrhea and the symptoms caused by hypokalemia. The major symptom of Verner–Morrison syndrome is diarrhea. There are three characteristics of the diarrhea seen in this syndrome. First, the watery nature of the diarrhea is the hallmark. This characteristic has earned it the term "pancreatic cholera." In fact, in areas where cholera is endemic, the diarrhea cannot be distinguished from cholera. (This may be a problem in the coastal area of Louisiana, where endemic pockets of cholera still exist.) The watery stool is dilute, often resembling weak tea. Second, the stool is *voluminous*, often exceeding 6 to 8 liters of stool a day. Even in mild cases, the volume is at least 2 liters a day. Third, the stool is *rich in electrolytes*, particularly potassium and bicarbonate. Continued losses of these electrolytes are responsible for several metabolic abnormalities such as hypokalemia, glucose intolerance, and metabolic acidosis.

The diarrhea of Verner–Morrison syndrome represents the most classic example of secretory diarrhea. Very few conditions mimic the type of diarrhea seen in Verner–Morrison Syndrome. These include infection with *Vibrio cholera*, the diarrhea seen with villous adenoma, and the humoral diarrheagenic syndromes caused by excessive secretion of gastrin or rarely serotonin. It is noteworthy that significant abdominal pain is not a frequent feature in patients with Verner–Morrison syndrome. The pain, when present, is in the nature of abdominal cramps of mild to moderate severity. Likewise, rectal bleeding is not a frequent feature of the syndrome. These two features are helpful in distinguishing the syndrome from the usual causes of infectious diarrhea and inflammatory bowel disease.

The next important symptom complex relates to hypokalemia. Thus, patients may complain of muscle weakness, parasthesias, abdominal cramps, and polyuria. The development of profound hypokalemia (often below 2.2. mEq), which is often extremely resistant to potassium replacement, is the leading cause of death in the fatal cases. The refractoriness of hypokalemia is consequent to the drastic losses of this electrolyte in the stool; the average patient with Verner–Morrison syndrome excretes 200–400 mEq K^+ daily in the stools. The long-term effects of chronic hypokalemia include tubular damage (hypokalemic nephropathy), glucose intolerance, and probably myocardial disease with congestive failure.

In addition to watery diarrhea and symptoms of hypokalemia, three additional facets of this syndrome have been described in the literature; these are flushing, psychotic behavioral changes, and hypoglycemic symptoms.

Episodes of flushing have been reported in patients with Verner–Morrison syndrome. These are usually episodic and are either patchy erythematous attacks or appear as urticarial flushing attacks. The cause of the flushing is not clear but is presumed to be, at least in some cases, related to serotonin or its metabolites.

Psychosis and abnormal behavior have been reported in 3% of cases with Verner–Morrison syndrome. It is not clear whether the psychosis is related to the metabolic problems of electrolyte depletion or if it is mediated by humoral factors.

Hypoglycemia has been reported in patients with Verner–Morrison syndrome, the etiology of which is unclear.

51.6.3. Diagnostic Studies

The diagnostic studies in the Verner–Morrison syndrome can be categorized as nonhormonal routine tests, hormonal studies, and localizational procedures.

51.6.3.1. Routine Nonhormonal Studies

These are the most impressively abnormal studies in patients with the watery diarrhea syndrome.

51.6.3.1a. Metabolic Abnormalities. Hypokalemia is invariably present in these patients, sometimes plummeting to dangerously low levels. Metabolic acidosis from bicarbonate loss is invariably noted.

51.6.3.1b. Stool Characteristics. The secretory diarrhea of this syndrome is evidenced by the massive losses of K, Na, and bicarbonate in the stools, which are voluminous. The stool cultures are sterile, indicating the noninfective nature of the watery diarrhea.

51.6.3.1c. Achlorhydria or Hypochlorhydria. Gastric hyposecretion is a feature of Verner–Morrison syndrome observed in 55% to 60% of patients with the disease. Hypochlorhydria is more frequent than absolute achlorhydria. In many patients, the abnormality is reversible following resection of the pancreatic tumor. This suggests a humoral etiology for the hypoacidity. More interesting is the observation that rebound gastric hypersecretion occurs in many patients, with the development of peptic ulcer in some instances, following resection of the pancreatic tumor. Although hypokalemia *per se* can inhibit gastric acid secretion, this does not seem to be a major mechanism, since in the majority of patients with Verner–Morrison syndrome, the gastric acid abnormalities persist even after correction of the hypokalemia.

51.6.3.1d. Hypercalcemia. The incidence of hypercalcemia in Verner–Morrison syndrome is approximately 25%. The hypercalcemia tends to be mild, nonparathormone mediated, and reverses following pancreatic tumor resection. The nature of the humoral mediator of hypercalcemia in this syndrome has not been established, although prostaglandins are favored.

51.6.3.1e. Glucose Abnormalities. Both glucose intolerance and hypoglycemia have been reported in this syndrome.

51.6.3.2. Hormonal Studies

As indicated earlier, the marker for Verner–Morrison syndrome is vasoactive intestinal polypeptide. The radioimmunoassay of VIP is limited to relatively few laboratories.

51.6.3.3. Localizational Studies

Since the pancreatic tumors that secrete VIP ("VIPoma") are small, the yield with computerized tomography is low. The success rate of visceral angiography has not been established in any large series. In most patients, exploratory laparotomy is the only means of localization.

51.6.4. Differential Diagnosis

The main differential diagnoses to consider are infective diarrheas (particularly shigellosis and cholera), fulminant ulcerative colitis, chronic laxative abuse, villous adenoma, and the humoral diarrheagenic syndromes resulting from hypersecretion of gastrin (ZES) and serotonin.

51.6.5. Course and Prognosis

In its mild form, Verner–Morrison syndrome can exist for years before the correct diagnosis is established. In its severe form, the disease is rapidly progressive and results in death as a consequence of dehydration and electrolyte imbalance.

51.6.6. Treatment

The supportive measures for Verner–Morrison syndrome are extremely important and include replacement of fluids and electrolytes, particularly potassium. Attention to fluid and electrolyte balance takes precedence over the performance of any diagnostic tests. Glucocorticoids have proven to be of some help in temporarily alleviating the diarrhea. The mechanism for steroid responsiveness is unclear, but almost half of all patients with Verner–Morrison syndrome experience considerable relief with intravenous or oral glucocorticoids. It should be noted that the hypokalemia (and the glucose intolerance seen in some patients) can be aggravated by steroid therapy.

The only definitive treatment for Verner–Morrison syndrome is removal of the pancreatic tumor that hypersecretes VIP. The attainment of a "complete" cure following removal of the tumor is seen in approximately 30–40% of patients. The reason for the relatively low cure rates is the malignant potential of these tumors, which may have metastasized by the time they are diagnosed. When a tumor is not identifiable, subtotal (or even total) resection of the pancreas is justifiably undertaken because of the high mortality of untreated Verner–Morrison syndrome. The cure rates are, of course, higher, since the bulk of the pancreas is removed. The surgery is major, with a significant operative mortality. Chemotherapy for malignant VIPoma with streptozotocin is unsatisfactory.

51.7. Glucagonoma

This is an extremely rare tumor, characterized by weight loss, glucose intolerance, a singularly impressive skin lesion, and a non-β-cell tumor.

51.7.1. Etiology

Glucagon-secreting tumors originate from the α islet cells. These tumors tend to possess a high malignant potential, metastasizing to the liver. In some cases the hyperglucagonemia is secondary to diffuse hyperplasia rather than adenoma or carcinoma of the islets.

51.7.2. Clinical Features

Glucagonomas typically occurs in elderly females. The clinical triad for glucagonoma is weight loss, a characteristic skin lesion, and diabetes.

51.7.2.1. Weight Loss

This feature is uniformly present in patients with glucagonoma and can be caused by several factors: metabolic effects because of the lipolytic effect of the hormone and anorexia from the underlying malignancy are the main reasons for the weight loss. Less frequently, diabetes is the major factor for weight loss. The weight loss may also be related to poor availability of amino acids for incorporation into protein, since hypoaminoacidemia is a consistent feature in this syndrome. Regardless of the mechanism, weight loss, often profound, dominates the clinical picture.

51.7.2.2. Skin Lesions

Nearly all patients with glucagon-secreting tumors present with a characteristic skin lesion. The skin lesion serves as a clinical marker to suspect this rare disease. The three characteristics of the skin lesions are incorporated in the descriptive term used by dermatologists to denote the lesions of glucagonoma: "necrolytic migratory erythema." The lesions start as erythematous areas and gradually become papular. Typically, they form blisters that rupture and "weep" with exudation of fluid, followed by healing. The lesions "migrate" and often coalesce. The preferred location is the groin and lower abdomen, although they can occur anywhere in the body. Stomatitis and encrusting of lips are frequent findings. The skin biopsy of affected areas demonstrates necrolysis with bulla formation. The reason for the skin lesion and for its remarkable association with hyperglucagonemia is unclear.

TABLE 117
Causes for
Hyperglucagonemia

Mild elevation
   Fasting
Moderate elevation
   Stress
   Burns
   Cirrhosis
   Portocaval shunting
   Hypermacroglucagonemia
   Diabetic ketoacidosis
Marked elevation
   Glucagonoma

51.7.2.3. Diabetes

Despite a phenomenal elevation in the level of circulating glucagon, the diabetes is mild. Ketoacidosis is rare, underscoring the dictum that elevated glucagon *per se* in the absence of insulin lack does not result in diabetic ketoacidosis. The only time the diabetes becomes severe is when the entire pancreatic tissue is replaced by the malignant tumor tissue.

51.7.3. Diagnostic Studies

When glucagonoma is suspected on the basis of the skin lesion and weight loss, the diagnosis can be readily established by measurement of glucagon levels in the plasma. Patients with glucagonoma characteristically demonstrate phenomenally elevated glucagon levels in the circulation, usually in the range exceeding 1000 pg/ml. In interpreting glucagon levels, other conditions that cause hyperglucagonemia should be kept in mind, although none of these result in the degree of elevation seen in glucagonoma (Table 117).

51.7.4. Prognosis

Glucagonoma is associated with a poor outcome because of its high malignant potential.

51.7.5. Treatment

The only treatment available for glucagonoma is surgical extirpation of the tumor. There is no satisfactory treatment for malignant glucagonoma.

Selected Readings

Ballard, H. S., Frame, B., and Hartsock, R. J.: Familial multiple endocrine adenoma—peptic ulcer complex, *Medicine* **43**:481, 1964.

Berson, S. A., and Yalow, R. S.: Nature of immunoreactive gastrin extracted from tissues of the gastrointestinal tract, *Gastroenterology* **60**:215, 1971.

Bloom, S. R., Polak, J. M., and Pearce, A. G. E.: Vasoactive intestinal peptide and watery diarrhea syndrome, *Lancet* **2**:14, 1973.

Bonfils, S., Landor, J. H., *et al.:* Results of surgical management in 92 consecutive patients with Zollinger Ellison syndrome, *Ann. Surg.* **194**:692, 1981.

Broder, L. E., and Carter, S. K.: Pancreatic islet cell carcinomas I. Clinical features in 52 patients, *Ann. Intern. Med.* **79**:101, 1973.

Broder, L. E., and Carter, S. K.: Pancreatic islet cell carcinoma II. Results of therapy with streptozotocin in 52 patients, *Ann. Intern. Med.* **79**:108, 1973.

Cherrington, A. D., Chiasson, J. L., *et al.:* The role of insulin and glucagon in the regulation of basal glucose production in the post absorptive dog, *J. Clin Invest.* **58**:1407, 1976.

Exton, J. H.: Gluconeogenesis, *Metabolism* **21**:945, 1972.

Fajans, S. S., and Floyd, J. C.: Fasting hypoglycemia in adults, *N. Engl. J. Med.* **294**:766, 1976.

Fausa, O., Fretheim, B., Elgjo, K., *et al.:* Intractable watery diarrhea, hypokalemia, and achlorhydria associated with non pancreatic retroperitoneal neurogenous tumor containing vasoactive intestinal polypeptide (VIP), *Scand. J. Gastroenterol.* **8**:713, 1973.

Friesen, S. R.: APUD tumors of the gastrointestinal tract, *Curr. Probl. Cancer* **1**(4): 1, 1976.

Freisen, S. R.: Tumors of the endocrine pancreas, *N. Engl. J. Med.* **306**:580, 1982.

Gorden, P., Roth, J., *et al.:* The circulating proinsulin-like components, *Diabetes* **21**:673, 1972.

Gutman, R. A., Lazarus, N. R., *et al.:* Circulating proinsulin like material in patients with functioning insulinomas, *N. Engl. J. Med.* **284**:1003, 1971.

Hansky, J.: Clinical aspects of gastrin physiology, *Med. Clin. North Am.* **58**:1217, 1984.

Higgins, G. A., Recant, L., and Fischman, A. B.: The glucagonoma syndrome: Surgically curable diabetes, *Am. J. Surg.* **137**:142, 1979.

Jensen, R. T., Gardner, J. D., Raufman, J. P., *et al.:* Zollinger–Ellison syndrome. Current concepts and management, *Ann. Intern. Med.* **98**:59, 1983.

Kane, M. G., O'Dorisio, T. M., and Krejs, G. J.: Production of secretory diarrhea by intravenous infusion of vasoactive intestinal polypeptide, *N. Engl. J. Med.* **309**:1482, 1983.

Malagelada, J. R., and Davis, C. S.: Laboratory diagnosis of gastrinomas: A prospective evaluation of gastric analysis and fasting serum gastrin levels, *Mayo Clin. Proc.* **27**:211, 1982.

Malagelada, J. R., Glanzman, S. C., and Go, V. L. W.: Laboratory diagnosis of gastrinoma II. A prospective study of gastrin challenge tests, *Mayo Clin. Proc.* **57**:219, 1982.

Mallinson, C. N., Bloom, S. R., Warin, A. P., *et al.:* A glucagonoma syndrome, *Lancet* **2**:1, 1974.

Matsumoto, K. K., Peter, J. B., Schultze, R. J., *et al.:* Watery diarrhea and hypokalemia associated with pancreatic islet cell adenoma, *Gastroenterology* **50**:231, 1966.

McCarthy, D. M.: Report on the United States experience with cimetidine in Zollinger–Ellison syndrome and other hypersecretory states, *Gastroenterology* **74**:453, 1978.

Mignon, M., and Vallot, T.: Ranitidine and cimetidine in Zollinger–Ellison syndrome, *Br. J. Clin. Pharmacol.* **10**:173, 1980.

Permutt, A.: Post prandial hypoglycemia, *Diabetes* **25**:719, 1976.

Polak, J. M., Stagge, B., Pierce, A. G. E., *et al.:* Two types of Zollinger–Ellison syndrome—immunofluorescent, cytochemical and ultrastructural studies of the antral and pancreatic gastrin cells in different clinical states, *Gut* **13**:501, 1972.

Reichlin, S.: Somatostatin, *N. Engl. J. Med.* **309**:1495, 1983.

Said, S. I., and Faloona, G. R.: Elevated plasma and tissue levels of vasoactive intestinal polypeptide in the watery diarrhea syndrome due to pancreatic, bronchogenic and other tumors, *N. Engl. J. Med.* **293**:155, 1975.

Scarlett, J. A., Mako, M. E., Rubenstein, A. H., *et al.:* Factitious hypoglycemia: Diagnosis by measurement of serum C-peptide immunoreactivity and insulin binding antibodies, *N. Engl. J. Med.* **297**:1029, 1977.

Schein, P. S., Delellis, R. A., Kahn, R., *et al.:* Islet cell tumors—Current concepts and management, *Ann. Intern. Med.* **79:**239, 1973.

Schmidt, M. G., Soergel, H. H., Hensley, G. T., *et al.:* Watery diarrhea associated with pancreatic islet cell carcinoma, *Gastroenterology* **69:**206, 1975.

Service, F. J., Dale, A. J., Elveback, L., *et al.:* Insulinoma: Clinical and diagnostic features in 60 consecutive cases, *Mayo Clin. Proc.* **51:**417, 1976.

Service, F. J., Rubenstein, A. H., and Horowitz, D.: C-peptide analysis in the diagnosis of factitious hypoglycemia in an insulin dependent diabetic, *Mayo Clin. Proc.* **50:**697, 1975.

Steiner, D. F., and Oyer, P. E.: The biosynthesis of insulin and a probable precursor of insulin by a human islet cell adenoma, *Proc. Nat'l. Acad. Sci. U.S.A.* **57:**473, 1967.

Unger, R. H., and Orci, L.: Physiology and pathophysiology of glucagon, *Physiol. Rev.* **56:**779, 1976.

Verner, J. V.: Endocrine pancreatic islet cell disease with diarrhea, *Arch. Intern. Med.* **133:**492, 1974.

Verner, J. V., and Morrison, A. B.: Islet cell tumor and a syndrome of refractory watery diarrhea and hypokalemia, *Am. J. Med.* **25:**374, 1958.

Verner, J. V., and Morrison, A. B.: Non β islet cell tumors and the syndrome of watery diarrhea, hypokalemia and hypochlorhydria, *Clin. Gastroenterol.* **3:**595, 1974.

Wermer, P.: Endocrine adenomatosis and peptic ulcer in a large kindred, *Am. J. Med.* **35:**205, 1963.

Zollinger, R. M., and Ellison, E. H.: Primary peptic ulceration of the jejunum associated with islet cell tumors of the pancreas, *Ann. Surg.* **142:**709, 1955.

52

Multiple Endocrine Adenomatosis

52.1. Introduction

Multiple endocrine adenomatosis is a familial disorder characterized by pluriglandular abnormalities, most commonly expressed as hypersecretory syndromes. The underlying histological abnormality consists of hyperplasia, adenoma, or even carcinoma.

52.2. Classification

The consistency with which certain patterns of association occur in the MEA syndromes has facilitated classification into three types (Table 118): MEA I (Wermer's syndrome) is characterized by abnormalities involving the parathyroids, pancreatic islet cells, and the pituitary gland; MEA II (Sipple's syndrome) consists of medullary carcinoma of the thyroid, pheochromocytoma, and hyperparathyroidism; MEA III (or MEA IIB) is also characterized by medullary carcinoma and pheochromocytoma but is highlighted by the presence of somatic abnormalities such as mucocutaneous neuromata and marfanoid habitus. The characteristics of the specific syndromes as well as the additional disorders that may be associated with each MEA type are discussed individually.

52.3. Etiology

There are several theories that have been put forward to explain the origin of multiple endocrine adenomatosis. These include the theory of mosaic pleiotropism, the theory of nesidioblastosis, and the theory of neuroectoder-

TABLE 118
Multiple Endocrine Adenomatosis

MEA type I	MEA type II	MEA type III
Parathyroids	Parathyroid hyperplasia of adenoma	Mucocutaneous neuromata, Marfanoid habitus
Pancreatic	Medullary carcinoma of thyroid	Medullary carcinoma of thyroid
Pituitary	Pheochromocytoma	Pheochromocytoma

mal dysplasia based on the APUD concept. Of the above, the bulk of embryological and physiological evidence favors the concept that MEA syndromes are expressions of neuroectodermal dysplasia.

52.3.1. The APUD Concept and Neuroectodermal Dysplasia

It is now recognized the neurosecretory activity is not limited to the hypothalamic–pituitary unit. The common characteristic of amine precursor uptake and decarboxylation (APUD) is shared by several tissues in addition to the brain and CNS. These tissues include cells of the stomach, duodenum, intestines, pancreatic islets, adrenal medulla, sympathetic ganglia, adenohypophysis, parafollicular cells of the thyroid, and melanoblasts. Cells containing APUD characteristics are also scattered within the respiratory tract and the urogenital tract. These diverse tissues, it is believed, are derived from the primitive neuroectoderm.

Elegant embryological studies based on ablative tissue graft techniques have convincingly demonstrated the migration of cells with histological and cytochemical characteristics of APUD cells to various organs such as the gastrointestinal tract, adrenal medulla, and the pancreas. The "neurosecretory code," it seems, is retained within these cells, which are capable of secreting biogenic amines. If a tumorogenic factor is incorporatated in the genome of the neuroectodermal precursor, it is conceivable that these diverse cells sharing a common embryological origin from the neuroectoderm would also carry this genome for tumor formation. This would explain the reason for tumor formation ("APUDomas") in widely different and distant tissues (such as the thyroid and adrenal medulla) as well as the occurrence of hypersecretory syndromes in widely scattered neuroendocrine cells involving several organs that share a common embryological origin. The one difficulty with the APUD concept is explaining the parathyroid involvement in MEA syndromes. The parathyroid glands do not hold membership in the "APUD club." The hyperparathyroidism seen in association with the MEA syndromes is thought to be, at least by some, a response to the hormonal milieu caused by the other constituents of the syndrome. Thus, the APUD concept, although offering the best explanation for the genesis of MEA syndromes, leaves some questions unanswered.

52.3.2. The Theory of Nesidioblastosis

The "nesidioblast" is the pancreatic islet stem cell. An inherited abnormality in the nesidioblast may result in proliferation of any type of islet cell, resulting in hypersecretion of insulin, glucagon, gastrin, etc. According to this theory, the hypersecretory syndromes of the other endocrine glands are a secondary response to the primary islet cell hypersecretion; for example, gastrin hypersecretion results in calcitonin excess, insulin hypersecretion results in growth hormone excess, serotonin hypersecretion results in ACTH excess, and so on. The limitations of the "nesidioblastosis theory" are twofold: first, hypersecretory states involving islet cell hormones are not invariably associated with reactive phenomena involving other glands; and second, tumors involving the pituitary and parathyroids in MEA I can and do occur in the absence of islet cell hypersecretion.

52.3.3. The Theory of "Mosaic Pleiotropism"

According to this theory, the genome for tumor formation is inherited by all endocrine glands, but "reactive factors" in each gland determine expression. The major drawback of this theory is that it fails to explain the consistency with which combination patterns occur.

In summary, the etiology for the development of MEA syndromes is not completely understood. The best explanation is offered by the APUD concept, which theorizes that these tumors are derived from cells with APUD characteristics, and the commonality between such widely scattered cells is their shared embryological origin from the neuroectoderm. Thus, MEA syndromes may be viewed as disorders resulting from neuroectodermal dysplasia. These syndromes are inherited by an autosomal dominant mode with high penetrance.

The clinical features of the three types of MEA syndromes are best viewed individually. Although the syndrome is variably expressed with characteristic pleiotropism, the expressions in members of a given family are usually identical.

52.4. Multiple Endocrine Adenomatosis Type I (Wermer's Syndrome)

The spectrum of expression of MEA I is outlined in Table 119. Several general comments apply, as they relate to the specific components of the MEA I syndrome.

1. The most frequently expressed facet of MEA I is hyperparathyroidism (80–85%). Histologically, hyperplasia of four glands and multiple

TABLE 119
Multiple Endocrine Adenomatosis I

Component	Manifestation
Parathyroids (85%) (adenoma or hyperplasia)	Hypercalcemia
Pancreatic neoplasia (80%) (adenoma, hyperplasia, or carcinoma)	
Gastrinoma	Peptic ulcer, diarrhea
Insulinoma	Hypoglycemia
VIPoma	Watery diarrhea (pancreatic cholera), hypokalemia, hypochlorhydria
Serotonin-secreting tumor	Carcinoid syndrome
Secretin-secreting tumor	Diarrhea, hypochlorhydria
Glucagonoma	Necrotizing skin rash, diabetes
Somatostatin	Dyspepsia, diarrhea, diabetes, gallstones
Pituitary neoplasms (50–64%)	
Chromophobe adenoma	Pituitary hypofunction
Hypersecretory micro- or macroadenoma	
Prolactin	Galactorrhea, amenorrhea, infertility, impotence
ACTH	Cushing's disease
HGH	Acromegaly, gigantism
TSH	Secondary hyperthyroidism
Rare associations	
Adrenal adenoma	Cushing's syndrome
Lipomatosis	Multiple "lumps"
Thyroid adenoma or hyperthyroidism	Nodular of diffuse thyromegaly

adenomas underlie the etiology in 50–60% of patients with familial hyperparathyroidism. This in sharp contrast to the nonfamilial, sporadic hyperparathyroidism, where chief-cell adenoma accounts for more than 85% of patients with the disease. Asymptomatic hypercalcemia is the main presentation in these patients.

2. Pancreatic islet cell hyperfunction runs a close second to parathyroid disease in terms of incidence (80%). Almost any pancreatic hormone can be hypersecreted, but the two that are most frequently encountered are hypergastrinemia and hyperinsulinism. The clinical, hormonal, and other laboratory features of hypergastrinemia are discussed in Section 51.4. Specifically, the hypergastrinemia of MEA I is most commonly caused by multiple tumors of hyperplasia. It is also believed that the pancreatic lesions tend to be more malignant

than the sporadic variety. There are no consistent clinical or laboratory parameters that permit distinction between the familial and nonfamilial varieties of gastrin-secreting islet cell tumors. Peptic ulcer symptoms represent the most frequent symptomology of the MEA I complex.

3. The incidence of insulin-secreting islet cell tumors (β cells) in the MEA I syndrome is approximately 35–40%. The features of islet cell tumors are discussed in Section 51.3.

4. Diarrheagenic syndromes represent an important symptom complex of the MEA I neoplasia. The humoral mediators of diarrhea in the MEA I syndrome are gastrin, serotonin, secretin, prostaglandins, and vasoactive intestinal polypeptide (VIP). The diarrhea in these circumstances is a classic example of osmotic diarrhea and is characterized by large volumes of stool, often watery. The tumors that secrete gastrin and serotonin are the ones that are mostly associated with diarrhea (Section 51.4), but rarely VIP is the diarrheagenic principle, as in the Verner–Morrison syndrome (Section 51.6.)

5. Carcinoids of the islet cells constitute an important subgroup of patients with familial islet cells tumors. In addition to serotonin, these tumors can secrete several peptide hormones that include growth hormone, ACTH, and insulin.

6. Glucagon hypersecretion is rare; the clinical features of it are discussed in Section 51.7.

7. The lastest addition to the hormones secreted by the islet cell tumors is somatostatin. The clinical expression of the somatostatinoma consists of dyspeptic symptoms, diabetes, diarrhea, cholelithiasis, and weight loss. The pansuppressive effects of somatostatin on growth hormone, TSH, prolactin, gastric acidity, insulin, glucagon, gastrin, and other gut hormones are evident on hormonal testing.

8. The pluripotentiality of familial islet cell tumors is evidenced by the frequent demonstration of increased circulating levels of several peptide hormones. Thus, a myriad of hormones can be hypersecreted by the same pancreatic tumor(s). Elevation of gastrin, VIP, insulin, secretin, serotonin, growth hormone, and even PTH may all be encountered as a consequence of secretion by a single or multiple pancreatic tumors. This pluripotentiality is shared by several APUD tissues.

9. Pituitary tumors are encountered in one-half to two-thirds of patients with MEA I, depending on the completeness of screening. Both, hypo- and hyperfunction may be encountered. It should be recognized that growth hormone, ACTH, and β-lipotropin can be "ectopically" secreted by islet cell tumors.

10. The rare associations of MEA I include multiple lipomatosis, adrenocortical adenomas with or without hyperfunction, thyroid adenomas, and hyperthyroidism.

52.5. Multiple Endocrine Adenomatosis Type II (Sipple's Syndrome)

Sipple's syndrome or MEA II is characterized by the combination of medullary carcinoma of the thyroid, pheochromocytoma, and hyperparathyroidism. All three facets may be evident at the same time or can be temporally separated. Multiple endocrine adenomatosis type II is also inherited as an autosomal dominant condition with a high degree of penetrance. Although the three aspects of Sipple's syndrome are equally important, the medullary carcinoma is the entity that is most completely expressed.

52.5.1. Medullary Carcinoma of the Thyroid

Although medullary carcinoma of the thyroid (MCT) accounts for fewer than 10% of all thyroid carcinomas, it has generated considerable interest for three reasons:

1. Medullary carcinoma of the thyroid represents the best-known example of a familial malignancy for which an autosomal dominant inheritance has been unequivocally demonstrated.
2. Medullary carcinoma of the thyroid is a prolific secretor of peptide hormones. This versatility in secretion is matched only by oat cell carcinoma of the lung. The substances secreted by medullary carcinoma of the thyroid include calcitonin, histaminase, dopa decarboxylase, serotonin, ACTH, and prostaglandins. Less commonly, this tumor secretes a nerve-growth-stimulating factor, catecholamines, and a prolactinlike substance.
3. In high-risk members, the diagnosis of this malignancy can be established even during the stage of C-cell hyperplasia, a stage when the malignancy is completely curable.

For the above reasons, medullary carcinoma has justifiably assumed an importance far outweighing its frequency.

Medullary carcinoma originates from the C-cells (parafollicular cells) of the thyroid, which secrete calcitonin. Although scattered throughout the thyroid, the C-cells are most densely populated at the junction of the upper and middle thirds of the lobe.

52.5.1.1. Clinical Features

There are three major presentations by which medullary carcinoma of the thyroid can manifest.

52.5.1.1a. Lump in the Neck (Thyroid Nodule). The most common symptom of MCT is a painless lump in the region of the thyroid. The rate of growth of the thyroid nodule can be quite rapid in some instances.

52.5.1.1b. Humoral Phenomena. In approximately 25–30% of patients with medullary carcinoma, diarrhea is a significant symptom, occasionally even antedating the appearance of the thyroid nodule. The humoral mediator of diarrhea in MCT is believed to be the prostaglandins, especially of the E series. Another humoral phenomenon, flushing, is inconsistently encountered in patients with MCT. Humoral phenomena occur in both the familial and the sporadic varieties of MCT.

52.5.1.1c. Hoarseness of Voice. This complication occurs as a consequence of recurrent laryngeal nerve involvement.

It should be noted that hypocalcemia is not a feature of MCT, although calcitonin is chronically hypersecreted. The compensatory response of PTH prevents the occurrence of hypocalcemia. Further, down-regulation of receptors in response to chronic hypercalcitonemia also serves as a protective mechanism against the development of hypocalcemia.

52.5.1.2. Diagnostic Studies

The diagnostic studies in medullary carcinoma can be classified into hormonal, isotopic, radiological, and cytological.

52.5.1.2a. Hormonal Studies. The marker for medullary carcinoma of the thyroid, a tumor of the parafollicular cells, is measurement of circulating levels of calcitonin in serum. The numerous causes of hypercalcitonemia should be kept in mind. These are outlined in Table 120.

The basal serum calcitonin level may be normal in early cases, especially when the disease is in the C-cell hyperplasia stage. In such instances, the response of calcitonin to an intravenous infusion of calcium or pentagastrin is characteristically exaggerated. This response helps to separate normals from those with early C-cell hyperplasia. This test is particularly useful in the evaluation of high-risk family members with normal basal calcitonin levels. The

TABLE 120
Causes for Elevated Basal Calcitonin Level

Condition	Mechanism
1. Medullary carcinoma of thyroid	Increased secretion by tumorous C-cells
2. Other neoplasms	Ectopic secretion by oat cell CA, carcinoid, breast, head and neck tumors
3. Pernicious anemia	Hypergastrinemia-induced calcitonin release
4. ZE syndrome	Hypergastrinemia-induced calcitonin release
5. Chronic renal failure	Decreased clearance of hormone
6. Subacute thyroiditis	Release of hormone into circulation from the inflamed gland

demonstration of an exaggerated serum calcitonin response to calcium infusion or pentagastrin strongly favors the diagnosis of early cancer; therefore, this test is a singularly useful screening test to detect the presence of a devastating disease at a stage when it is totally curable.

Serum histaminase levels are markedly elevated in patients with metastatic medullary carcinoma. Combination of serum calcitonin and serum histaminase after total thyroidectomy provides an excellent means of detecting local recurrence and distant metastases of this cancer.

Carcinoembryonic antigen (CEA) levels are elevated in patients with MCT, but not consistently enough to permit its use as a humoral marker for the disease.

Finally, all patients with MCT must undergo intensive screening to exclude the presence of pheochromocytoma.

52.5.1.2b. Isotopic. The thyroid scan (performed with radioiodine or technetium) characteristically reveals hypofunction of the palpated nodule ("cold nodule"). The appearance of MCT on conventional radionuclide scans is indistinguishable from adenoma, cysts, and differentiated thyroid cancer.

The recent discovery that MCT tumors concentrate the isotope dimercaptosuccinic acid (DMSA) tagged with technetium while the normal thyroid, as well as differentiated tumors of the thyroid, do not, may find future diagnostic application in detecting the presence of MCT in thyroid nodules.

52.5.1.2c. Radiological Studies. In 25–30% of patients with MCT, the plain film of the neck may reveal characteristic dense, clumpy, aggregate calcification. Demonstration of bilateral disease is indicative of familial MCT. The calcification may also be evident in the lymph nodes and even the mediastinum. The high content of amyloid within the tumor is probably the reason for the irregular calcification.

52.5.1.2d. Cytological Studies. The diagnostic yield of MCT by aspiration biopsy cytology is lower than that of papillary and follicular carcinoma. The low yield is probably a reflection of the cells "stuck" to the amyloid and thus not being shed for aspiration.

52.5.1.3. Complications

Medullary carcinoma is an aggressive malignancy. Metastasis to the cervical lymph nodes is evident in one-third to half the number of patients undergoing surgery. The carcinoma also spreads by local invasion and dissemination by bloodstream to distant sites such as lungs, liver, and the bones.

52.5.1.4. Prognosis

The prognosis of medullary carcinoma is highly variable. The inconsistencies of the biological behavior of MCT in part account for this variability. The familial forms of MCT (particularly the ones associated with MEA III) tend to be more aggressive, with a tendency to disseminate. Bilateral disease, lymph node involvement, and markedly elevated serum histaminase levels are associated with a poorer outcome. The basal levels of calcitonin and the response of calcitonin to stimulation have no bearing on the prognosis. The demonstration of increased calcitonin staining in the excised tumor tissue may have some predictive value. The higher the index for calcitonin staining, the more differentiated is the tumor, and the better is the outcome.

52.5.1.5. Treatment

The treatment of medullary carcinoma of the thyroid is total thyroidectomy coupled with *en bloc* removal of the lymph nodes. This cancer is not responsive to radiation, radioactive iodine, or chemotherapy. It is crucial to exclude pheochromocytoma before surgery in order to avoid a surgical catastrophe.

52.5.2. Familial Pheochromocytoma

The second component of the Sipple syndrome is the pheochromocytoma. There are several features unique to the pheochromocytoma of the Sipple's syndrome:

1. The pheochromocytomas tend to be multiple and bilateral. Even when unilateral, the opposite "uninvolved" medulla may still show medullary hyperplasia, a harbinger of tumor formation.
2. The pheochromocytomas associated wtih MCT tend to be "silent" clinically until provoked by stress, usually surgical. In such a setting, it is not uncommon for the first manifestation of the pheochromocytoma to be the last one.
3. The pheochromocytomas associated with MCT tend to be smaller, thus eluding visualization by ultrasonography or computerized tomography.
4. Routine biochemical screening with VMA, metanephrine, normetanephrine, and total urinary catecholamines may not provide the diagnosis of pheochromocytoma associated with MCT. One reason for this may be the rapid turnover of catecholamines within the tumor. This is conducive to missing the diagnosis even when screened.
5. Provocative tests to "unmask" the"silent tumor" are generally less successful in the familial pheochromocytomas than in the sporadic variety.
6. Familial pheochromocytomas, especially the ones associated with MCT, tend to preferentially secrete more epinephrine, at times constituting 70% of the total plasma catecholamines. Thus, measurement of epinephrine (fractionation of catecholamines) provides a superior screening method to detect these tumors.
7. The incidence of malignancy in the pheochromocytoma associated with MCT is higher than the incidence of malignancy in the sporadic pheochromocytoma.
8. Rarely, catecholamine secretion can be secondary to direct secretion by the medullary carcinoma of the thyroid. The only method to doc-

ument this phenomenon is by measuring catecholamine levels in the effluent from the thyroid veins.

The clinical features, laboratory evaluation, and treatment of pheochromocytoma are discussed in Chapter 31.

52.5.3. Hyperparathyroidism

The third facet of Sipple's syndrome is the hyperparathyroidism. In contrast to the sporadic variety of hyperparathyroidism, hyperplasia of all four glands predominates as the etiology of hyperparathyroidism associated with MCT. Although it is tempting, based on the hyperplasia, to ascribe a "reactive" etiology for the hyperparathyroidism, three lines of evidence suggest that the hyperparathyroidism is not merely an adaptive response to the calcitonin excess and that it is a separately inherited genetic entity. First, although less common, adenoma of a single parathyroid accounts for the hyperparathyroidism in at least a minority of cases. Second, the hyperparathyroidism may be expressed in the absence of medullary carcinoma of the thyroid or pheochromocytoma. Finally, the incidence of hyperparathyroidism in familial medullary carcinoma is approximately 40–50%. If the hyperparathyroidism of Sipple's syndrome were to be ascribed as secondary to hypercalcitonemia *per se,* one would expect a much higher, almost universal, incidence of hyperparathyroidism in familial MCT. Such is not the case.

The clinical features, laboratory evaluation, and treatment of hyperparathyroidism are discussed in Chapter 22.

52.6. Multiple Endocrine Adenomatosis Type III

Multiple endocrine adenomatosis type III is viewed by many investigators as a variant of MEA II and consequently is also termed MEA IIB; MEA III is characterized by medullary carcinoma of the thyroid, pheochromocytoma, and somatic stigmata. There are four noteworthy features of MEA III:

1. The somatic stigmata are invariably present and consist of a Marfanoid habitus and the presence of mucocutaneous neuromata, which are mostly evident in the lips, tongue, and eyelids. These neuromata can be internal, particularly in the mucosa of the large intestine (ganglioneuromatosis). This can result in constipation or diarrhea. The reason for the development of mucocutaneous neuromata is not completely understood, but it is believed to be secondary to elaboration of a nerve-growth-stimulating factor by the MCT tissue.
2. The medullary carcinoma of the thyroid in MEA III follows a more aggressive course in comparison to the MCT of MEA II or the sporadic variety. Local invasion as well as lymph node and distant metastases occur earlier and more extensively in the course of the MCT associated with MEA III. This ominous prognostic fact is compounded by the

fact that the medullary cancer of MEA III expresses itself earlier in life (often in childhood or young adulthood) than the medullary cancer of MEA II.

3. The expression of pheochromocytoma in MEA III is more complete, approaching an 80% incidence. These pheochromocytomas are more often symptomatic and are readily detectable by conventional assays for catecholamines and their methylated products.

4. Hyperparathyroidism is negligibly expressed in MEA III, the incidence being approximately 1–2%.

Selected Readings

Andrew, A.: The APUD concept: Where has it led us? *Br. Med. Bull.* **38:**221, 1982.

Ballard, H. S., Frame, B., and Hartsock, R. J.: Familial multiple endocrine adenoma–peptic ulcer complex, *Medicine* **43:**481, 1964.

Baylin, S. B.: Medullary carcinoma of the thyroid gland. Symposium on endocrine surgery, *Surg. Clin. North Am.* **54:**309, 1974.

Baylins, S. B., Beaven, M. A., and Keiser, H. R.: Serum histaminase and calcitonin levels in medullary carcinoma of the thyroid, *Lancet* **1:**455, 1972.

Birkenhager, J. C., and Upton, G. V.: Medullary thyroid carcinoma: Ectopic production of peptides with ACTH like, CRF like and prolactin production stimulating activity, *Acta Endocrinol.* **83:**280, 1976.

Chong, G. C., Beahrs, O. H., Sizemore, G. W., *et al.*: Medullary carcinoma of the thyroid gland, *Cancer* **35:**695, 1975.

Deftos, L. J: Radioimmunoassay for calcitonin in medullary thyroid carcinoma, *J.A.M.A.* **227:**403, 1974.

Flectcher, J. R.: Medullary (solid) carcinoma of the thyroid gland. A review of 249 cases, *Arch. Surg.* **100:**257, 1970.

Friesen, S. R.: APUD tumors of the gastrointestinal tract, *Curr. Probl. Cancer* **1**(4):1, 1976.

Friesen, S. R.: Tumors of the endocrine pancreas, *N. Engl. J. Med.* **306:**580, 1982.

Frohman, L. A.: Ectopic hormone production, *Am. J. Med.* **70:**995, 1981.

Gordon, P. R., and Huvos, A. G.: Medullary carcinoma of the thyroid gland, *Cancer* **31:**915, 1973.

Hamilton, B. P., Landsberg, L., and Levine, R. J.: Measurement of urinary epinephrine in screening for pheochromocytoma in multiple endocrine neoplasia type II, *Am. J. Med.* **65:**1027, 1978.

Hennessy, J. F., Wells, S. A., Ontjes, D. A. *et al.*: A comparison of pentagastrin injection and calcium infusion as provocative agents for the detection of medullary carcinoma of the thyroid, *J. Clin. Endocrinol. Metab.* **39:**489, 1974.

Hill, C. S., Ibanex, M. E., Samaan, N. A., *et al.*: Medullary carcinoma of the thyroid gland, *Medicine* **52:**141, 1973.

Keiser, H. R., Beaven, M A., Doppman, J., *et al.*: Sipple syndrome—medullary thyroid carcinoma, pheochromocytoma, and parathyroid disease, *Ann. Intern. Med.* **78:**561, 1973.

Khairi, M. R. A., Dexter, R. N., Burzynski, N. J., *et al.*: Pheochromocytoma and medullary thyroid carcinoma: Multiple endocrine neoplasia type III, *Medicine* **54:**89, 1975.

Lips, K. J. M., Veer, J. V. S., Struyuenberg, A., *et al.*: Bilateral occurrence of pheochromocytoma in patients with multiple endocrine neoplasia syndrome 2-A (Sipple syndrome), *Am. J. Med.* **70:**1051, 1981.

Melvin, K. E. W., and Tashjian, A. H.: Studies in familial thyroid carcinoma, *Recent Prog. Horm. Res.* **28:**399, 1972.

Melvin, K. E. W., Miller, H. H., and Tashjian, A. H.: Early diagnosis of medullary carcinoma of thyroid gland by means of calcitonin assay, *N. Engl. J. Med.* **285:**1115, 1971.

Patel, Y. C., Ganda, O. P., and Benoit, R.: Pancreatic somatostatinoma: Abundance of somatostatin - 28 (1–12)-like immunoreactivity in tumor, *J. Clin. Endocrinol. Metab.* **57:**1048, 1983.

Reichlin, S.: Somatostatin, *N. Engl. J. Med.* **309:**1495, 1983.

Sipple, J. H.: The association of pheochromocytoma with carcinoma of the thyroid gland, *Am. J. Med.* **31:**163, 1961.

Soderstrom, N., Telenius- Berg, M., and Akerman, M.: Diagnosis of medullary carcinoma of the
thyroid by fine needle aspiration biopsy, *Acta Med. Scand.* **197:**71, 1975.

Tashjian, A. H., Howland, B. G., Melvin, K. E. W., *et al.:* Immunoassay of human calcitonin, *N. Engl. J. Med.* **283:**890, 1970.

Valk, T. W., Frager, M. S., Gross, M. D., *et al.:* Spectrum of pheochromocytoma in multiple
endocrine neoplasia, *Ann. Intern. Med.* **94:**762, 1981.

Welbourn, R. B.: Current status of the apudomas, *Ann. Surg.* **185:**1, 1977.

Wermer, P.: Endocrine adenomatosis and peptic ulcer in a large kindred, *Am. J. Med.* **35:**205, 1963.

Williams, E. D., and Morales, A. M.: Thyroid carcinoma and Cushing's syndrome, *J. Clin. Pathol.* **21:**129, 1968.

53

Carcinoid Tumors

53.1. Introduction

Carcinoid tumors originate from the enterochromaffin cells. These cells contain granules and stain with silver salts. Embryologically, these cells are derived from neurectoderm and are found throughout the gastrointestinal tract.

53.2. Classification

According to their embryological origin, carcinoids can be derived from the foregut (bronchial, pancreatic, and duodenal carcinoids), midgut (ileal and probably gonadal carcinoids), or hindgut (rectal carcinoids). The salient aspects of carcinoids from various locations are summarized below:

53.2.1. Appendicial Carcinoids

These are almost always benign, are found incidentally at appendectomy, and never cause the carcinoid syndrome.

53.2.2. Rectal Carcinoids

These tend to be multicentric, often benign, and generally are nonfunctional.

53.2.3. Ileal Carcinoids

These are mostly in the distal ileum and often cause intestinal obstruction either on a mechanical basis or because of metastatic involvement of the bowel wall. Ileal carcinoids are the ones most likely to cause the "classic carcinoid syndrome" with cardiovascular, pulmonary, gastrointestinal, and striking vasomotor phenomena. They metastasize to the liver and less frequently to the bones. When the carcinoid syndrome is seen, hepatic metastases are usually present.

53.2.4. Bronchial Carcinoids

These can be benign or malignant. The "classic" carcinoid syndrome and hepatic metastases are less common. The four pathognomonic features of bronchial carcinoid, when present, are:

1. There is sustained, severe "livid" flush, often with marked hypotension, volume depletion, and even shock.
2. They are highlighted by their proclivity to secrete ectopic hormones such as ACTH or growth hormone. Thus, the presentation may be that of Cushing's disease or acromegaly even at a stage when the carcinoid is occult.
3. Left-sided heart lesions may occur alone or in combination with right-sided lesions.
4. There is hypertension in between attacks.

53.2.5. Gastric Carcinoids

These rare tumors produce a characteristic flush with urticarialike features (wheallike with brownish borders) and itching. Thus, the condition can masquerade as a skin disorder for several years. These tumors are also characterized by an increase in circulating serotonin and histamine in plasma.

53.2.6. Pancreatic Carcinoids

These can present as islet cell tumors and can secrete a variety of hormones (insulin, ACTH, etc.) and often metastasize to the liver.

53.2.7. Ovarian or Testicular Carcinoids

These are seen with teratomas and are unique in that they can cause carcinoid syndrome in the absence of hepatic metastases (whereas intestinal carcinoids do so only after extensive hepatic metastases). This is because the gonads are drained by the general circulation and not by the portal vein.

53.3. Clinical Features

The clinical features of carcinoid tumors can be divided into three categories: those caused by local effects, those resulting from the carcinoid syndrome, and those consequent to metastatic disease (Table 121).

TABLE 121
Comparative Analysis of Various Carcinoids

Feature	Ileal carcinoid	Gastric carcinoid	Bronchial carcinoid
Flush	Transient, "cyanotic flush"	Bright red, urticarialike; serpentine borders	Prolonged, livid red; severe with systemic symptoms
Metastases	Liver	Liver	Liver and bone (osteoblastic)
Valvular	Right-sided	Unusual	Left-sided (pulmonary edema may occur)
Other associations	Unusual	Peptic ulcer disease	Ectopic secretion of growth hormone or ACTH
Urine 5-HIAA	Elevated in more than 90–95%	May be normal	Elevated in nearly all cases
Plasma 5-hydroxy-tryptamine (serotonin)	Often normal	Elevated	Elevated

53.3.1. Clinical Features Caused by Local Effects

These depend on the location of the tumor. Carcinoid tumors in the ileum may cause intestinal obstruction or slow, occult gastrointestinal bleeding. Bronchial carcinoids may present with partial or complete bronchial obstruction with atelectasis or with hemoptysis. Testicular carcinoid presents as a rapidly growing testicular mass.

53.3.2. Clinical Features Resulting from the "Carcinoid Syndrome"

The syndrome is caused by circulating humoral mediators secreted by the tumor. Hepatic metastases are usually present when the carcinoid syndrome has developed. The humoral mediator of the carcinoid syndrome is serotonin. The other substances secreted by carcinoid tumors such as vasoactive kinins, histamine, prostaglandins, and other polypeptide hormones play only a peripheral role, if any, in causing the symptomatology.

The features of the complete carcinoid syndrome outlined below consist of vasomotor, cardiovascular, pulmonary, gastrointestinal, and dermatological manifestations. It should be realized that the complete spectrum is seldom present, and at times the manifestations can be subtle enough to be missed.

The cardinal vasomotor manifestation is the "carcinoid flush." Unfortunately, in one-third of patients the flush may be absent or so minimal that it is often overlooked. The bronchial carcinoid flush is livid red, sustained, and severe and may be associated with systemic symptoms such as anxiety, tremulousness, lacrimation, fever, diaphoresis, and even hypotension.

The classic (or ileal) flush is characterized by being transient with a reddish to purplish hue ("cyanotic flush"), and the gastric carcinoid causes more of a pruritic, urticarialike, bright red flush. The attacks may be unprovoked and spontaneous or may be precipitated by food, alcohol, or emotion. The flushing seen in carcinoid syndrome and systemic mastocytosis share several similarities, but the carcinoid flush can be precipitated by a small dose of epinephrine, as opposed to the flushing of mastocytosis. However, such testing is neither necessary nor recommended, since it can precipitate vascular collapse.

The cardiovascular features of the syndrome include right-sided heart lesions (pulmonary stenosis, tricuspid stenosis or insufficiency) and chronic right heart failure. These lesions are fibroproliferative in nature, ocurring predominantly on the undersurface of the valves, and are presumed to be a result of altered serotonin metabolism. Left-sided valve lesions occur in bronchopulmonary carcinoids, as does hypertension in between attacks.

The gastrointestinal features of carcinoid syndrome are abdominal pain, cramps, diarrhea, and weight loss. The mediator of diarrhea and intestinal hypermotility is serotonin. Steatorrhea is often encountered in the carcinoid syndrome and contributes to the weight loss. Acute abdominal crisis can occur in the carcinoid syndrome and is characterized by fever, abdominal pain, leukocytosis, and thrombocytosis. This is said to be caused by necrosis of the hepatic metastases when the neoplastic lesions outgrow their vascular supply. Rarely, abdominal pain can occur as a consequence of fibrotic lesions in the peritoneum or the mesentery causing adhesions.

The pulmonary abnormalities can take two forms of presentation: episodic wheezing (asthmalike attacks) or a more chronic dyspnea on exertion. In the chronic form, the pulmonary function tests may reveal obstructive lung disease, improving after bronchodilators. These findings occur in 20–30% of patients and can lead to the mistaken diagnosis of asthma or chronic bronchitis. The abnormal pulmonary function tests can be a result of fibrosis of the small airways or may be caused by serotonin. Occasionally, the asthmalike symptoms can precede the recognition of carcinoid syndrome by months to years.

Finally, dermatological features may be apparent in some patients with prolonged flushing. These include thickening of the facial skin fold, telangiectasia, and a nasal appearance indistinguishable from a rhinophyma.

In addition to the above, hypermetabolism, weight loss, and niacin deficiency may contribute to the clinical presentation. Thus, carcinoid syndrome can mimic a multisystem disease. When deficiency of niacin becomes severe, a clinical syndrome similar to pellagra may develop. The mechanism of nicotinic acid deficiency in the carcinoid syndrome is as follows. Normally, the sites of serotonin synthesis in the body are the gastrointestinal mucosa, brain, and platelets. These tissues synthesize serotonin from the amino acid tryptophan. This is obtained from the diet and also serves as the substrate for nicotinic acid (niacin) via the kyneurinine pathway. When carcinoid tumors secrete excessive serotonin, they do so by shunting the available tryptophan away from niacin synthesis, causing vitamin deficiency.

53.3.3. Clinical Features Resulting from Metastases

Malignant carcinoids should be considered in the differential diagnosis of hepatic metastases. This is especially important when the primary source is not evident, because malignant carcinoid tumors can be very small and occult. The primary carcinoids that metastasize to the liver usually originate in the ileum, pancreas, stomach, or gonads. The carcinoid syndrome may or may not be clinically expressed in these cases, but urinary levels of serotonin metabolites are often found to be elevated. Bronchial carcinoids may also cause osteoblastic bone lesions.

53.4. Diagnostic Studies

The 24-hr urinary excretion of 5-hydroxyindoleacetic acid (5-HIAA) is elevated in 90% of patients with the carcinoid syndrome. The 24-hr 5-HIAA is the product of serotonin metabolism. Normally, the amino acid tryptophan is converted into 5-hydroxytrypotophan, which is further decarboxylated to 5-hydroxytryptamine (or serotonin). This is inactivated by monoamine oxidase and aldehyde dehydrogenase to form 5-hydroxyindoleacetic acid (5-HIAA). Since almost all of the serotonin is converted to 5-HIAA, it is a remarkably good index of serotonin secretion in normal as well as abnormal states. The normal 24-hr excretion of 5-HIAA is less than 9 mg.

A simple bedside test can be performed on a spot urine for the qualitative determination of excess 5-HIAA. When nitrosonaphthol reagent is added to urine, a reddish-brown color reaction will occur if the 5-HIAA in the urine is in excess of 30 mg. The test, however, will be negative in the case of a carcinoid tumor with 15 to 20 mg excretion of 5-HIAA and will be falsely positive when the patient is on glyceryl guaicolate, mephenesin, or on a diet rich in bananas or nuts. The test will also be falsely negative when patients are on phenothiazine therapy. Therefore, as good as the "spot" test is for screening, it should not substitute for the formal 24-hr collection for 5-HIAA in an acidified, dark container, and on a specific diet free of bananas, tomatoes, or walnuts ("VMA diet").

Plasma serotonin (5-HT) levels may help in patients with gastric carcinoids in whom the 5-HIAA levels may not always be elevated. This measurement is unlikely to be of use in classic carcinoid syndrome, since almost 99% of serotonin is converted into 5-HIAA.

Tissue biopsy (metastatic or the primary carcinoid) would reveal a characteristic histology consisting of islands of epithelial tumor cells with small dark nuclei and a pale granular cytoplasm. The granules stain positive for the argentaffin stain (Fontana–Masson stain).

53.5. Course and Prognosis

Malignant carcinoids have a variable, often protracted and indolent course. Some patients with metastatic liver disease with the carcinoid syndrome have survived 5 to 8 years. Of course, the quality of life is markedly compromised and burdened by nutritional problems, diarrhea, vasomotor phenomena, and eventually by hepatic failure. The prognosis is fair for ileal carcinoids and very poor for malignant bronchial carcinoids.

53.6. Treatment

Surgical therapy with resection of the tumor is recommended when the tumor is "resectable."

Medical therapy is indicated mostly to control the troublesome symptoms of carcinoid syndrome. Specifically, medical therapy is necessary to control the flushing and the diarrhea. There are several drugs that can be tried for flushing. Antiadrenergic drugs (especially those with α-blocking activity), glucocorticoids, serotonin antagonists, and even prostaglandin inhibitors (indomethacin) have all been tried with varying degrees of success. In general, the flushing episodes are best prevented, since they are difficult to control once they have occurred. Prevention of attacks depend on avoiding precipitating factors such as alcohol and stress. Phenothiazines with α-adrenergic blocking activity like chlorpromazine (25 to 50 mg q.i.d.) or prochlorperazine (5 to 10 mg q.i.d.) are useful to reduce the frequency of the flushing episodes. If these drugs fail to abort an attack, or if the attacks persist with these drugs, phenoxybenzamine, a potent α blocker, in doses of 10 to 50 mg a day may be tried and can be very effective. When the flushing is severe, sustained, and causes hypotension (as in bronchial carcinoids), glucocorticoids (prednisone, 10 to 50 mg daily) with intravenous fluids are necessary to prevent oliguria and renal failure. Serotonin antagonists are, in general, more useful for treating the gastrointestinal symptoms of carcinoid syndrome than the vasomotor symptoms.

The treatment of diarrhea in this disorder can be frustrating. After the conventional medications (kaolin, etc.) fail opiates can be tried, failing which serotonin antagonists such as cyproheptadine or methysergide may be employed. The long-term use of methysergide can result in fibrotic complications, an unwelcome adverse effect, since patients with carcinoid syndrome already have a predisposition for myocardial fibrosis.

The drug parachlorphenylalanine is an inhibitor of the enzyme tryptophan hydroxylase, the enzyme responsible for the conversion of tryptophan into serotonin. In the doses of 2–3 g daily, this drug is an effective modality to reduce serotonin synthesis. The drug works best in the control of diarrhea when all the other modalities have failed.

Considerable attention has to be paid to treating the patient's nutritional status, which can be greatly compromised by the anorexia (seen as part of the malignancy), the hypermetabolic state (caused by serotonin and the other bioamines), and aggravated by the diarrhea, malabsorption, the niacin deficiency, and the result of surgery in some patients. These patients must have supplementation of vitamins (especially niacin) and minerals.

Chemotherapy with streptozotocin is at best palliative. The decision to use this chemotherapeutic agent should take into consideration the general condition of the patient and the potential benefits of the drug. Initial claims of enthusiasm as to the beneficial effects of this drug are now questioned when the data are reviewed critically. Addition of 5-fluorouracil and more recently adriamycin has not been critically evaluated to justify routine use.

Selected Readings

Davis, Z., Moertel, C. G., and McIlrath, D. C.: The malignant carcinoid syndrome, *Surg. Gynecol. Obstet.* **137**:637, 1973.

Engelman, K.: The carcinoid syndrome, in Wyngaarden, J. B., and Smith, L. H. (eds.): *Cecil's Textbook of Medicine.* Philadelphia, W. B. Saunders, 1982.

Engelman, K., Lovenberg, W., and Sjoerdsma, A.: Inhibition of serotonin synthesis by parachlorphenylalanine in patients with the carcinoid syndrome, *N. Engl. J. Med.* **277**:1103, 1967.

Godwin, J. D.: Carcinoid tumors: An analysis of 2837 cases, *Cancer* **36**:560, 1975.

Grahame-Smith, D. G.: The biosynthesis of 5-hydroxytryptamine in carcinoid tumors and intestine, *Clin. Sci.* **33**:147, 1967.

Grahame-Smith, D. G.: *The Carcinoid Syndrome.* London, Heineman, 1972.

Kazi, M. U., and Grover, V.: Carcinoid tumors and the carcinoid syndrome, *J. Am. Geriatr. Soc.* **17**:807, 1969.

Malafosse, M.: Carcinoid tumors: Surgical problems, *Clin. Gastroenterol.* **3**(3):711, 1974.

Melmon, K. L., Sjoerdsma, A., and Mason, D. T.: Distinctive clinical and therapeutic aspects of the syndrome associated with bronchial carcinoid tumors, *Am. J. Med.* **39**:568, 1965.

Williams, E. D., and Sandler, M.: The classification of carcinoid tumors, *Lancet* **1**:238, 1963.

Index